ANNALS OF THE NEW YORK ACADEMY OF SCIENCES

Volume 348

LIPOPROTEIN STRUCTURE

Edited by Angelo M. Scanu and Frank R. Landsberger

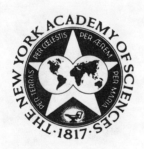

The New York Academy of Sciences
New York, New York
1980

PCP

Printed in the United States of America
ISBN 0–89766–082–X (cloth)
0–89766–083–8 (paper)

ANNALS OF THE NEW YORK ACADEMY OF SCIENCES

VOLUME 348

June 29, 1980

LIPOPROTEIN STRUCTURE *

Editors and Conference Chairmen
ANGELO M. SCANU AND FRANK R. LANDSBERGER

———◆———

CONTENTS

* This series of papers is the result of a conference entitled *Conference on Lipoprotein Structure,* held by The New York Academy of Sciences on September 10–12, 1979.

Part IV. Structure–Function Relationships: Lipoproteins, Apolipoproteins, Enzymes, Exchange Proteins, and Receptors

Part V. Structure of Plasma Lipoproteins

Part VI. Lipoprotein Models

Part VII. Poster Session Papers

Financial assistance was received from:

- AMERICAN HEART ASSOCIATION
- AYERST
- BECKMAN INSTRUMENTS, INC.
- BOEHRINGER INGELHEIM LTD.
- CHICAGO HEART ASSOCIATION
- ELI LILLY AND COMPANY
- HOFFMANN-LA ROCHE INC.
- MERCK SHARP & DOHME RESEARCH LABORATORIES
- NATIONAL HEART, LUNG, & BLOOD INSTITUTE
- NATIONAL INSTITUTE OF GENERAL MEDICAL SCIENCES
- NORWICH-EATON PHARMACEUTICALS

INTRODUCTORY REMARKS

Angelo M. Scanu

University of Chicago
Pritzker School of Medicine
Chicago, Illinois 60637

First of all, I wish to take this opportunity to thank the many people that made this Conference possible: the Conference Committee of the New York Academy of Sciences; Mrs. Helen Marks, the Conference Director, and her staff—she really provided excellent help; all the members of the Advisory Committee of this Conference; and needless to say, all of the speakers and participants. I should also say that this Conference would not be possible without the active work by the Co-chairman, Frank Landsberger. He took care of many problems and was always ready with encouragement and advice.

We are here to discuss plasma lipoproteins and related areas, a field which has become important and exciting as attested by the number of laboratories engaged in this type of research and by the number of accounts that are published every year.

I do hope that this Conference will provide a forum for putting these new developments into focus and encourage an active interaction among participants. A few days ago, while reading the September issue of the magazine *The Sciences* published by the New York Academy of Sciences, I encountered an article written by Stevan Harnad. He approaches the very interesting question as to whether scientists should always agree on scientific issues. His theory is that they should not. He feels that anything that is an established fact, and thus is agreed upon, becomes history and, perhaps, less fun. He considers ongoing research as something current and vital, consisting of active and often heated interactions of data, ideas, and minds—what he calls creative disagreement.

I do hope that this philosophy will prevail during this meeting and that you feel free to participate, express your ideas, and hopefully have fun.

THE PLASMA LIPOPROTEINS: HISTORICAL DEVELOPMENTS AND NOMENCLATURE *

Frank T. Lindgren

Division of Biology and Medicine
Lawrence Berkeley Laboratory
University of California
Berkeley, California 94720

INTRODUCTION

It is my pleasure and honor to be here today to offer a few thoughts, recollections, and conclusions on the historical developments and nomenclature of the serum lipoproteins. As is usually the case, new methodology and technical improvements preceded and were necessary for applications and breakthroughs. The first landmark was in 1924, when Svedberg and Rinde invented the ultracentrifuge with application to the study of particle size of gold colloids.[1] Later, in 1927, Svedberg and Lysholm developed a higher speed oil turbine analytic ultracentrifuge for protein analysis, which allowed detection of migrating boundaries by an optical system. FIGURE 1 shows one of the first low-speed direct-drive electrical analytic ultracentrifuges. Thereafter, there were many improvements and refinements.[2]

About the same time, Macheboef[3] performed the first chemical separation of a horse serum lipoprotein. The definition was, as in later years, operational, i.e., "coenapse precipitated by acid" or CA using half-saturated ammonium sulfate. Much later in 1944, after electrophoresis had been developed, he reported it to be an α_1 globulin, which now would indicate this first isolated lipoprotein to be a high-density lipoprotein (HDL).

EARLY ANALYTIC ULTRACENTRIFUGATION

Application of the analytic ultracentrifuge to lipoproteins began in 1935 with McFarlane's early studies of normal and pathological serum.[4] The serum protein boundaries as obtained by tedious manual plots using the Lamm scale method[5] are shown in FIGURE 2. Note the suggestion of multicomponents and distortions in the region of the albumin boundary. These shapes changed with time and were influenced by salt concentration and dilution. Because of its apparent labile nature, this lipid-containing component, thought to be sedimenting in the region of the albumin boundary, was called the "X protein." Others such as Mutzenbecher and Pederson later verified these observations.[2] However, there was no definitive study and explanation of these conflicting findings.

During World War II there was large scale fractionation of human plasma at Harvard. Here Cohen, Oncley, Edsall, and their group isolated two distinctly

* This work was supported in part by Grant 5-PO1-HL-18574 from the National Heart, Lung, and Blood Institute and by the Health Effects research component, United States Environmental Protection Agency Project No. RPIS 308.

1

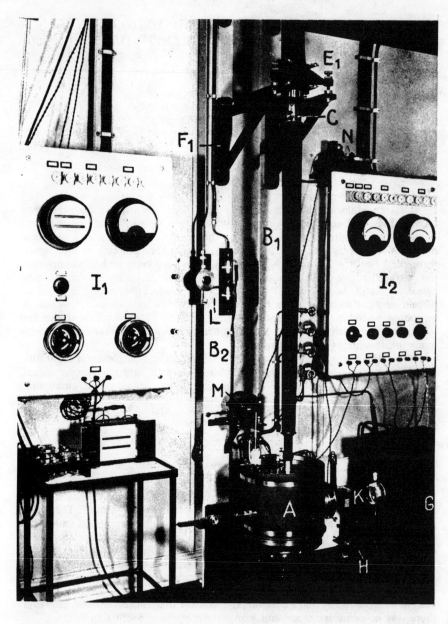

FIGURE 1. Low-speed analytic ultracentrifuge, Institute of Physical Chemistry, Upsala, Sweden. Main components are: A, ultracentrifuge chamber; C, D, E, and D, optical system and camera; H, optical bench; H, K, and G, optical bench and light source; L, hydrogen atmosphere control; I_1 and I_2, control panels. (From Svedberg & Pedersen.[2] By permission of Clarendon Press.)

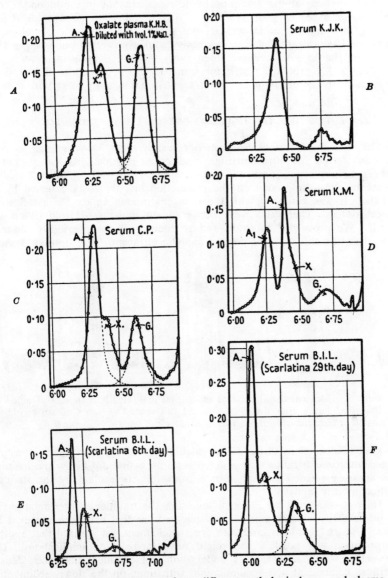

FIGURE 2. Sedimentation diagrams from different pathological sera and plasma. In the region of the albumin boundary note the appearance of two components in all but Serum K.M. where distortion and three components might be resolved. (From McFarlane.[4] By permission of the *Biochemical Journal*.)

different lipid-containing fractions by low-salt ethanol precipitation.[6] These were characterized as a dense (1.10 g/ml) α lipoprotein and a low-density (1.03 g/ml) high-molecular-weight (1.3×10^6) β lipoprotein. Simultaneous with these studies were Pederson's extensive studies on serum published in 1945 as a small book.[7] All evidence then suggested the β lipoprotein to be the troublesome "X protein," which for some 15 years seemed to defy rational explanation for its behavior in the ultracentrifugal analysis of serum.

RESOLUTION AND THE DEVELOPMENT OF LIPOPROTEIN FLOTATION

This was the status of lipoprotein research some 31 years ago as John Gofman started his ultracentrifugal and other physical-chemical studies at Donner Laboratory. There was one new electrically-driven Spinco analytic ultracentrifuge—the second off the production line that was designed by Ed Pickels.[8] It was equipped with the new continuous dn/dx Philipot-Svenson optical system. There also were two graduate students—Harold Elliott and myself. We proceeded to study and reproduce all the previously observed anomalies with this new commercial analytic ultracentrifuge. FIGURE 3 shows

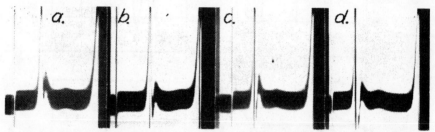

FIGURE 3. Ultracentrifugal patterns of normal undiluted human sera obtained approximately 2 hours after the rotor attained full speed. (From Gofman et al.[9] By permission of the *Journal of Biological Chemistry.*)

the kind of distortions observed in which there usually developed, after prolonged ultracentrifugation of undiluted sera, an actual dip below the baseline. This anomaly seemed difficult, if not impossible, to explain by the standard multicomponent analysis.

Then at one point we began to question the traditional interpretations of the ultracentrifugal diagrams of schlieren patterns that had been accepted for some 15 years. Suddenly, and with great excitement, we realized that another interpretation was possible and might have far-reaching implications. This explanation was that instead of undergoing true sedimentation, the "density sensitive" component was accumulating, with time, on the slowly sedimenting albumin boundary. Also, with this explanation it was thought for theoretical reasons that, for macromolecules like the X protein, the albumin itself contributed a density increment, changing with time and (of course) with buffer solvent dilution. FIGURE 4 shows the concept of pile-up with a resultant explanation of the "dip phenomenon." In addition, this hypothetical analysis clearly indicated that a floating component should give an "inverse" peak, rising from the base of the cell. Additional confirmation that this analysis was the correct one is given in FIGURE 5. Here, by changing the position of the pile-up on the

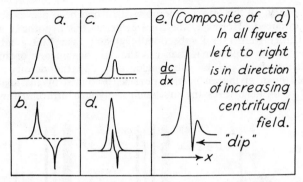

FIGURE 4. Pile-up analysis and the resulting "dip" phenomenon that is observed ultracentrifugally. (From Gofman *et al.*[9] By permission of the *Journal of Biological Chemistry*.)

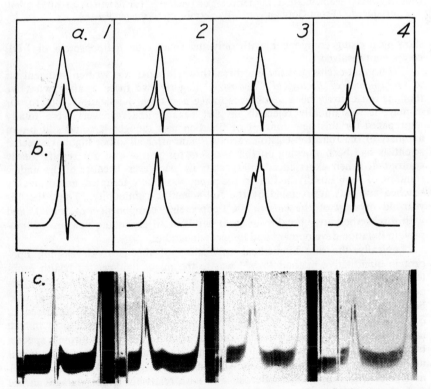

FIGURE 5. Variation in ultracentrifugal patterns with variations in the location of the lipoprotein pile-up on the albumin concentration gradient. (From Gofman *et al.*[9] By permission of the *Journal of Biological Chemistry*.)

albumin boundary, all the bizarre anomolies that had been previously observed could be reproduced. However, the final proof of this hypothesis was that if the serum density were raised substantially greater than 1.03 g/ml (the estimated density of the X protein), then (1) the dip phenomenon or any albumin boundary distortion would be eliminated, and (2) the density-sensitive X protein would float, giving an inverse peak as predicted by the analysis given in FIGURE 4. FIGURE 6 gives the first such analytical ultracentrifuge flotation

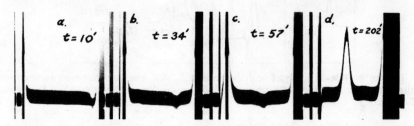

FIGURE 6. Progressive flotation of lipoprotein in a serum containing 7.8% added NaCl ($\rho_{26}=1.063$ g/ml). To distinguish flotation in the ultracentrifuge, as contrasted with traditional sedimentation, the term S_f, or svedbergs (of flotation) at 1.063 g/ml, was introduced. (From Gofman et al.[9] By permission of the publisher.)

showing a rising component, with only the small total β lipoprotein or LDL component resolved.

With great excitement the first breakthrough paper was written and sent off to the *Journal of Biological Chemistry*. Eagerly, we three awaited what we thought must surely be a quick acceptance and rapid publication. But to our dismay, it was initially rejected, in part because the reviewers were totally unprepared for this new concept of flotation and thought it could still be an anomaly of the Johnston-Ogston variety;[10] and after all, other highly respected scientists had been working on this problem for years—and our results totally contradicted their experienced interpretations. However, because of the understanding of John Edsall, the Editor, the paper was finally accepted, and it quickly reached and was appreciated by the full scientific community. Thus, the 15-year-old mystery of the elusive "X lipoprotein" component was solved, and with this methodology breakthrough, it heralded an expanding new era of lipoprotein flotation development and lipoprotein studies.

Logically, the first biomedical application of this newly-developing lipoprotein quantitative methodology[11] was to the major lipid-related health problem, atherosclerosis, and coronary artery disease particularly. Therefore, repeating the classical Anitschkow cholesterol-feeding studies,[12] Gofman et al.[13] began to identify more closely the actual macromolecules that increased in concentration with the development of experimental atherosclerosis in the rabbit. However, these early studies did not evaluate the full lipoprotein spectra but concentrated only on the major portion of the low-density class. The initial findings are given in FIGURE 7, showing increase in the S_f 10–30 class (IDL) molecules with rabbit atherosclerosis and with relatively minor changes in the S_f 5–8 class (LDL). Comparable components were to be found in the human. Later pathological human studies[14] began to focus and identify the S_f 12–20 class as the most "atherogenic class" portion of the total LDL-IDL spectra.

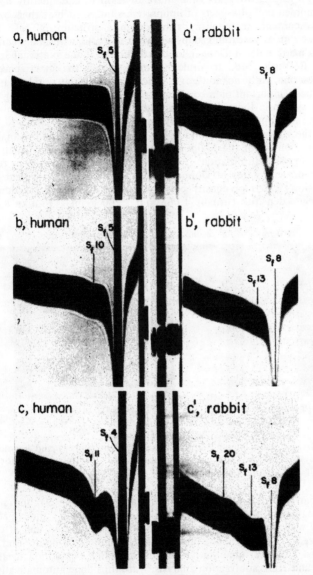

FIGURE 7. Ultracentrifugal flotation diagrams of lipoproteins of the human, the normal rabbit, and the rabbit developing atherosclerosis. During cholesterol induction of atherosclerosis, the rabbit develops additional components of the S_f 10–30 class (b′ and c′). All runs were of the isolated $d > 1.063$ g/ml total low-density class lipoproteins. (From Gofman et al.[18] By permission of Science.)

During the past 30 years there have developed subsequently and with increasing momentum all aspects of lipoprotein studies, such as their composition, apoprotein content, metabolism, function, and structure. These have been conducted by many research groups all over the world, with many early pioneering efforts made both at Donner and particularly at the National Institutes of Health in Bethesda, Md. It would be impossible in the short space available here to describe, fully acknowledge, or even outline the number, nature, and scope of these important biomedical contributions. However, among books and the recent symposia there are several that can provide much of this historical information for appreciation and evaluation.[15-21]

From the viewpoint of technique, we began by describing the analytic ultracentrifugal anomaly of the X lipoprotein, and later its solution with the introduction of lipoprotein flotation. Perhaps it may be worthwhile to recapitulate briefly the present status at Donner of this developed and refined technique. Presently, low- and high-density preparative ultracentrifuge fractions are run at appropriate densities (usually 1.063 and 1.200 g/ml). FIGURE 8 shows the

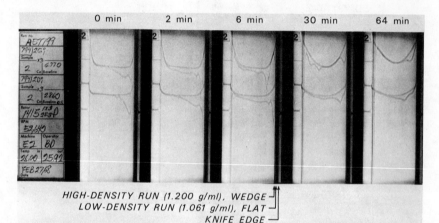

HIGH-DENSITY RUN (1.200 g/ml), WEDGE ⌉
LOW-DENSITY RUN (1.061 g/ml), FLAT ⌉
KNIFE EDGE ⌐

FIGURE 8. Selected schlieren patterns used for high- (upper) and low-density lipoprotein analysis. A card photograph identifies all necessary information for each run. (From Lindgren.[22] By permission of Bi-Science Publishing Division.)

schlieren patterns that are used for the tracing (FIGURE 9) and subsequent computer calculation.[22] Although initially done manually, these patterns are now traced with a sonic digitizer, fed into a small computer, and after editing, then analyzed using a telephone line to a larger memory computer and program. All standard graphical quantitative output, including population means, difference plots, and HDL subfraction analysis,[23] are thus done automatically. Potential new features of this analytic ultracentrifugal methodology will include similar curve resolution of LDL and a completely on-line computer availability with almost instant hard copy output of the corrected schlieren patterns by means of a cathode-ray tube and hard copier.

FIGURE 10 summarizes the major lipoprotein components now characterized by analytic ultracentrifugation. This is, of course, incomplete since there exist an unknown number of VLDL components as well as at least six separable S_f 2–12 (LDL$_2$) subfractions.[24] Further, the complexity and interrelationships

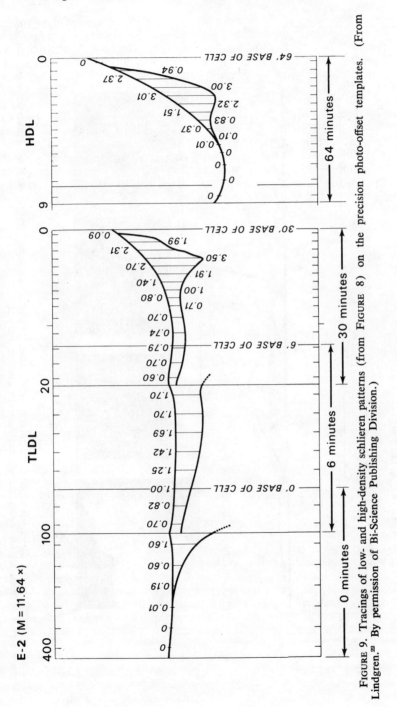

FIGURE 9. Tracings of low- and high-density schlieren patterns (from FIGURE 8) on the precision photo-offset templates. (From Lindgren.[22] By permission of Bi-Science Publishing Division.)

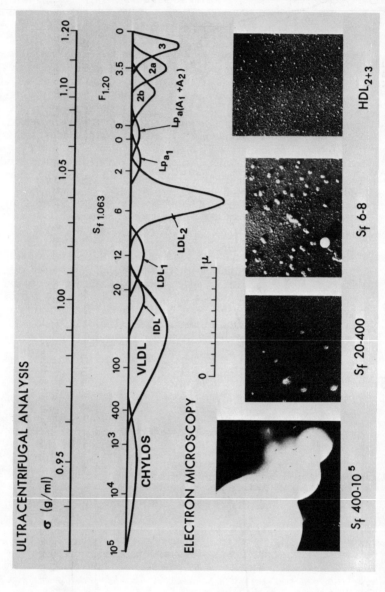

FIGURE 10. Summary of major lipoprotein components subfractionated and characterized by the analytic ultracentrifuge. The Lpₐ components exist at relatively low concentration and normally are not resolved.

among these lipoprotein subfractions as well as their metabolism and inter-conversion present challenges for future lipoprotein research related to health and disease.

CONCLUSIONS

Finally, I would like to offer a few thoughts and conclusions in perspective regarding the historical developments of lipoprotein fractionation and their characterization. First, technical problems, inadequate methodology, and mis-interpretation of data can long stand in the way of scientific progress. What began as a bizarre distortion of the albumin peak delayed for years utilization of ultracentrifugal techniques for lipoprotein isolation and characterization. However, once solved, it seemed simple, and there was a natural flow of de-velopments in all forms of lipoprotein work by increasing numbers of investiga-tors in ever-larger numbers of laboratories, particularly at the National Institutes of Health. These included the important clinical, metabolic, pathologic, and structural aspects of the serum lipoproteins.

The present ultracentrifugal characterization shown in FIGURE 10 involves many more components than were conceived back in 1949 when the first flota-tion of LDL (FIGURE 6) was observed. Claude Bernard summed it up well when he said, "Every advance in science is first preceded by an advance in technique." This was one important advance in technique. But we needed the invention and development of the ultracentrifuge by Svedberg. We needed the preliminary studies by McFarlane and Pederson, because the anomalous distor-tion, however vexing, held the key to further lipoprotein studies. We also needed the practical commercial developments by Ed Pickels [8] that have made ultracentrifuges available to thousands of laboratories today. And finally, we needed the correct interpretations of the ultracentrifuge data with the introduc-tion of lipoprotein flotation by Gofman et al. [9]

It would be impossible in this short time to detail the wealth of lipoprotein contributions made by others since this initial breakthrough. But I have taken my text mainly from what I have considered the highlights of these early historical ultracentrifugal landmarks.

This initial lipoprotein work was not done by a large research group with a big budget and a fixed agenda of experiments. It was done by one dedicated and visionary scientist in his prime and by two enthusiastic, excited half-time graduate students. We frequently worked 18 hours a day and even slept on the one analytic ultracentrifuge during the runs, which were done around the clock.

But times have changed, and many of us now find ourselves in relatively large, goal-oriented research groups. I hope that even within this changed system, especially for the younger scientists, there can be more smaller-scale, independent, basic biomedical-science-oriented research support. This would be particularly important for these younger scientists during their potentially most creative years. Such support, with freedom, is needed for dedicated and inspired research.

Finally, there are still important discrepancies, frontiers, and opportunities in lipoprotein research, and this important Symposium on Lipoprotein Structure will shortly discuss them. In considering lipoprotein history, let us remember two ultracentrifugal pioneers for their contribution and impetus toward findings that may be the ultimate characterization and nomenclature of lipoproteins, namely, their full physical-chemical definition and complete structure. Svedberg provided the ultracentrifuge and Gofman helped show how it could be effectively used. A scientist's immortality surely is to be found in his creative work.

ACKNOWLEDGMENTS

We thank Sonja Coffey for preparation of the manuscript. Special thanks to Dr. P. Alaupovic for proper description of Lp_a for preparation of FIGURE 10.

REFERENCES

1. SVEDBERG, T. & H. RINDE. 1924. J. Am. Chem. Soc. **46:**2677.
2. SVEDBERG, T. & K. PEDERSON. 1940. The Ultracentrifuge. R. H. Fowler and P. Kapitza, Eds. International Series of Monographs on Physics. Clarendon Press, London.
3. MACHEBOEF, M. 1929. Bull. Soc. Chem. Biol. **11:**268.
4. McFARLANE, A. S. 1935. Biochem. J. **29:**1175.
5. LAMM, O. 1933. Nature **132:**820.
6. ONCLEY, J. L. & F. R. N. GURD. 1953. The lipoproteins of human plasma. Chap. 1. *In* Blood Cells and Plasma Proteins. J. L. Tullis, Ed. Academic Press, New York, N.Y.
7. PEDERSON, K. O. 1945. Ultracentrifugal Studies on Serum and Serum Fractions. Almquist and Wiksells, Uppsala, Sweden.
8. PICKELS, E. G. 1950. Ultracentrifugation. *In* Biophysical Research Methods. R. M. Uber, Ed. Interscience Publishers, New York, N.Y.
9. GOFMAN, J. W., F. T. LINDGREN & H. ELLIOTT. 1949. J. Biol. Chem. **179:**973.
10. JOHNSTON, J. P. & A. G. OGSTON. 1946. Trans. Faraday Soc. **42:**789.
11. DE LALLA, O. & J. W. GOFMAN. 1954. Ultracentrifugal analysis of serum lipoproteins. *In* Methods of Biochemical Analysis. D. Glick, Ed. Vol. 1: 459–478. Interscience, New York, N.Y.
12. ANTSCHKOW, N. 1933. *In* Arteriosclerosis. E. V. Gowdry, Ed. MacMillan, New York, N.Y.
13. GOFMAN, J. W., F. T. LINDGREN, H. ELLIOTT, W. MANTZ, W. HEWITT, B. STRISOWER, V. HERRING & T. P. LYON. 1950. Science **111:**166.
14. GOFMAN, J. W., O. DE LALLA, F. GLAZIER, N. K. FREEMAN, F. T. LINDGREN, A. V. NICHOLS, B. STRISOWER & A. R. TAMPLIN. 1954. Plasma **2:**413.
15. LINDGREN, F. T. & A. V. NICHOLS. 1960. Structure and function of human serum lipoproteins. *In* Plasma Proteins. F. W. Putnam, Ed. Vol. 2:1–58. Academic Press, New York, N.Y.
16. TRIA, E. & A. M. SCANU, Eds. 1969. Structural and Functional Aspects of Lipoproteins. Academic Press, Inc., New York, N.Y.
17. NELSON, G. J., Ed. 1972. Blood Lipids and Lipoproteins. John Wiley-Interscience, New York, N.Y.
18. PEETERS, H., Ed. 1978. The Lipoprotein Molecule (NATO ASI). Plenum Publishing Corp., New York, N.Y.
19. LINDGREN, F. T., A. V. NICHOLS & F. M. KRAUSS, Eds. 1978. Symposium on High Density Lipoproteins. I. Structure, Function and Analysis; II. Clinical, Epidemiological and Metabolic Aspects. American Oil Chemists' Society, Champaign, Ill.
20. GOTTO, A. M., L. C. SMITH & B. ALLEN, Eds. 1980. Atherosclerosis V. Proceedings of the 5th International Symposium on Atherosclerosis, Houston, 1979. Springer-Verlag, New York, N.Y.
21. LIPPEL, K., Ed. 1979. Report of the HDL Methodology Workshop. NIH Publication No. 79–1661. National Institutes of Health, Bethesda, Md.

22. LINDGREN, F. T. 1974. Serum lipoproteins: Isolation and analysis with the preparative and analytical ultracentrifuge. *In* Fundamentals of Lipid Chemistry. R. M. Burton & F. C. Guerra, Eds. 2nd edit. pp. 470–510. Bi-Science Publishing Division, Webster Groves, Mo.

23. ANDERSON, D. W., A. V. NICHOLS, S. S. PAN & F. T. LINDGREN. 1978. Atherosclerosis **29:**161.

24. SHEN, M. S., R. M. KRAUSS, F. T. LINDGREN & T. FORTE. 1978. Circulation **50**(Suppl.):11–39, 142.

DISCUSSION OF THE PAPER

DR. N. PAPADOPOULOS (*National Institutes of Health, Bethesda, Md.*): While the ultracentrifuge has brought forth a lot of information, I think that it is important to name some limitations of this technique: the ultracentrifugal force, the addition of salt, and the time of analysis, all of which may introduce certain artifacts to the lipoproteins molecules. These molecules, as you know, are large labile, constantly undergoing changes and exchanges. Those of us who work with high resolution agarose gel electrophoresis have made certain observations, some of which agree with the ultracentrifugal data, but others which point at artifacts introduced by ultracentrifugation.

DR. F. T. LINDGREN: I could not agree more. I think Dr. Papadopoulos has brought up one of the frontiers that I alluded to. I would amplify it by simply saying that one of the major artifacts may result from the high g-forces that are commonly used in ultracentrifugal separations and analyses. We have data that some of you may have already seen, namely, that LDL subfractions are influenced by the g-force. At the lower g-forces you get higher flotation rates, and this is significant. For instance, between runs at 53,000 and 37,000 rpm you will get as much as one svedberg difference in flotation rates using moving boundary techniques. If we consider LDL a spherical molecule and try to figure out what is happening, that is, why the molecule is moving slower at the higher g-forces, we just do not have a clear explanation. This is one of the frontiers in need of exploration. We are all using ultracentrifuges almost with impunity now, and it is quite possible that these molecules are distorted in the ultracentrifugal field. This distortion may lead to the formation of asymmetrical particles such as prolate or oblate ellipsoids and may be a factor in lipoprotein degradation. Higher g-forces may also affect HDL and many investigators have observed some degradation of these particles in the ultracentrifuge.

DR. A. M. GOTTO, JR. (*Baylor College of Medicine, Houston, Texas*): Dr. Lindgren, do you want to comment on the pressure effects?

DR. LINDGREN: Pressure effects may only be part of the explanation for the change in shape. Other factors would be differential pressure, differential compression of the lipoprotein as opposed to the salt solution. With smectic cholesteryl ester changes one would expect $\bar{v}$ might change, and this in turn could give additional discrepancies. Thus, in the ultracentrifuge the lipoproteins may distort with possible $\bar{v}$ changes.

DR. J. C. OSBORNE, JR. (*National Institutes of Health, Bethesda, Md.*): I would like to just carry the issue of pressure effects a little bit further. These effects of pressure in the ultracentrifuge are not necessarily expressed by the beating up of the LDL or other plasma lipoproteins. For instance, if the sample is heterogeneous, i.e., the species in that sample have different partial specific volumes, then association or dissociation phenomena can occur as a function of the ultracentrifugal force. We have observed such phenomena with lipid-free apoA-I as I will discuss later in this Conference.

DR. LINDGREN: Yes, I believe that this has also been observed in other nonlipoprotein macromolecules by Vinograd and others. Pressure can affect the association constant.

DR. A. M. SCANU: On the issue of heterogeneity, in the case of HDL, besides the ultracentrifugal documentation of the heterogeneity of this lipoprotein class, investigators have reported on as many as 10 to 13 species in HDL by using the technique of isoelectric focusing. It would be important to validate this observation by independent techniques.

On the question of artifacts, I would like to ask whether the distortions due to g-forces, pressure effects, or other factors are reversible. In other words, when ultracentrifugation is over, is the shape of the lipoprotein molecule returning to that before centrifugation?

DR. LINDGREN: I think that we are dealing with both reversible and irreversible processes. By and large, however, the shape changes appear to be reversible.

DR. GOTTO: One of the real early pioneers in the field of lipoprotein chemistry is with us today, Dr. John Oncley. I have not alerted him that we would call on him, but I wonder whether or not he would like to make any historical remarks or other comments.

DR. J. L. ONCLEY (University of Michigan, Ann Arbor, Mich.): I would like to point out that, although I consider myself as something of a ultracentrifuge man, I think that my own ideas about lipoproteins have been more strongly affected by quite a few other things, some of which Dr. Lindgren did not mention.

Generally, it is hard to get rid of old ideas. And, I think that this also is true in lipoproteins. Certainly, the work by Macheboeuf was almost completely neglected for some 10 or 15 years. I myself entertained Macheboeuf in my home around the end of the late forties; I never knew a nicer scientist than him and I think that he never got the credit that he should have for pointing out that lipids were truly associated with proteins.

I think some of this occurred because it really was not until Dr. Scatchard studied the osmotic pressure of albumin in World War II that we got the concept of protein binding. The first binding studies were between sodium chloride and serum albumin; later a number of investigators, but particularly Robert Gordon and Vincent Dole showed that the fatty acid binding of serum albumin was of great importance in energy production all over the body, with particular regard to the oxidation of fatty acids.

Another thing which from the historical viewpoint was not mentioned is the work by Gordon Gould showing that cholesterol is bound by these lipoproteins in a labile fashion. Until that time I thought of cholesterol as a nice, stable molecule that was undoubtedly important in membranes and that probably went there to spend its lifetime in a particular spot. But now we know, of course, that practically all of the lipids are equally labile.

I just like to mention these earlier biochemical observations in the context of the biophysical outlook on the structure of lipoproteins to remind you that when you look at those studies today it is easy to think how foolish those early scientists were.

DR. GOTTO: In addition to his important work on the fractionation of lipoproteins, which was initiated at Harvard in collaboration with Dr. Cohn, I believe that Dr. Oncley was the first to introduce the term apoprotein, of which we shall hear more in this Conference.

DR. ONCLEY: I forgot to mention that the earliest papers I published in this field recognize the collaboration particularly of Frank Gurd. I do not know if he is here or not. He was my first graduate student and also my best graduate student.

LIPOPROTEIN BIOSYNTHESIS AND METABOLISM *

Richard J. Havel

Cardiovascular Research Institute and Department of Medicine
University of California, School of Medicine
San Francisco, California 94143

LIPOPROTEIN BIOSYNTHESIS AND METABOLISM

It is generally accepted that the protein and some of the lipid components of the plasma lipoproteins are synthesized in the parenchymal cells of the liver and the absorptive cells of the small intestine. Most of the detailed research in this area has been performed in rats, but some important information has been obtained in humans as well. The sites of removal of lipoprotein components are for the most part, uncertain. Major attention in recent years has attached to the role of the liver in the "terminal" catabolism of lipoproteins. The mechanisms of biosynthesis and terminal catabolism have also received attention. This review summarizes some recent research on the sites and mechanisms of biosynthesis and terminal catabolism of lipoproteins in rats and humans. FIGURE 1 summarizes some major features of lipoprotein-lipid metabolism and transport.

LIPOPROTEIN BIOSYNTHESIS

Sites of Apolipoprotein Biosynthesis in the Rat

In the rat, all of the apoprotein components investigated to date have been found to be synthesized in the liver, whereas the small intestine evidently synthesizes some, but not others (TABLE 1).[2] The B apoprotein evidently is an essential component of triglyceride-rich lipoproteins, but the molecular properties of this complex protein as secreted from the liver may differ from those of the intestinal component.[3, 4] Very-low-density lipoproteins (VLDL) secreted from the liver contain, in addition, the various C apolipoproteins (apoC) and the arginine-rich protein (apolipoprotein E). By contrast, large chylomicrons secreted from the mucosal cells of the small intestine during absorption of dietary fat, as well as small chylomicrons (also called intestinal VLDL) secreted under other conditions, contain apolipoproteins of the A group (mainly apoA-I and apoA-IV) and little or no varieties of apoC or apoE.[2]

The liver also secretes apoA-I and apoA-IV, but almost all of these proteins appear in perfusates of isolated livers as components of high-density lipoproteins (HDL). A substantial amount of apoE is also found in HDL of these perfusates. The fraction of apoprotein E that is secreted in association with VLDL and HDL is difficult to assess because this protein readily dissociates from lipoproteins during centrifugation.[5] This problem has also made it difficult to

* The personal work cited herein was supported by grants from United States Public Health Service: HL-14237 (Arteriosclerosis SCOR) and HL-06285.

16

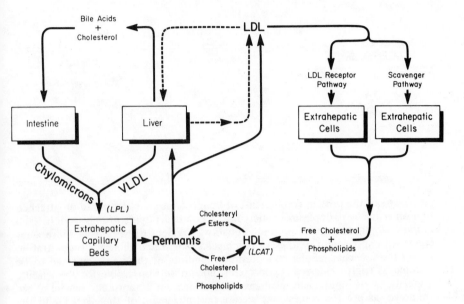

FIGURE 1. Pathways for lipid transport in plasma lipoproteins.[1] Triglycerides synthesized in intestine and liver are transported in chylomicrons and VLDL, respectively, together with cholesteryl esters synthesized in these organs. The triglycerides are mainly delivered to extrahepatic tissues through the action of endothelial lipoprotein lipase (LPL) to yield remnant lipoproteins that are taken up by the liver or ultimately converted to LDL. Most cholesteryl esters in blood plasma arise from the action of LCAT in HDL and are largely transferred (at least in humans) to triglyceride-rich lipoproteins or their remnant products. The free cholesterol substrate for LCAT arises both from the surface of remnant lipoproteins and from the membranes of body tissues. LDL are catabolized in extrahepatic tissues by receptor-dependent and independent pathways and also to an uncertain extent in the liver. Plasma cholesteryl esters can be delivered to the liver as components of remnant lipoproteins, as components of LDL or (not shown) as components of HDL, providing several routes for the ultimate excretion of cholesterol in the bile. The immediate sources of lipoprotein cholesterol (free or esterified) and the sites at which lipoprotein cholesterol is removed from the blood have not been quantified. (From Havel et al.[1] By permission of W. B. Saunders Co.)

determine the extent to which intestinal A apoproteins are normally secreted separately from chylomicrons.[6] Our own studies suggest that much of the A apoproteins found in HDL of intestinal lymph of rats are either ultracentrifugal artifacts of reflect the entry of HDL into lymph from blood plasma.[7]

Mechanisms of Lipoprotein Biosynthesis

Research on the mechanisms of lipoprotein biosynthesis has progressed slowly during the past few years. Much of our present information is based upon experiments in which electron microscopy has figured importantly.[8] The

TABLE 1

SITES OF APOLIPOPROTEIN BIOSYNTHESIS IN THE RAT

Apoprotein	Liver	Intestine
B	+	+
A-I	+	+
A-II	?	?
A-IV	+	+
C's	+	±
E	+	±

precursors of the protein components of lipoproteins are synthesized on attached ribosomes in the endoplasmic reticulum. Lipoprotein-lipids are also synthesized in the endoplasmic reticulum, but probably in regions distinct from those associated with apoprotein synthesis. The mechanisms responsible for sequestration within the cisternae of the endoplasmic reticulum of the lipids destined to be secreted as triglyceride-rich lipoproteins, and those responsible for the specific associations of lipids and proteins in the nascent lipoprotein particles are unknown, as are the forces that dictate the movement of the particles to the Golgi apparatus. These problems remain general ones for cell biology, to which research on lipoprotein biosynthesis and secretion can contribute. As with many plasma proteins,[9] some of the protein components of lipoproteins are progressively glycosylated as they move through the endoplasmic reticulum and Golgi apparatus. These modifications of the structure of the proteins, as well as modifications of the protein backbone, may contribute to the directed movement of nascent lipoproteins through the cell, including the process of secretion from secretory vesicles of the Golgi apparatus by emiocytosis.

Structure of Nascent Rat Lipoproteins

Whereas it is now clear that the triglyceride-rich lipoproteins are largely formed as spherical "pseudomicellar" particles within the cell of origin, this is not the case for HDL. Lipoproteins in this density range appear in perfusates of isolated livers as discoidal particles in which a bilayer of glycerophosphatides is stabilized by apoproteins of the A group or apoprotein E.[10] Whereas nascent VLDL isolated from the Golgi apparatus of rats contain virtually the same complement of triglycerides and cholesteryl esters (core lipids) as plasma VLDL, these components are scarce in nascent HDL isolated from liver perfusates. Although the form in which the protein components of HDL are secreted from the hepatocyte is unknown, the nascent HDL do not appear to arise as ultracentrifugal artifacts from newly secreted VLDL. Thus, the amount and properties of HDL that accumulate in perfusates of livers from orotic-acid-fed rats are not materially different from those of normally fed rats, even though secretion of triglyceride-rich lipoproteins is almost completely inhibited by the pyrimidine.[11]

Under ordinary conditions, almost all of the B apoprotein is secreted from liver perfusates in lipoproteins that float in the ultracentrifuge at a nonprotein solvent density of 1.006 g/ml. However, perfused livers from cholesterol-fed rats appear to secrete appreciable amounts of this protein in a triglyceride-poor form that has a higher density.[12] Under some conditions, it therefore seems possible that the liver can contribute directly to plasma LDL, although virtually all LDL are normally derived from the catabolism of triglyceride-rich lipoproteins, especially VLDL.

Rates of Lipoprotein Synthesis in the Rat

Most of the information about hepatic lipoprotein secretion has been obtained from experiments with isolated, perfused rat livers. Although very useful for some purposes, this technique has important limitations, especially for estimating rates of secretion. One limitation arises from removal of the liver from influences that normally regulate lipoprotein synthesis. This can be overcome, in part, by including in the perfusate critical components normally present in blood plasma. Another limitation arises from the fact (described below) that the liver takes up and catabolizes the lipoproteins that it secretes. With certain technical limitations, this problem can be obviated by use of "single pass" rather than recirculating perfusions. In general, results obtained from experiments with perfused livers are likely to underestimate secretion rates. The limitations for perfused livers apply as well to experiments with isolated, perfused small intestinal preparations. Much of the information on intestinal lipoprotein secretion has been obtained in intact rats in which the main intestinal lymph duct has been cannulated.[2] Some of the problems inherent to perfused preparations are thereby avoided, but it is difficult to maintain such animals in a steady state, and direct measurements of secretion rates are not possible owing to transfer of lipoproteins from the blood into the lymph. For this reason, isotopic techniques have been devised to estimate the rate of intestinal synthesis.[13] Isotopic techniques in intact animals can also be used to provide some information about relative contributions of the liver and small intestine to lipoprotein biosynthesis. From such studies it appears that the intestine makes a large contribution to the synthesis of the A apolipoproteins but that the others are synthesized primarily in the liver.[14]

Less is known about factors regulating apolipoprotein biosynthesis. Available evidence suggests that the content of apoprotein B is constant among chylomicrons and VLDL of varying size. If so, it follows that augmented triglyceride secretion can result from synthesis of larger lipoproteins, with no change in synthesis of this protein. This evidently occurs in the liver when rats are fed carbohydrate-rich diets.[15] Similarly, the size of chylomicrons increases during absorption of dietary fat with relatively little increase in secretion of B or A apolipoproteins.[13] In the intestine in particular, recruitment of more absorptive cells in the process of fat absorption after fat feeding may be required for the generation of more lipoprotein particles and their associated proteins. Our knowledge of the regulation of the hepatic synthesis of lipoproteins other than apoprotein B is even more fragmentary. Cholesterol feeding in guinea pigs stimulates the accumulation of discoidal HDL and apoprotein E in liver perfusates,[16] and accumulation of apoprotein A-I is increased in perfusates of livers from cholestatic rats.[17]

From the methods described, important information has been obtained concerning the contribution of the liver and intestine to the secretion of the proteins as well as the core components of chylomicrons and VLDL. However, little is yet known about the contribution of these tissues to the synthesis of the polar (surface) lipid components, especially cholesterol. Both *in vivo* and in perfusion systems in which blood cells are present, cholesterol found in secreted lipoproteins may be derived from the formed elements. Nascent VLDL isolated from the Golgi apparatus of rat livers contain less cholesterol than plasma VLDL,[18] suggesting an extrahepatic origin of some cholesterol in this lipoprotein. Most of the cholesteryl esters of rat chylomicrons and VLDL evidently are synthesized in cells producing these lipoproteins but almost all of the cholesteryl esters in plasma HDL, and much of those in plasma LDL are derived from the action of lecithin-cholesterol acyltransferase (LCAT) upon HDL in blood plasma.[19] Inasmuch as the ultimate source of the cholesterol substrate for LCAT is uncertain, we remain ignorant of the site(s) from which much of the lipoprotein-cholesterol arises. The problem is not readily susceptible to attack with radio-labeled cholesterol because of the ready exchangeability of cholesterol among lipoproteins and between lipoproteins and most cells.

Lipoprotein Biosynthesis in Humans

From catheterization studies, we know that chylomicrons and VLDL are produced in humans as they are in the rat from small intestine and liver. Information on the sites of apolipoprotein biosynthesis is, however, derived solely from immunofluorescent studies and immunoassays in *in vivo* systems. For the most part, these show good correspondence with results obtained in rats.[20-23] The inference that LDL are derived primarily from VLDL in humans is based entirely upon isotopic precursor-product studies.[24] As in the rat, LDL may, however, be produced directly under abnormal circumstances, as shown in individuals with homozygous familial hypercholesterolemia.[25] Apolipoprotein A-IV, first identified in the rat plasma HDL[26] and lymph chylomicrons,[6] has now been found as well in human plasma[27] and lymph.[28] These homologies provide encouragement for those who use the rat as an experimental model. However, much evidence indicates that important quantitative differences exist between the two species in some aspects of lipoprotein biosynthesis or catabolism: (1) In humans, the fatty acid composition of cholesteryl esters of VLDL resembles that of HDL and LDL, suggesting that the former are derived mainly from LCAT rather than hepatic biosynthesis as in the rat. (2) The concentration of LDL is much lower in rats than humans, presumably owing to a lesser conversion of components (especially apoprotein B) of VLDL to LDL in the rat.[29] (3) The concentration of apoprotein E is considerably higher in rats than in humans. This is especially the case for the concentration of this protein in HDL. Rat plasma contains an appreciable fraction of HDL as particles in which apoprotein E is the major protein component,[5] whereas apoprotein E comprises only about 1% of the total apoprotein complement of human HDL.[30] It is not known whether this difference arises from different rates of biosynthesis or catabolism.

LIPOPROTEIN METABOLISM

General Features

In principle, several mechanisms can be envisioned for the metabolism of plasma lipoproteins. First, lipoproteins may be subject to processes that occur within the circulating blood. Second, lipoproteins may interact with endothelial cells, or, after transport through the endothelium, they may interact with tissue cells in various ways: (1) They may be subjected to enzymatic attack at the cell surface. (2) They may be taken up into the cell by pinocytosis, either nonspecifically (bulk fluid pinocytosis) or specifically (adsorptive, receptor-mediated pinocytosis). (3) They may interact with the cell surface so as to lead to uptake of one or more components into the cell, without uptake of the entire particle.

Within the blood compartment, certain changes occur rapidly after lipoproteins are secreted. These include various net transfers or exchanges of components among lipoprotein particles of the same or different species. In some cases, these transfers are reciprocal, tending to preserve the mass of surface and core components. When like species transfer reciprocally, this amounts to a simple exchange, with no change in chemical or physical properties. For esterified lipids, reciprocal transfers can involve compounds with different fatty acyl residues, leading to altered properties. Transfers can also occur between differing surface residues (i.e., protein for phospholipids [6] or core components (i.e., triglycerides for cholesteryl esters).[31] Such transfers will evidently be limited by certain physical constraints. However, under some conditions, transfers may occur in concert with enzymatic reactions that produce metastable particles, as described below. In addition, enzymatic reactions are generally followed by component-transfers, as in the transfer of cholesteryl esters produced in HDL by LCAT to VLDL or LDL.

Perhaps the best characterized interaction of plasma lipoproteins with a cell surface is that associated with the action of endothelial lipoprotein lipase.[32] By removing core triglycerides from lipoproteins the enzymatic reaction is thought to lead to a redundance of surface material on the residual lipoprotein, producing a metastable particle from which surface components then dissociate. At least under some circumstances, these surface materials accumulate in HDL to produce another metastable particle,[7] lipid components of which are acted upon by LCAT, followed by transfer of product cholesteryl esters to other lipoproteins and of product lysolecithin to albumin. It appears that any cellular reaction that consumes one component of a stable lipoprotein particle will produce a less stable particle, generating a series of events that eventually yields a new population of stable, but different particles.

The specific interaction of lipoproteins with enzymes and with cells evidently depends upon specific determinants on or near the lipoprotein surface. With respect to enzymatic interactions, both lipid and protein composition may be important.[32, 33] We now have strong evidence for a physiological function in the lipoprotein lipase reaction for one of the proteins (apoprotein C-II), from the discovery of a genetically determined deficiency of the protein.[34] ApoC-II increases the velocity of triglyceride hydrolysis in lipoproteins by lipoprotein lipase, whereas other C apoproteins as well as other apoproteins inhibit the reaction.[32] We presently have no persuasive evidence that these inhibitory proteins normally regulate this reaction. Another possible regulatory function of C apoproteins has come to light from research on hepatic lipoprotein catabolism. The isolated perfused rat liver takes up and catabolizes hepatogenous VLDL (obtained from liver perfusates) as well as small chylomicrons from intestinal lymph.[35] As compared with plasma VLDL and plasma chylomicrons these newly secreted lipoproteins are deficient in C apolipoproteins and acquire them from HDL when they enter the blood. This modification can be produced by briefly incubating the triglyceride-rich lipoprotein with the density >1.006 g/ml fraction of rat serum.[6] The modified VLDL and small chylomicrons thus produced are no longer effectively removed by the liver.[35] This result is consistent with the hypothesis that one function of C apolipoproteins is to prevent the interaction of newly secreted triglyceride-rich lipoproteins with a hepatic receptor, thereby contributing to the delivery of triglycerides to extrahepatic tissues, where they are acted upon by lipoprotein lipase.

The "LDL Pathway"

In various cultured cells and in freshly obtained blood leucocytes, LDL are taken up by receptor-dependent adsorptive pinocytosis and transferred to lysosomes where they are catabolized by acid hydrolases. This "LDL pathway" and its regulation have been delineated in some detail in cultured cells, particularly human fibroblasts.[36] The LDL receptor in human fibroblasts recognizes not only lipoproteins or lipid–phospholipid complexes containing the B apoprotein, but also lipoproteins or complexes containing apoprotein E. The affinity of the receptor for apoprotein E, estimated per unit mass of protein, exceeds that of apoprotein B.[37] A physiological role for the LDL receptor in humans is strongly supported by the diminished fractional rate of catabolism of the B apoprotein of LDL in receptor-deficient or defective familial hypercholesterolemia.[1] Other evidence for functioning LDL receptors in vivo is limited, but, in addition to freshly isolated leucocytes, the receptor has been demonstrated in membranes from fresh tissue in bovine steroid-secreting endocrine glands and adipose tissue, but not in other tissues, including the liver.[38]

Hepatic Lipoprotein Catabolism

The rat liver can catabolize the protein moiety of several classes of lipoproteins, including triglyceride-rich lipoproteins,[39] LDL,[40] and HDL.[41] The mechanism of lipoprotein uptake by the liver and the importance of the liver in lipoprotein catabolism, especially of LDL and HDL, are subjects of active investigation in several laboratories. The best established role of the liver in lipoprotein catabolism is in the uptake of triglyceride-rich lipoproteins that have been partially degraded by lipoprotein lipase in extrahepatic tissues ("remnant" lipoproteins). Such lipoproteins, isolated from plasma of functionally hepatectomized rats, are rapidly removed from the blood of intact rats and are also rapidly taken up and catabolized by isolated, perfused rat livers.[35, 42, 43] Remnants of chylomicrons and VLDL have several common characteristics.[44] They range from 350 to about 1000 Å in diameter and retain the surface-core characteristics of typical pseudomicellar lipoproteins. Their protein components include the original complement of apoprotein B and probably apoprotein E and they are deficient in A and C apoproteins. As described above, the rate of uptake of nascent triglyceride-rich lipoproteins (small chylomicrons from intestinal lymph and VLDL from perfused livers) by perfused livers is inhibited when the content of C apoproteins in the lipoproteins is increased. This can be achieved not only by incubation of the lipoproteins with the density >1.006 g/ml infranatant fraction of rat plasma (which results in transfer of C apoproteins from HDL) but also by incubating the triglyceride-rich lipoproteins with isolated C apoproteins. In a similar manner, incubation of apoprotein E with small chylomicrons from intestinal lymph increases the amount of this protein on the triglyceride-rich particles. These modified chylomicrons are taken up by the perfused liver at a rapid rate, similar to that of chylomicron remnants.[45] These results suggest that the amount of apoprotein E relative to apoprotein C may critically determine the interaction of the triglyceride-rich particle with a hepatic surface component (receptor).[35] Some evidence for such a receptor has been obtained in studies of perfused livers [42, 43] and isolated hepatocytes.[46] ApoE-HDL$_C$, a lipoprotein isolated from the plasma of cholesterol-fed dogs, has recently been found to be rapidly taken up by the liver of rats after intravenous administration.[47] Inasmuch as apoprotein E is virtually the only protein component of this lipoprotein, this observation is consistent with the hypothesis [1] that the remnant receptor recognizes apoprotein E. The mechanism of remnant uptake is uncertain, but available evidence suggests that endocytosis of the lipoprotein particle [29, 43, 48] is followed by lysosomal catabolism.[49] Such an endocytic pathway must have a minor role in the case of human VLDL, the B protein component of which is mainly converted to LDL.[24] A role for the liver in the VLDL-LDL conversion is not firmly established.

The mechanism by which the liver normally takes up and catabolizes LDL and HDL is unknown. Recent studies in rats treated with massive amounts of estrogens have provided some clues in the case of LDL and some species of HDL.[50] Within a few days such rats develop profound hypolipidemia that involves all classes of lipoproteins. Perfused livers from these rats take up and catabolize the protein moiety of rat and human LDL at rates several-fold greater than those observed in livers from untreated animals. Livers from treated animals also take up and catabolize HDL that contain apoprotein E (but no apoprotein B) at increased rates. HDL containing only A and C apoproteins are catabolized at rates comparable to those found in livers from untreated animals. Crude membrane fractions (obtained by centrifugation of liver homogenates between 10,000 and 100,000 g) from livers of estrogen-treated rats specifically bind LDL.[51] This binding resembles that of the LDL receptor in cultured fibroblasts in that it recognizes human LDL but not HDL, requires calcium ion, and is prevented by methylation of the B apoprotein. However, the affinity of the hepatic receptor for LDL is much lower than that of the fibroblast receptor. Likewise, the augmented catabolism of LDL in perfused livers from estrogen-treated rats is abolished by chemical modification of arginyl residues of apoprotein B and the enhanced catabolism continues to increase at concentrations of LDL in the perfusate that would easily saturate the LDL receptor in cultured fibroblasts.[50]

The receptor activity demonstrable in membranes from livers of estrogen-treated rats has not been reliably demonstrated in membranes from untreated rats. Hence, despite certain similarities, the relationship between the normal mechanism of catabolism of LDL in perfused rat livers and that observed in livers from estrogen-treated rats is uncertain. Livers from estrogen-treated rats also catabolize triglyceride-rich lipoproteins at an increased rate.[45] Inasmuch as these lipoproteins contain both apoprotein B and E, as do their remnant products, the estrogen-induced receptor could constitute the putative "remnant" receptor. If this is so, the receptor must normally recognize remnant lipoproteins preferentially.

The existence of a regulated pathway for hepatic uptake and catabolism of human LDL could explain certain well-established phenomena.[1] For example, the accelerated catabolism of LDL produced by administration of bile acid-sequestrants could result from increased receptor activity owing to the increased conversion of cholesterol to bile acids with consequent drain upon hepatic cholesterol. The increased production of apoprotein B (largely in the form of LDL) in patients with homozygous familial hypercholesterolemia could also be explained if the hepatic receptor were a product of the gene coding for the LDL receptor in cultured fibroblasts, given the added assumption that apoB synthesis is regulated by hepatic uptake of apoB in LDL.

Autoradiographic studies in livers from rats given estrogen suggest that LDL are taken up and catabolized mainly by parenchymal cells.[52] However, several covalent modifications of the protein moiety of LDL lead to rapid and apparently exclusive uptake of LDL into Küpffer cells.[47, 53, 54] Such covalent modifications also lead to rapid uptake of some other, similarly modified plasma proteins.[53, 54] There is presently no evidence that covalent modifications normally precede hepatic catabolism of LDL or other plasma proteins, but neither are there data available to exclude a significant role for such a process. Uptake of modified LDL into Küpffer cells is also receptor-dependent,[53] providing another example of the critical role of protein structure in specifying both the site and rates of catabolism.

Sites of LDL and HDL Catabolism

The relative importance of the liver in the normal catabolism of the cholesterol-rich lipoproteins is uncertain. From experiments with perfused rat livers, it has been estimated that the liver accounts for only a minor fraction of the catabolism of the protein moiety of LDL and HDL.[40, 41] A new approach to this problem has been to utilize LDL covalently labeled with radioactive sucrose (in a manner that does not affect the interaction of LDL with its receptor in cultured fibroblasts) to evaluate pinocytotic uptake of LDL *in vivo*.[55] The labeled sucrose, presumably carried with the LDL to lysosomes, remains within the cell for substantial periods following enzymatic degradation of the lipoprotein components, thereby serving as a marker of the site of uptake. Studies with this method indicate hepatic uptake on the order of 50% of injected [³H]sucrose-LDL in intact rats and swine.[56]

Pinocytotic uptake of LDL in rat liver can account for only a small fraction of the catabolism of LCAT-derived plasma cholesteryl esters.[41] Thus in this species, direct hepatic uptake of HDL or, alternatively, uptake of remnant lipoproteins is likely to be responsible for delivery of such cholesteryl esters to the liver. If, as suggested from experiments with perfused livers [41] and partially hepatectomized rats,[57] the liver has a minor role in HDL catabolism, HDL could participate in the delivery of cholesterol to other tissues that require it for synthesis of membranes or steroid hormones. However, the importance of the liver in the catabolism of the apoE-containing HDL found in rat plasma has not been evaluated. In humans, LDL rather than HDL are probably the major vehicles for the catabolism of LCAT-derived cholesteryl esters.[1] These cholesteryl esters in LDL are derived either directly from HDL or via VLDL. Transfer of cholesteryl esters from human HDL to VLDL and LDL has been shown to be mediated by a specific apoprotein, presumably apoprotein D.[31] This discovery provides yet another role for apolipoproteins in lipoprotein metabolism.

One or more functions can now be ascribed to most of the known apolipoproteins (TABLE 2). Further research seems certain to uncover additional functions and thereby to increase our understanding of plasma lipid transport and its regulation.

TABLE 2

FUNCTIONS OF APOLIPOPROTEINS IN LIPOPROTEIN METABOLISM

Function	Apolipoprotein(s)
Lipoprotein biosynthesis/secretion	B
Lipoprotein-lipid metabolism	
Lipoprotein lipase activity	C-II
Lecithin-cholesterol acyltransferase activity	A-I
Cholesteryl ester transfer	D
Recognition of lipoproteins by cell receptors	
Cultured cells, leucocytes, adrenal cortex, gonads	B and E
Liver	B and E
Inhibition of cellular uptake, liver	C's

ACKNOWLEDGMENTS

The recent research on hepatic lipoprotein metabolism summarized here was carried out principally by Y.-S. Chao and E. Windler. R. L. Hamilton and J.-L. Vigne have made important contributions to recent studies of metastable lipoproteins.

REFERENCES

1. HAVEL, R. J., J. L. GOLDSTEIN & M. S. BROWN. 1979. In Disease of Metabolism. 8th edit. P. K. Bondy & L. E. Rosenberg, Eds. W. B. Saunders Company, Philadelphia, Pa. In press.
2. HAVEL, R. J. 1978. In High Density Lipoproteins and Atherosclerosis. A. M. Gotto, Jr., N. E. Miller & M. F. Oliver, Eds. :21–35. Elsevier/North-Holland Biomedical Press, Amsterdam, The Netherlands.
3. KRISHNAIAH, K. V., J. ONG, L. F. WALKER, J. BORENSZTAJN & G. S. GETZ. 1978. Fed. Proc. 37:257(241A).
4. KANE, J. P., D. A. HARDMAN & H. E. PAULUS. 1980. Proc. Natl. Acad. Sci. USA. In press.
5. FAINARU, M., R. J. HAVEL & K. IMAIZUMI. 1977. Biochem. Med. 17:347–355.
6. IMAIZUMI, K., M. FAINARU & R. J. HAVEL. 1978. J. Lipid Res. 19:712–722.

7. HAVEL, R. J., R. L. HAMILTON & J.-L. VIGNE. Unpublished data.
8. HAMILTON, R. L. & H. J. KAYDEN. 1974. *In* The Liver: Normal & Abnormal Function (Part A). The Biologic Chemistry of Disease. F. F. Becker, Ed. Vol. 5: 531–572. Marcel Dekker, New York, N.Y.
9. LEBLOND, C. P. & G. BENNETT. 1977. *In* International Cell Biology 1976–1977. B. R. Brinkley & K. R. Porter, Eds. pp. 326–336. Rockefeller University Press. New York, N.Y.
10. HAMILTON, R. L., M. C. WILLIAMS, C. J. FIELDING & R. J. HAVEL. 1976. J. Clin. Invest. **58:**667–680.
11. HAMILTON, R. L., Y.-S. CHAO & R. J. HAVEL. Unpublished observations.
12. NOEL, S.-P., L. WONG, P. L. DOLPHIN, L. DORY & D. RUBINSTEIN. 1979. J. Clin. Invest. **64:**674–683.
13. IMAIZUMI, K., R. J. HAVEL, M. FAINARU & J.-L. VIGNE. 1978. J. Lipid Res. **19:** 1038–1046.
14. WU, A.-L. & H. G. WINDMUELLER. 1979. J. Biol. Chem. **254:**7316–7322.
15. WITZTUM, J. L. & G. SCHONFELD. 1978. Diabetes **27:**1215–1229.
16. HAMILTON, R. L., R. OSTWALD, L. S. S. GUO & R. J. HAVEL. Unpublished observations.
17. FELKER, T. E., R. L. HAMILTON, J.-L. VIGNE & R. J. HAVEL. 1979. J. Am. Oil Chem. Soc. **56:**200(199A).
18. HAVEL, R. J. 1975. Adv. Biochem. Med. Biol. **63:**37–59.
19. FAERGEMAN, O. & R. J. HAVEL. 1975. J. Clin. Invest. **55:**1210–1218.
20. RACHMILEWITZ, D., J. J. ALBERS, D. R. SAUNDERS & M. FAINARU. 1978. Gastroenterology **75:**677–682.
21. ASSMANN, G., E. SMOOTZ & A. CAPURSO. 1978. *In* High Density Lipoproteins and Atherosclerosis. A. M. Gotto, Jr., N. E. Miller & M. F. Oliver, Eds. pp. 77–89. Elsevier/North-Holland Biomedical Press, Amsterdam, The Netherlands.
22. GLICKMAN, R. M., P. H. R. GREEN, R. LEES & A. R. TALL. 1978. N. Engl. J. Med. **299:**1424–1427.
23. WALTON, K. W., G. V. H. BRADBY & C. J. MORRIS. 1978. *In* International Conference on Atherosclerosis, Milan, 1977. L. A. Carlson, *et al.*, Eds. pp. 303–310. Raven Press, New York, N.Y.
24. SCHAFER, E. J., S. EISENBERG & R. I. LEVY. 1978. J. Lipid Res. **19:**667–687.
25. THOMPSON, G. R., A. K. SOUTAR & N. B. MYANT. 1976. Circulation **54** (Suppl. 2):26.
26. SWANEY, J. B., H. REESE & H. A. EDER. 1974. Biochem. Biophys. Res. Commun. **59:**513–519.
27. BEISIEGEL, U. & G. UTERMANN. 1979. Eur. J. Biochem. **93:**601–608.
28. WEISGRABER, K. H., T. P. BERSOT & R. W. MAHLEY. 1978. Biochem. Biophys. Res. Commun. **85:**287–292.
29. FAERGEMAN, O., T. SATA, J. P. KANE & R. J. HAVEL. 1975. J. Clin. Invest. **56:** 1396–1403.
30. HAVEL, R. J., L. KOTITE, J.-L. VIGNE, J. P. KANE & P. TUN. Unpublished observations.
31. CHAJEK, T. & C. J. FIELDING. 1978. Proc. Natl. Acad. Sci. USA **75:**3445–3449.
32. FIELDING, C. J. & R. J. HAVEL. 1977. Arch. Pathol. Lab. Med. **101:**225–229.
33. FIELDING, C. J., V. G. SHORE & P. E. FIELDING. 1972. Biochim. Biophys. Acta **270:**513–518.
34. BRECKENRIDGE, W. C., J. A. LITTLE, G. STEINER, A. CHOW & M. POAPST. 1978. N. Engl. J. Med. **298:**1265–1273.
35. WINDLER, E., Y.-S. CHAO & R. J. HAVEL. 1980. J. Biol. Chem. In press.
36. GOLDSTEIN, J. L. & M. S. BROWN. 1977. Ann. Rev. Biochem. **46:**897–930.
37. INNERARITY, T. L. & R. W. MAHLEY. 1978. Biochemistry **17:**1440–1447.
38. KOVANEN, P. T., J. R. FAUST, M. S. BROWN & J. L. GOLDSTEIN. 1979. Endocrinology **104:**599–609.

39. HAVEL, R. J. 1977. *In* Atherosclerosis. G. W. Manning & M. Daria Haust, Eds. pp. 406–412. Plenum Press, New York, N.Y.
40. SIGURDSSON, G., S.-P. NOEL & R. J. HAVEL. 1978. J. Lipid Res. **19:**628–634.
41. SIGURDSSON, G., S.-P. NOEL & R. J. HAVEL. 1979. J. Lipid Res. **20:**316–324.
42. SHERRILL, B. C. & J. M. DIETSCHY. 1978. J. Biol. Chem. **253:**1859–1867.
43. COOPER, A. D. & P. Y. S. YU. 1978. J. Lipid Res. **19:**635–643.
44. MJØS, O. D., O. FAERGEMAN, R. L. HAMILTON & R. J. HAVEL. 1975. J. Clin. Invest. **56:**603–615.
45. WINDLER, E., Y.-S. CHAO & R. J. HAVEL. Unpublished observations.
46. FLOREN, C. H. & A. NILSSON. 1978. Biochem. J. **174:**827–838.
47. MAHLEY, R. W., K. H. WEISGRABER, T. L. INNERARITY & H. G. WINDMUELLER. 1979. Proc. Natl. Acad. Sci. USA **76:**1746–1750.
48. NAITO, M. & E. WISSE. 1978. Cell Tiss. Res. **190:**371–382.
49. STEIN, O., D. RACHMILEWITZ, L. SANGER, S. EISENBERG & Y. STEIN. 1974. Biochim. Biophys. Acta **360:**205–216.
50. CHAO, Y.-S., E. E. WINDLER, G. C. CHEN & R. J. HAVEL. 1979. J. Biol. Chem. **254:**11360–11366.
51. KOVANEN, P. T., M. S. BROWN & J. L. GOLDSTEIN. 1979. J. Biol. Chem. **254:** 11367–11373.
52. CHAO, Y.-S., A. L. JONES, E. WINDLER & R. J. HAVEL. Unpublished observations.
53. GOLDSTEIN, J. L., Y. K. HO, S. K. BASU & M. S. BROWN. 1979. Proc. Natl. Acad. Sci. USA **76:**333–337.
54. CHAO, Y.-S., G. C. CHEN, E. WINDLER, J. P. KANE & R. J. HAVEL. 1979. Fed. Proc. **38:**896(3516A).
55. PITTMAN, R. C. & D. STEINBERG. 1978. Biochem. Biophys. Res. Commun. **81:** 1254–1259.
56. STEINBERG, D. 1979. Ann. N.Y. Acad. Sci. This volume.
57. VAN TOL, A., T. VAN GENT, F. M. VAN'T HOOFT & F. VLASPOLDER. 1978. Atherosclerosis **29:**439–448.

DISCUSSION OF THE PAPER

DR. A. M. GOTTO, JR.: Dr. Havel, one point about the perfused system you were using—what exactly did you mean by hepatic VLDL?

DR. R. J. HAVEL: We use a recycling system that contains no plasma components but does contain washed rat erythrocytes. Recirculation goes on for 1 to 4 hours. In the experiments I showed, we harvest VLDL from the system. They are very similar to plasma VLDL, but they are relatively depleted in free cholesterol and proteins and somewhat enriched in phospholipids.

DR. GOTTO: The VLDL incubated with the *d* 1.019 bottom—was that hepatic or what?

DR. HAVEL: In that case, the hepatic VLDL were mixed with plasma depleted of VLDL to simulate what happens in the circulation. We have done, as I have mentioned, the same thing with chylomicrons and the results in the liver system were identical.

DR. D. STEINBERG (*University of California at San Diego, La Jolla, Calif.*): It was a very nice review. We appreciated hearing that. I wanted to make one comment and ask one question. The comment is that studies which Miss Sharon Pangborn has done in our laboratory and which she reported at the Gordon

Conference also point to the presence, at least in the pig liver cell, of a high-affinity receptor for LDL. The studies in rat liver, I think, have been somewhat confusing, at least in our laboratory and I think in others, particularly when one uses human LDL. And, when one uses rat LDL, which people have not often used because it is so difficult to get enough to do experiments with, then the results, I think, clearly show a high-affinity receptor.

I would like to urge that in the discussion here, in relationship to this interesting paper and others, that we keep in mind the possibility that there is species specificity. Indeed, as we learn more about the rather narrow ranges of specificity, the small variations in molecular charge and possibly shape can alter the interaction of lipoproteins with their receptors. It is not then really so surprising that lipoproteins of different species interact differently. Certainly, it has been our impression with rat liver cells, pig liver cells, rat fibroblasts, and human fibroblasts. The differences are quite remarkable.

The only other question I would like to ask is in relationship to the perfusion studies. Our *in vivo* studies, as you know, showed that the rat liver, using our sucrose labeling technique, takes up a lot of LDL. Your normal values, i.e., the control values, seem to be small, or at least let me ask you—the 10% value in 4 hours was 10% of what? Also, would you comment on the rate of degradation of LDL in the control animals and address the issue of whether total TCA-soluble iodide, which we also use, is a true measure of degradation.

DR. HAVEL: In the original studies with Gunnar Sigurdson we were unable to show distinct difference in the rates of hepatic catabolism in the perfused liver system with human and rat LDL. But, as you may have seen on one of the slides, the current results show about a two- or threefold difference in the rates, the values being higher in the case of rat LDL than in the case of human LDL.

Now, as you mentioned, it is very difficult to isolate satisfactorily rat LDL from the standpoint of their protein content, if one uses as an operational definition a lipoprotein that contains apoB as a sole protein component. Now, one can almost achieve this in the case of narrow cut human LDL. One can never achieve it in the case of rat LDL, which, in our hands, always contain 5%–10% of non-apoB proteins; about half of those are apoE, and apo E certainly has an influence upon the system you are studying. So, the differences in rates may be due to species differences in apoB, but could also reflect the amount of apoE present in our rat system.

The rates of 10% in 4 hours are somewhat higher than those recorded in the paper by Sigurdson, about two- or threefold higher. So, they would yield an uptake in the liver which would amount to about 15% to 20% of the total LDL catabolism.

The question about the iodide is difficult to answer. I must say that with the accelerated catabolism stimulated by estrogens we found no change in the proportions of iodotyrosine and radiodide produced. There is about 60% iodo-tyrosine and about 40% iodide, no matter what the rate is. If iodide production did not reflect catabolism it would be unlikely to remain in the same proportion under those widely difficult conditions. We, of course, added unlabeled iodo-tyrosine to the system to dilute the effects of nonspecific deiodination.

DR. M. S. BROWN (*University of Texas, Dallas, Texas*): The possibility that the C apoproteins may modulate the interaction of the lipoprotein particles with the liver is really fascinating and obviously of great importance. I remember that Dr. Gotto's group reported that VLDL isolated by zonal ultracentrifugation, from hyperlipidemic patients, bound to the LDL receptor in fibroblasts, but did not do so when isolated from normal subjects. Is is known what the difference in the C content of these two particles is?

DR. GOTTO: We have not measured the C content in the particles in that system.

DR. G. J. GETZ (*University of Chicago, Chicago, Ill.*): I would like to ask for two points of clarification. First, you mentioned, I think, that the lower-density LDLs also show an increment of uptake after estrogen treatment. Have you been able to correlate this increase in the uptake with the differential composition with respect to B and E apoproteins?

Second, in your first chart you suggested—although I am not sure you suggested—that the remnants derived from chylomicrons and hepatic VLDL may be regarded as equivalent with particular reference to the origin of plasma LDL. I wonder whether you really believe that?

DR. HAVEL: I should first mention that there was a paper by Hay and Getz showing that estrogen stimulated catabolism of LDL. The particular LDL they used were more contaminated, I believe, with remnant particles than ours.

With respect to the first question, we have not looked at the apoE content of the different LDL subclasses in detail. We have shown, however, that the uptake of isolated rat apoE as a complex with phospholipids is very rapid and markedly stimulated in the livers of estrogen-treated rats.

In regard to the second question, I think that I said that human VLDL is converted to LDL. Now, there are no direct conclusive studies that I am aware of on the conversion of human chylomicrons to LDL, but there are some calculations one can make which indicate that if there was retention of apoB in the chylomicron particles as there appears to be in the VLDL particle, the conversion to LDL is possible. But, the amount of cholesteryl esters in the chylomicron remnant, at least in the case of the rats, is many-fold greater per particle than that which is present in LDL. So, if chylomicrons are a precursor, there has to be much greater modification than in the case of VLDL, which also contained more cholesteryl ester molecules per particle than LDL.

DR. P. S. ROHEIM (*Louisiana State University, New Orleans, La.*): We are also studying the mechanism of estrogen action and our approach is to use ovariectomized rats. The major feature of these animals is that after ovariectomy the remnant particles containing apoB and apoE markedly increase. So, we are very much in agreement with your findings, although we use a different model.

PLASMA LIPOPROTEIN CONVERSIONS: THE ORIGIN OF LOW-DENSITY AND HIGH-DENSITY LIPOPROTEINS *

Shlomo Eisenberg

Lipid Research Laboratory
Department of Medicine B
Hadassah University Hospital
Jerusalem, Israel

A concept that some of the plasma lipoproteins are products of triglyceride transport in chylomicrons and very-low-density lipoproteins (VLDL) rather than primary secretory products of cells, has been recently suggested by us.[1, 2] The concept involves the low- and high-density lipoproteins (LDL and HDL) of the blood plasma and is based on experimental data and theoretical considerations. It is the purpose of the present report to describe the data and provide the hypotheses that support this concept.

THE INTRAVASCULAR ORIGIN OF LDL

Several years ago it became apparent that LDL, the major transport vehicle of plasma cholesterol, is a final breakdown product of VLDL metabolism.[3–9] The process of LDL formation—designated also the VLDL-LDL interconversion—was studied in detail *in vivo* and *in vitro*.

Evidence from in Vivo Studies

Conversion of VLDL constituents to LDL has been established for the apolipoprotein B (apoB) moiety of the lipoprotein.[3–9] Other LDL constituents, i.e., cholesterol esters, phospholipids, and remaining triglycerides presumably also originate from VLDL. The VLDL-LDL interconversion occurs through multiple steps of delipidation of the triglyceride-rich VLDL and IDL particles. The essential enzymatic reaction is triglyceride hydrolysis and removal of the hydrolytic products [10, 11] at extrahepatic sites. This reaction is dependent on the presence and activity of the endothelial bound extrahepatic lipoprotein lipase.[12, 13] Indeed, LDL is almost completely absent from the plasma of humans with a severe defect of lipoprotein lipolysis (Type I hyperlipoproteinemia [14] or apoC-II deficiency [15]). In normal humans a complete conversion of VLDL to LDL takes about 12 hours.[9] Each interaction of a VLDL particle with lipoprotein lipase results in shrinkage of the core volume of the particle, and a decrease of the diameter and increase of the particle's density. The spectrum of VLDL, IDL, and LDL particles found in the plasma represents

* The author's research cited herein was supported by research grants (219 and 1189) from the U.S.–Israel Binational Science Foundation, and a research grant (HL23864–01) from the U.S. Public Health Service.

30

most probably release of partially degraded lipoproteins along the VLDL → LDL delipidation path. The key observation along the VLDL → LDL interconversion was the demonstration that one and only one product particle is formed from each precursor particle.[5] Thus, either fission or fusion of particles during the interconversion process is ruled out.

Formation of LDL from VLDL, however, cannot be equated with triglyceride hydrolysis. This is evident when the lipid and protein composition of one VLDL particle is compared to that of one LDL particle (FIGURE 1). Major

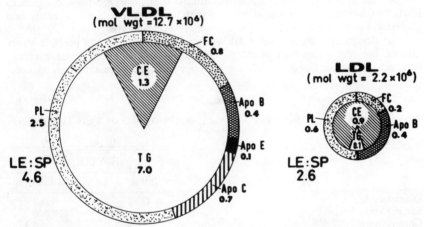

FIGURE 1. VLDL → LDL interconversion. Mass contribution of lipids and proteins to the mass of one VLDL particle (mol wt: 12.7×10^6) and one LDL particle (mol wt: 2.2×10^6). Data compiled from Eisenberg et al.[5] and presented as 10^6 daltons: TG, Triglyceride; CE, cholesterol esters; PL, phospholipids; LE, Lecithin; SP, Sphingomyelin; FC, free cholesterol.

changes in all constituents—with the exception of apoB—are apparent. In the figure, we have elected to present the different constituents at their respective location in the particles, surface (phospholipids, unesterified cholesterol, and proteins) and core (triglycerides and cholesterol esters). About 75% of the phospholipids, 85% of the unesterified cholesterol, and almost all of the apoC and apoE molecules have been deleted from the lipoprotein surface during the interconversion. Most of the triglycerides (>98%) were hydrolyzed and removed from the particle. By calculation, even some of the cholesterol ester molecules might have been deleted from the particle during the delipidation process. It thus seems that concomitantly with triglyceride hydrolysis, many other constituents are deleted from the VLDL and IDL particles. The metabolic pathways responsible for these changes, however, could not be ascertained in the *in vivo* experiments. Therefore, we have turned to *in vitro* systems.

Evidence from in Vitro Studies: Formation of IDL

The possibility to form and characterize products of VLDL lipolysis in the test tube provides a means to study in detail metabolic events that take place during the VLDL → LDL interconversion. In our initial experiments we have characterized a partially lipolyzed VLDL particle isolated after incubation of VLDL with lipoprotein-lipase-rich (postheparin) rat plasma.[16, 17] The main features of the precursors and product particles are shown in TABLE 1. It is evident that apoC, apoE, phospholipids, unesterified cholesterol, and even some cholesterol ester molecules are deleted from the VLDL concomitantly with the hydrolysis of triglycerides. ApoC removed from the VLDL was found in HDL.[16] Phospholipids were removed by two different pathways: (a) hydrolysis of glycerophosphatides to lyso compounds with subsequent transfer of the lyso compounds to albumin, and (b) distribution of unhydrolyzed phospholipids to HDL.[18] Cholesterol was found mainly with HDL.[18] The fate of apoE and cholesterol esters could not be followed in these experiments.

The design of the experiment allowed us to speculate on the possible structure of the precursors and product particle.[17] To this end, we have reconstructed the two main domains of the lipoprotein, i.e., the surface and core.

TABLE 1

PHYSICAL AND CHEMICAL FEATURES OF INTACT AND POSTLIPOLYSIS VERY-LOW-DENSITY LIPOPROTEIN (VLDL)

	VLDL	
	Intact	Postlipolysis
Diameter, Å	427	269
Surface area, Å^2	573,000	227,000
Core volume, 10^{-6}, Å^3	30.3	6.3
Average S$_f$ rate	115.0	30.5
Particle weight, $\times 10^{-6}$	23.1	7.0
Composition, mg/100 mg lipoprotein		
Apoproteins	14.3	19.0
ApoB, % of total protein	21.5	57.0
ApoVS-2, % of total protein	22.7	33.8
ApoC, % of total protein	55.7	9.2
Triglycerides	62.0	46.4
Phospholipids	14.5	20.1
Cholesterol	9.2	14.5
Unesterified/esterified cholesterol, molar ratio	2.45	1.34
Lipid and protein † composition, mole/mole lipoprotein		
ApoB	70	73
ApoE ‡	24	15
ApoC	180	12
Triglycerides	15,660	3,440
Phospholipids	4,373	1,813
Unesterified cholesterol	3,700	1,375
Cholesterol esters	1,600	1,092

* Adapted from Eisenberg and Rachmilewitz.[16, 17]

† ApoB and apoC expressed as molecular weight units of 10,000.

‡ Defined operationally as the second protein peak emerged by gel filtration on Sephadex G-151.

TABLE 2

THE CORE AND SURFACE OF VLDL AND POSTLIPOLYSIS VLDL PARTICLES *

	VLDL	
	Intact	Postlipolysis
The lipoprotein core, $Å^3 \times 10^{-6}$		
Calculated core volume	30.3	6.3
Volume of triglycerides	25.1	5.5
Volume of cholesteryl esters	1.7	1.2
Total volume of lipids	26.8	6.7
The lipoprotein surface, $Å^2 \times 10^{-3}$	573	227
Molecules/10^5 $Å^2$ surface area		
ApoB	12	34
ApoE	4	7
ApoC	31	6
Phospholipids, total	760	850
Unesterified cholesterol	644	648

* Adapted from Eisenberg and Rachmilewitz.[16, 17]

We have calculated the concentration of apoproteins, phospholipids, and un-esterified cholesterol at the surface of the lipoproteins, and the volume of the core constituents, triglycerides, and cholesterol esters (TABLE 2). The data show that the volume of core constituents is in excellent agreement with the calculated core volume of the two particles and that the concentration of surface constituents at the outer shell of the two particles remained essentially unchanged. These observations indicated that a relationship exists between the decrease of the core volume and the surface area of the VLDL during triglyceride hydrolysis. We envision that the primary event is the decrease of the particle's volume followed by a coordinated deletion (or exclusion) of surface constituents.[11] The possible mechanisms for deletion of surface constituents from lipolyzed VLDL particles are discussed in the second part of this article.

Formation of LDL in the Test Tube

This experiment was carried out with human plasma VLDL, and purified lipoprotein lipase.[19] LDL particles produced *in vitro* were isolated at the density interval of 1.019–1.063 g/ml and were compared to LDL isolated at the same density from the plasmas of the VLDL donors (TABLE 3). The similarities between the two are striking, but there are also some differences. The results therefore provided us with the unique opportunity to differentiate between effects that are due to triglyceride hydrolysis only, (as observed *in vitro*), and those that may require the activity of other pathways. The formation of LDL obviously requires nearly complete hydrolysis of triglyceride, and that could be accomplished with lipoprotein lipase of extrahepatic origin. LDL thus is a collapsing core-remnant of the residual core-constituents of VLDL. With this one reaction we have also identified the following alterations of the VLDL:lipid composition, lipid-to-protein ratio, apoprotein profile, and the organization of lipids in the lipoprotein. Most of the apoC and apoE were deleted from the particle. The lecithin to sphingomyelin ratio (4.0 in VLDL) decreased to that found in the circulating LDL, of 2.4. The main difference between the *in vitro* produced LDL and the circulating lipoprotein was the greater core volume, a reflection of the two-fold excess of cholesterol esters in the former particle. We interpret this finding as an indication for the presence of excess cholesterol ester in VLDL particles than is necessary for the formation of LDL. Cholesterol esters should therefore be deleted from the lipolyzed VLDL as the particle is converted to LDL. Although the pathways for removal of cholesterol esters from lipoproteins are unknown, there are at least two reports on preferential

TABLE 3

PHYSICAL AND CHEMICAL PROPERTIES OF CIRCULATING AND *in Vitro* LOW-DENSITY LIPOPROTEINS (LDL) *

	LDL	
	Circulating	*In vitro*
Diameter, Å	215	270
Flotation Rate, S_f	4.2	7.2
Core volume, $Å^3 \times 10^{-6}$	3.05	6.37
Molecular weight, $\times 10^{-6}$	2.5	5.0
Lipid and protein † composition, moles/mole lipoprotein		
ApoB	63	90 ‡
Cholesterol esters	1,388	2,738
Triglycerides	192	161
Phospholipids	743	1,787
Unesterified Cholesterol	538	1,308

* Adapted from Deckelbaum *et al.*[19]
† Apoproteins expressed as molecular weight units of 10,000.
‡ The increase of apoB in the *in vitro* LDL is probably artifactual (see Reference 19).

removal of cholesterol esters from lipoproteins either in the perfused rat heart[20] or the liver.[21] Another difference between the *in vitro* produced LDL and the circulating lipoprotein is an excess of surface constituents relative to core constituents. This excess, although a small fraction of the original VLDL surface coat, requires explanation. A contamination with surface fragments (see next section) is possible, but not enough to explain the discrepancy. Apparently, the presence of plasma or tissue constituents is necessary for the formation of the native LDL. Such constituents may include phospholipid exchange proteins,[22, 23] cholesterol ester exchange proteins,[24, 25] lipoproteins, enzymes (the hepatic triglyceride hydrolase, and the lecithin:cholesterol acyl-hydrolase) as well as tissue cells. The exact role, if any, of these interactions in LDL formation, remains to be established.

Structure–Function Relationship in LDL Formation

The LDL-forming system as described above reflects predominantly the process of triglyceride transport where LDL is the final product of VLDL metabolism. Yet, the system also provides important clues for cholesterol transport and the metabolism of apoB-containing lipoproteins. That was first suggested by us when we have observed that the apoB moiety of VLDL remained associated with the core-constituents along the VLDL → LDL conversion path.[17] Assuming that apoB is located at the outer shell of the lipoprotein particle, it can be calculated that the concentration of apoB at the surface of the lipoprotein increases along the delipidation path. Simultaneously, the concentration of apoC decreases. The initial analysis of apoB and apoC concentration at lipoprotein surfaces were confined to the *in vitro* produced IDL.[17] Recently, seven VLDL subfractions were prepared and fully characterized.[26] When analyzed, the data indicated that the slope of the increased concentration of apoB at the surface of the lipoprotein, and the slope of the decreased concentration of apoC are not linear.[11] Rather, a sharp increase of apoB concentration and a sharp decrease of apoC concentration occurred at a molecular weight of about 10–15 million. If the interactions of the particles with lipoprotein lipase are dependent on the surface concentration of apoC, and those with tissue cells on the surface concentration of agoB, one might expect a change of the biological behavior of the particles when they cross that molecular weight point. That indeed this is the case has been shown in several experiments. Small VLDL particles (S_f 20–60, mol wt ~ 10^7) accumulate in plasma immediately after the injection of heparin to humans.[5] The further delipidation of these small particles is considerably retarded, presumably due to the lower content of apoC at the particles' surface. Small VLDL particles ("VLDL-remnants") are cleared by the liver from rats' serum at an extremely fast rate,[27, 28] presumably reflecting enhanced interaction between the apoB-rich remnants and hepatic receptors.[29] Small VLDL particles suppress the activity of 3-hydroxy-3-methylglutaryl coenzyme A in fibroblasts, similar to LDL, whereas larger particles do not.[30] These, as well as other examples (see Reference 11 for a detailed discussion) indicate that the LDL receptor pathway and the VLDL → LDL interconversion pathway may be related. Indeed, only when the two pathways are considered together, as demonstrated in FIGURE 2, is it possible to describe some of the fundamental features of fat transport in lipoproteins.

INTRAVASCULAR ORIGIN OF HDL

In the previous section it has been repeatedly demonstrated that VLDL-intermediates and LDL conform with the general core-lipid model of lipoproteins. The process of VLDL delipidation therefore, should account for a pathway—or pathways—for the removal and further metabolism of surplus surface constituents released from VLDL (and chylomicrons) during triglyceride transport. It is our hypothesis that HDL in fact is the final metabolic product of the surface constituents of triglyceride-rich lipoproteins. We would like, moreover, to suggest that this part of HDL formation may serve as the major source of circulating HDL.

Triglyceride Transport and HDL: in Vivo Studies

Earlier studies have shown enrichment of HDL lipids—cholesterol and phospholipids—during accelerated fat transport, i.e., after a fatty meal [32, 33] or following injection of heparin.[34, 35] La Rosa and his associates were the first to demonstrate an enrichment of HDL-apoC immediately after the injection of heparin to humans.[35] To study this phenomenon in detail, we have determined the distribution of labeled apoproteins in human plasma following the injection of ^{125}I-labeled VLDL and heparin.[5] Labeled apoC-II and apoC-III

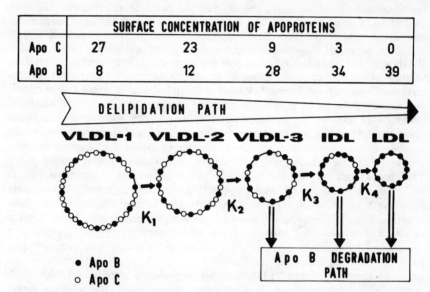

	SURFACE CONCENTRATION OF APOPROTEINS				
Apo C	27	23	9	3	0
Apo B	8	12	28	34	39

FIGURE 2. A proposed relationship between the VLDL delipidation path and the apoB catabolism (LDL receptor) path. Calculated concentrations of apoB and apoC molecular weight units (10^4 daltons) are presented as units per 10^5 square angstroms of surface area. K_1, K_2, K_3, and K_4 represent rates of delipidation of different intermediates along the VLDL → LDL conversion. It is suggested that as the particle becomes smaller and contains fewer apoC molecules per unit surface area, the rates of delipidation are slower, i.e., $K_1 > K_2 \gg K_3 \gg K_4$. Concomitantly, as the surface concentration of apoB increases, the particles start to interact with the LDL receptor.

distributed from the VLDL to HDL within 15–45 min of the heparin injection. Six hours later, and when newly secreted VLDL particles appeared in the plasma, some of the labeled apoC molecules distributed back to VLDL. Essentially identical results were reported later for rats.[16, 18] In another study, distribution of apoC (measured as lipoprotein lipase activator) between chylomicrons and HDL was demonstrated during induction and clearance of chylomicronemia in humans.[33] These data suggested that HDL plays a role in triglyceride transport being a flexible reservoir in plasma for the physiologically important apoC molecules.[10, 36] However, we soon started to suspect that this role of HDL in triglyceride transport, although essentially correct, was only a first approximation of a more complex situation. We therefore again returned to *in vitro* experiments.

Formation of "Nascent" HDL in Vitro

Our initial study was carried out specifically to determine whether the presence of HDL was obligatory for the removal of apoC from lipolyzed VLDL particles. To this end, we have followed the distribution of labeled apoC during lipolysis of VLDL carried out in the absence of plasma.[37] Without lipoprotein lipase, 80%–90% of the labeled apoC were isolated with VLDL. In the presence of the enzyme, however, increasing amounts of labeled (and unlabeled) apoC redistributed to higher density fractions, including that of HDL ($d = 1.04$–1.21 g/ml) and of $d > 1.21$ g/ml. The distribution of apoC to the density of HDL in the absence of plasma indicated that a high-density lipoprotein particle originated from the lipolyzed VLDL. Subsequent studies carried out during perfusion of the isolated rat heart with labeled VLDL [38] or during *in vitro* incubation [39] have substantiated the earlier observations. In these experiments, furthermore, we followed the fate of all lipid constituents of the VLDL labeled biosynthetically with [14C]palmitic acid, [3H]cholesterol, and [32P]phospholipids. Some glycerophosphatides were hydrolyzed to lyso compounds. Unhydrolyzed phospholipids (lecithin and sphingomyelin) and unesterified cholesterol were freed from the lipolyzed VLDL and accumulated together with apoC at the HDL density range. We therefore concluded that an HDL precursor was generated as a by-product of VLDL lipolysis.[1, 2]

The Nature of "Nascent" HDL Particles

The morphology of the HDL precursors generated during VLDL lipolysis was investigated by electron microscopy. As expected, these were discoidal lipoproteins, about 250×60 Å in diameter, indistinguishable from other nascent HDL particles (see below). More recently, however, and while using other albumin preparations, we have identified a greater variety of morphologically different surface fragments generated during VLDL lipolysis. All were of HDL density, but while some were discoidal, others were vesicular or elongated unilamellar fragments.

Nascent HDL particles have been observed in several experimental systems. Initially, discoidal lipoproteins of HDL density were identified in the perfusate during rat liver perfusion.[40] It is, however, not yet known whether these nascent particles are primary secretory products of the liver cells or are formed in the perfusion medium following a physical or a metabolic reaction. More recently, discoidal HDL particles were found in intestinal lymph and were partially characterized.[41-43] Also discoidal HDL particles can be formed in the test tube following interaction of phospholipids with the different isolated apolipoproteins.[31] Whether such interactions may occur *in vivo* is doubtful.

A comparison of the features of the hepatic and intestinal nascent HDL and the nascent HDL generated during VLDL lipolysis reveals that the three have similar lipid composition but are very different in apoprotein profile. The hepatic particles contain predominantly apoE,[40] the intestinal HDL contain apoA-I [41-43] and apoA-II, whereas the HDL produced during lipolysis contain predominantly apoC. These differences, however, are reconciled when the nature of the triglyceride-rich lipoprotein included—or present—in each of the three systems is considered: the hepatic VLDL contains predominantly apoE,[40] the intestinal chylomicrons apoA-I [41-44] and the VLDL, apoC. Is it then possible that in each system the nascent HDL are produced from the triglyceride-rich lipoproteins? This question cannot be answered at the present time. Neither in the liver perfusion experiment nor in intestinal lymph has it been demonstrated that the nascent HDL are primary secretory particles of liver and intestinal cells. It is of course unknown whether the conditions created in the test-tube lipolysis experiment ever exist *in vivo*. Yet, as discussed later in this article, there exists enough circumstantial evidence to assume that "surface remnants" generated during lipolysis of triglyceride-rich lipoproteins are a major source of the circulating HDL lipids and proteins.

Effects of Lipolysis on Circulating HDL

In the experiments discussed so far, we have chosen to study VLDL degradation in the simplest possible system, i.e., the one containing VLDL, buffer, albumin, and lipoprotein lipase. To study the effects of lipolysis on HDL, we have modified the experimental procedure and have included HDL subfractions (HDL$_3$ or HDL$_2$) in an *in vitro* lipolysis system.[45, 46] In our first experiment we have studied the effects of lipolysis on the HDL$_3$ and used ultracentrifugation in a zonal rotor for the analysis of the reaction products.[45] With this system we have consistently observed that phospholipids, unesterified cholesterol, and apoC freed from the lipolyzed VLDL distributed to the existing HDL$_3$ particles. Since the combined density of the VLDL surface constituents transferred to the HDL$_3$ was lower than that of the acceptor lipoprotein, the density of the HDL$_3$ decreased towards that of HDL$_2$. Thus, a conversion of HDL$_3$ to HDL$_2$-like particles was achieved in the test tube. The HDL$_2$-like particles produced in the test tube were isolated and further characterized. As expected, they contained the phospholipids, unesterified cholesterol and apoC freed from the lipolyzed VLDL, as well as the amounts of these constituents initially present in the HDL$_3$. The increment of cholesterol esters was minimal and there was no change of the HDL triglyceride content. Under the conditions used, almost all of the apoA proteins present initially in the HDL$_3$ were retained in the modified particle. The modified particle was stable even when stored in buffer for several weeks. Gel filtration demonstrated that the dimensions of the HDL$_3$ and HDL$_2$-like particles were similar, and this impression was confirmed by electron microscopy. When HDL$_2$ replaced the HDL$_3$ in the system, it also served as an acceptor for the surface constituents freed from the lipolyzed VLDL.[46] The density of the HDL$_2$, however, almost did not change, and we have not observed fission of the large HDL$_2$ particles to HDL$_3$. Thus, plasma HDL$_3$ is a possible precursor of plasma HDL$_2$. The experiment moreover indicated that HDL$_2$ may accumulate in plasma when triglyceride transport is accelerated. As discussed below, this suggestion is compatible with many clinical observations on the relationships between triglyceride transport, lipoprotein lipase levels, HDL levels, and the ratio between plasma HDL$_2$ to plasma HDL$_3$.

TRIGLYCERIDE TRANSPORT AND PLASMA LDL AND HDL: AN INTEGRATED APPROACH

The data described above allow the formulation of an integrated view of the lipoprotein system. This view assumes that the basic function of the plasma lipoproteins is triglyceride transport. Accordingly, it is assumed that chylomicrons and VLDL are the two triglyceride-rich particles that are synthesized in cells and are secreted from cells. It is furthermore assumed that both LDL and HDL are products of the process of triglyceride transport, the former being the final "core remnant," and the latter the final "surface remnant" of the triglyceride-rich lipoproteins.

The hypothesis concerned with the origin of LDL seems to be established. In part, this reflects the relatively long time (8–9 years) that passed since it has been suggested that LDL is a final metabolic product of VLDL degradation.[3] Numerous studies carried out in several different species and under a variety of experimental conditions have supported that view. It is therefore quite surprising that the exact molecular events that take place during the VLDL → LDL interconversion are still obscure. Our own studies have demonstrated that all the constituents necessary to form LDL are present in VLDL and that under proper experimental conditions LDL-like particles can indeed be formed from VLDL.[19] Yet, many details of this pathway are unknown. For example, the following problems have not been satisfactorily resolved:

What pathway is responsible for deletion of cholesterol esters from lipolyzed VLDL particles? At what stage of the interconversion process and by what mechanism are the apoE molecules removed from the particles? Do all, or only a subfraction of the VLDL particles serve as potential precursors of LDL? Do intestinal triglyceride-rich lipoproteins, and in particular chylomicrons, contribute to the circulating LDL? Is some of the LDL (or IDL) secreted as such in normal or pathological conditions? What is the exact role of lipoproteins, plasma exchange proteins, and enzymes in the process of LDL formation, if any? It is only when answers will be available to these and many other questions, that a more complete understanding of the interconversion process will be reached.

Hardly any evidence is available to support the second part of our hypothesis, that HDL is the final product of the metabolism of surface constituents of triglyceride-rich lipoproteins. This uncertainty undoubtedly reflects the shorter period of time that has passed since the initial observations, suggesting that HDL precursors may be formed as a by-product of lipolysis, were presented and published.[1, 2] This pathway should thus be regarded as a working hypothesis. The essential features of the hypothesis are presented in FIGURES 3 and 4 and are described below.

Before discussing the hypothesis, however, it is necessary to define the circulating HDL and in particular the nature of the two subfractions, HDL_2 and HDL_3. When properly isolated, the HDL range (1.063–1.21 g/ml) can be separated into two or even three discernible populations.[47–49] Using zonal centrifugation, the HDL_2 and HDL_3 can be separated completely from one another, with a minimum between the two.[47] The isolation of discernible HDL subpopulations contrasts with the situation in either VLDL or LDL, where particles of different densities distribute around a mean density. Also, HDL_2 and HDL_3 are affected differently by metabolic processes. For example, in a population study[48, 49] it was reported that HDL_3 levels were similar in all

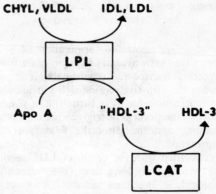

FIGURE 3. A proposed pathway for the origin in plasma of HDL₃. The source of apoA, as discussed in the text, is probably triglyceride-rich lipoprotein of intestinal origin, and the apoA is freed after their initial interaction with lipoprotein lipase. The source of the lipids is continued lipolysis of the chylomicrons and VLDL. For the sake of simplicity, apoA is shown here independent of chylomicrons and VLDL degradation. "HDL₃" designates the complex of apoA, phospholipids and unesterified cholesterol generated during the lipolytic process, and is interchangeable with the terms "HDL precursors," or "nascent HDL." The conversion of HDL₃ to the circulating spherical HDL₃ particles is dependent on LCAT activity.

individuals and were not related to total HDL levels. HDL₂ levels in contrast differed markedly between individuals and accounted for the variability of the levels of total HDL. The hypothesis concerning the origin of HDL must explain these variabilities.

    The composition of the two HDL subfractions, expressed as moles of apoproteins and lipids/mole of lipoprotein, is presented in TABLE 4. The main difference between the two HDL subfractions is the lipid-to-protein ratio, which

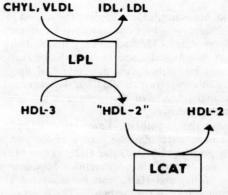

FIGURE 4. A proposed pathway for the conversion in plasma of HDL₃ to HDL₂. The symbols used are similar to those described in FIGURE 3. It is proposed that HDL₃ particles acquire lipids and C proteins generated from lipolyzed triglyceride-rich lipoproteins, is transformed to HDL₂-like particles ("HDL₂"), which are converted to circulating HDL₂ after interacting with the LCAT system.

is an integral parameter of the difference in diameter, volume, and molecular weight. The 3-fold increase in the core volume of HDL_2 as compared to HDL_3 results in tripling the number of cholesterol ester molecules per particle. In contrast, the number of A proteins increased only by 50%. Therefore, *HDL₂ carries about twice as much cholesterol ester molecules per mole of A proteins.* If the efficiency of fat transport in lipoproteins is indeed the number of lipid molecules carried by a mole of proteins, then HDL_2 is twice as efficient in fat transport as HDL_3. This analysis suggests that HDL_2 levels should increase when the cholesterol transport in HDL increases without a proportional increase of apoA synthesis. Again, hypotheses concerning the origin of HDL must explain this phenomenon.

Let us now consider the pathways that may operate during the formation of HDL from surface fragments of lipolyzed triglyceride-rich lipoproteins. We first assume that the origin of the A proteins and of the HDL lipids is inde-

TABLE 4

PHYSICAL AND CHEMICAL PROPERTIES OF HDL_2 AND HDL_3

	HDL_2	HDL_3
Diameter, Å	100	80
Core diameter, Å	60	40
Core volume, Å³	113,040	33,490
Density, g/ml	1.10	1.15
Molecular weight	200,000	400,000
Lipid and protein composition, moles/mole lipoprotein		
ApoA-I	4–5	3
ApoA-II	1–2	1
ApoC	1	±
Phospholipids	137	51
Unesterified cholesterol	50	13
Cholesterol ester	90	32
Cholesterol/apoA, mole/mole	20–28	11

pendent (FIGURE 3). It has recently been shown that apoA-I and apoA-II are synthesized and secreted by intestinal absorptive cells and are associated with the triglyceride-rich lipoproteins in the intestinal lymph.[41-44] Apparently, most of the apoA comes off the chylomicrons only after they circulate in plasma,[50] presumably following their interaction with lipoprotein lipases. Most of the HDL lipids (phospholipids and unesterified cholesterol), however, originate from the continued metabolism of chylomicrons and from lipolyzed VLDL. We suggest that the A proteins and the lipid-rich surface fragments become associated in the HDL density range to form true HDL precursors. These precursors are an ideal substrate for the lecithin-cholesterol acyltransferase (LCAT) reaction and are transformed to spherical HDL particles. We further assume that the amount of apoA and of phospholipids generated from triglyceride transport are such that the initial HDL particles formed are of the HDL_3 subpopulation. This assumption is based on the amount of apoA synthesized per day [51] and the amount of unhydrolyzed phospholipids generated per day from triglyceride transport, corrected for the lecithinase activity of the lipoprotein lipase and the LCAT activity.

The situation described above, however, may vary between individuals and during physiological and pathological perturbations of the fat transport system. The main two variables will be the amount of apoA synthesized per day, and the amount of phospholipids and unesterified cholesterol generated by the lipolytic systems. A situation where the amount of phospholipids and unesterified cholesterol generated per day exceeds the capacity of the A proteins to form HDL_3 is depicted in FIGURE 4. Under this situation we suggest that the existing HDL_3 particles are transformed to HDL_2, thus increasing the capacity of the HDL to carry and transport cholesterol molecules. We suggest that the initial event is the formation of HDL_2-like particles, similar to those formed by us in the *in vitro* system. These particles will acquire one or two additional molecules of apoA-I and, through the LCAT reaction, will be transformed to circulating HDL_2 particles. Since the relatively large apoA-I molecules (mol wt about 27000) are added to the particles as a quantum of protein (it is of course impossible to add half a molecule), the molecular weight distribution of HDL particles also changes in a quantum fashion, accounting for the two (or three [48, 49]) discernible HDL subpopulations found in the circulation.

As stated above, the views presented here with regard to the origin of HDL are largely speculative and are based on only a few experiments. Yet, it is interesting to note that many observations—both clinical and experimental—heretofore unexplained, are compatible with the hypothesis. Surface fragments originating from triglyceride-rich lipoproteins have been consistently observed in two genetic diseases when either HDL is absent from the plasma (Tangier disease [52, 53] or when there is a congenital deficiency of the LCAT system [54, 55]). Such fragments were also observed in plasma after the injection of heparin to hypertriglyceridemic humans [56] and after toxic damage to the rat liver by galactosamine and the ensuing LCAT deficiency.[57]

HDL levels, and in particular HDL_2 levels, are moreover highly correlated with lipoprotein lipase activity and triglyceride transport, in many circumstances. These include diabetes mellitus,[58] estrogen administration,[59] male-female comparisons,[60] alcohol consumption,[61] physical activity,[62] and others. Conversely, HDL levels are extremely low, and HDL_2 is absent, from the plasma of patients with lipoprotein lipase deficiency [14] or apoC-II deficiency.[15] In this last situation, HDL levels promptly increase after administration of the apoC-II.[15] Inasmuch as all these and other examples support the hypothesis, they do not prove it. Only by further research will it be possible to prove—or disprove—the hypothesis, and to delineate the various pathways involved with the origin of HDL and the regulation of the circulating levels of the lipoprotein.

REFERENCES

1. EISENBERG, S., T. CHAJEK & R. DECKELBAUM. 1978. J. Am. Oil Chem. Soc. **55:** A256.
2. EISENBERG, S., T. CHAJEK & R. J. DECKELBAUM. 1978. Pharmacol. Res. Commun. **10:**729–738.
3. BILHEIMER, D. W., S. EISENBERG & R. I. LEVY. 1972. Biochim. Biophys. Acta **260:**212–221.

4. EISENBERG, S., D. W. BILHEIMER & R. I. LEVY. 1972. Biochim. Biophys. Acta **280:**94–104.
5. EISENBERG, S., D. W. BILHEIMER, F. T. LINDGREN & R. I. LEVY. 1973. Biochim. Biophys. Acta **326:**361–377.
6. SIGURDSSON, G., A. NICOLL & B. LEWIS. 1975. J. Clin. Invest. **56:**1481–1490.
7. REARDON, M. F., N. H. FIDGE & P. J. NESTEL. 1978. J. Clin. Invest. **61:**850–860.
8. PACKARD, C. J., J. SHEPHERD, A. M. GOTTO & O. D. TAUNTON. 1977. Clin. Res. **25:**396A.
9. BERMAN, M., S. EISENBERG, M. H. HALL, R. I. LEVY, D. W. BILHEIMER, R. D. PHAIR & R. H. GOEBEL. 1978. J. Lipid Res. **19:**38–56.
10. EISENBERG, S. & R. I. LEVY. 1975. Adv. Lipid Res. **13:**1–89.
11. EISENBERG, S. 1979. Progr. Biochem. Pharmacol. **15:**139–165.
12. ROBINSON, D. S. 1970. Compr. Biochem. **18:**51–116.
13. SMITH, L. C. & R. O. SCOW. 1979. Prog. Biochem. Pharmacol. **15:**109–138.
14. FREDRICKSON, D. S., R. I. LEVY & F. T. LINDGREN. 1968. J. Clin. Invest. **47:** 2446–2457.
15. BRECKENRIDGE, W. C., J. A. LITTLE, G. STEINER, A. CHOW & M. POAPST. 1978. New Engl. J. Med. **298:**1265–1273.
16. EISENBERG, S. & D. RACHMILEWITZ. 1975. J. Lipid Res. **16:**451–461.
17. EISENBERG, S. 1976. *In* Lipoprotein Metabolism. M. Greten, Ed. pp. 32–43. Springer, Heidelberg, West Germany.
18. EISENBERG, S. & D. SCHURR. 1976. J. Lipid Res. **17:**578–587.
19. DECKELBAUM, R. J., S. EISENBERG, M. FAINARU, Y. BARENHOLZ & T. OLIVECRONA. 1979. J. Biol. Chem. **254:**6079–6087.
20. FIELDING, C. J. 1978. J. Clin. Invest. **62:**141–151.
21. SNIDERMAN, A., D. THOMAS, D. MARPOLE & B. TENG. 1978. J. Clin. Invest. **61:** 867–873.
22. EISENBERG, S. 1978. J. Lipid Res. **19:**229–236.
23. BREWESTER, M. E., J. IHM, J. R. BRAINARD & J. A. K. HARMONY. 1978. Biochim. Biophys. Acta **529:**147–159.
24. CHAJEK, T. & C. J. FIELDING. 1979. Proc. Natl. Acad. Sci. USA **75:**3445–3449.
25. PATTNAIK, N. M. & D. B. ZILVERSMIT. 1979. J. Biol. Chem. **254:**2782–2786.
26. PATSCH, W., J. R. PATSCH, G. M. KOSTNER, S. SAILER & H. BRAUNSTEINER. 1978. J. Biol. Chem. **253:**4911–4915.
27. EISENBERG, S. & D. RACHMILEWITZ. 1973. Biochim. Biophys. Acta **326:**378–390.
28. FAEGERMAN, O., T. SATA, J. P. KANE & R. J. HAVEL. 1975. J. Clin. Invest. **56:** 1396–1403.
29. STEIN, O., D. RACHMILEWITZ, L. SANGER, S. EISENBERG & Y. STEIN. 1974. Biochim. Biophys. Acta **360:**205–216.
30. GIANTURCO, S. H., A. M. GOTTO, JR., R. L. JACKSON, J. R. PATSCH, H. D. SYBERS, O. D. TAUNTON, D. L. YESHURUN & L. C. SMITH. 1978. J. Clin. Invest. **61:**320–328.
31. MORRISETT, J. D., R. L. JACKSON & A. M. GOTTO. 1977. Biochim. Biophys. Acta **472:**93–133.
32. HAVEL, R. J. 1957. J. Clin. Invest. **36:**848–854.
33. HAVEL, R. J., J. P. KANE & M. L. KASHYAP. 1973. J. Clin. Invest. **52:**32–38.
34. LINDGREN, F. T., A. V. NICHOLS & N. K. FREEMAN. 1955. J. Physical Chem. **59:**930–938.
35. LAROSA, J. C., R. I. LEVY, W. V. BROWN & D. S. FREDRICKSON. 1971. Am. J. Physiol. **220:**785–791.
36. HAVEL, R. J. 1975. Adv. Exp. Med. Biol. **63:**37–59.
37. GLANGEAUD, M. C., S. EISENBERG & T. OLIVECRONA. 1977. Biochim. Biophys. Acta **486:**23–35.
38. CHAJEK, T. & S. EISENBERG. 1978. J. Clin. Invest. **61:**1654–1665.
39. EISENBERG, S. & T. OLIVECRONA. 1979. J. Lipid Res. **20:**614–623.

40. HAMILTON, R. L., M. C. WILLIAMS, C. J. FIELDING & R. J. HAVEL. 1976. J. Clin. Invest. **58:**667–680.
41. GLICKMAN, R. M. & P. H. R. GREEN. 1977. Proc. Natl. Acad. Sci. USA **74:** 2569–2573.
42. GREEN, P. H. R., A. R. TALL & R. M. GLICKMAN. 1978. J. Clin. Invest. **61:** 528–534.
43. GREEN, P. H. R., R. M. GLICKMAN, C. D. SANDEK, C. B. BLUM & A. R. TALL. 1979. J. Clin. Invest. **64:**233–242.
44. IMAIZUMI, K., R. J. HAVEL, M. FAINARU & J. L. VIGNE. 1978. J. Lipid Res. **19:** 1038–1046.
45. PATSCH, J. R., A. M. GOTTO, T. OLIVECRONA & S. EISENBERG. 1978. Proc. Natl. Acad. Sci. USA **75:**4519–4523.
46. EISENBERG, S., J. R. PATSCH, H. F. HOFF, A. M. GOTTO & T. OLIVECRONA. In preparation.
47. PATSCH, J. R., S. SAILER, G. KOSTNER, F. SANDHOFER, A. HOLASEK & H. BRAUNSTEINER. 1974. J. Lipid Res. **15:**356–366.
48. ANDERSON, D. W., A. V. NICHOLS, T. M. FORTE & F. T. LINDGREN. 1977. Biochim. Biophys. Acta **493:**55–68.
49. ANDERSON, D. W., A. V. NICHOLS, S. S. PAN & F. T. LINDGREN. 1978. Atherosclerosis **29:**161–179.
50. SCHAEFER, E. J., L. L. JENKINS & H. B. BREWER. 1978. Biochem. Biophys. Res. Commun. **80:**405–411.
51. BLUM, C. B., R. I. LEVY, S. EISENBERG, M. HALL, R. H. GOEBEL & M. BERMAN. 1977. J. Clin. Invest. **60:**795–807.
52. ASSMAN, G., P. N. HERBERT, D. S. FREDRICKSON & T. FORTE. 1977. J. Clin. Invest. **60:**242–252.
53. HERBERT, P. N., T. FORTE, R. J. HEINEN & D. S. FREDRICKSON. 1978. New Eng. J. Med. **299:**519–522.
54. FORTE, T., K. R. NORUM, J. A. GLOMSET & A. V. NICHOLS. 1971. J. Clin. Invest. **50:**1141–1148.
55. GLOMSET, J. A., K. R. NORUM, A. V. NICHOLS, W. C. KING, C. D. MITCHELL, K. R. APPLEGATE, E. L. GONG & E. GJONE. 1975. Scand. J. Clin. Lab. Invest. **35**(Suppl. 142):3–30.
56. FORTE, T., R. M. KRAUSS, F. T. LINDGREN & A. V. NICHOLS. 1977. Circulation **51**(Suppl. 3):94.
57. SABESIN, S. M., L. B. KNIKEN & J. B. RAGLAND. 1975. Science **190:**1302–1304.
58. NIKKILA, E. A. 1978. *In* High Density Lipoproteins and Atherosclerosis. A. M. Gotto, N. E. Miller & M. F. Oliver, Eds. pp. 177–192. Elsevier, North-Holland Biomedical Press, New York, N.Y.
59. SCHAEFER, E. J., R. I. LEVY, L. L. JENKINS & H. B. BREWER. 1977. Proc. 6th Int. Symp. Drugs Affecting Lipid Metabolism. Abst. p. 82.
60. NICHOLS, A. V. 1967. Adv. Biol. Med. Phys. **11:**110–158.
61. DANIELSSON, B., R. EKMAN, G. FEX, B. G. JOHANSSON, H. KRISTENSSON, P. NILSSON-EHLE & J. W. WADSTEIN. 1978. Scand. J. Clin. Lab. Invest. **38:**113–119.
62. KRAUSS, R. M., F. T. LINDGREN, P. O. WOOD, W. L. HASKELL, J. J. ALBERS & M. C. CHEUNG. 1977. Circulation **56**(Suppl. 3):4.

DISCUSSION OF THE PAPER

DR. A. M. GOTTO, JR.: Thank you very much, Dr. Eisenberg. One of the precepts that is taught at the Harvard Business School to all future executives of major U.S. corporations is that they should require their employees and associates to condense the most complex information on no more than one sheet of paper. So, I congratulate you for summarizing your ideas on one slide. This paper is open for discussion.

DR. A. R. TALL (*Columbia University, New York, N.Y.*): I am going to ask you to comment on something that obviously you must have thought about before. Your modified HDL_3 particle, which you call an HDL_2 in inverted commas and which you see after you incubate VLDL with HDL_3 and then isolate it in the zonal rotor—I wonder if you would consider the possibility that it might be equivalent to what is called an HDL_{2A} particle? If one looks at the compositional results obtained by Anderson and co-workers based on equilibrium density ultracentrifugation of the whole human HDL fraction, one sees that the HDL_{2A} subclass—that is, the one between *d* 1.121–1.125, differs from HDL_3 primarily by having an increased number of phospholipids and by having probably an additional apoA-I molecule. The number of all constituents, inclusive of the number of cholesteryl ester molecules, is almost exactly the same in the two particles.

In addition, some data that I shall be talking about later in this Conference indicate that if you incubate phospholipids (egg yolk phosphatidylcholine) vesicles with HDL_3 to a saturation level, the phosphatidylcholine inserts into the surface of HDL_3 and, at saturating amounts, produces a particle of density 1.115; that is similar in density and in composition to what is called HDL_{2A}. I wonder if you would comment on the possibility that your modified HDL_2, which is not exactly like the whole HDL_2 fraction may, in fact, be HDL_{2A}?

DR. S. EISENBERG: First, of course, it is very dangerous to compare the modified lipoprotein that we made *in vitro* to the lipoprotein that is isolated from the circulation. Inasmuch as they may have very similar composition, they may have very different meaning. First of all, *in vitro* we have an artifactual lipoprotein. My own gut feeling is that *in vivo* the transformation of HDL_3 to HDL_2 occurs through an increase in constituents, namely, phospholipids and cholesterol partially generated from tissues. At the end of the particle this would probably reflect some chemical and physical stability. We have discussed this issue with Dr. Scanu about a year ago. I would like to hear his comments sometime at one point or another. My feeling is that during the interconversion you have a metastable lipoprotein structure. In HDL, for example, to me what would dictate the stability of this particle is the fact that the apoA-I is added as a quantum phenomenon. You cannot have half an apoA-I. In other words, you cannot have a particle with three and a half apoA-I molecules. It has to be either three or four.

Now, if you have four apoA-I molecules and you put on phospholipids and free cholesterol, what would you get? Would you get HDL_{2A}? And, then if you have apoA-I would you obtain HDL_{2B}? I cannot answer this question and you may be in the position of answering it better. If this is a one-stage or a two-stage transformation, I do not know. It is very possible that we are dealing with a two-stage transformation.

DR. GOTTO: Thank you. I do not have Dr. Patsch's data with me and, unfortunately, he was unable to come to the meeting, but I know that he feels very strongly, Dr. Tall, that the HDL_2 "particle formed" is not the same as Anderson's HDL_{2A}.

DR. J. D. MORRISETT (*Baylor College of Medicine, Houston, Texas*): It appeared to me from down here that the LDL that you generated *in vitro* had in the DSC curve an endotherm had occurred at a temperature a little bit higher than for native LDL, and I just wonder whether it could be attributed to the smaller amount of triglyceride that is present and that makes the cholesterol esters melt a little bit higher. This observation has obvious metabolic ramifications in terms of lipoprotein removal, I think.

DR. EISENBERG: I completely agree. Our interpretation is that the high transition temperature is due to the smaller amount of triglycerides in LDL. We did not, unfortunately, assess it because in order to really do so we should have made, say, 10 or 20 different particles *in vitro* with different cholesterol–triglyceride ratios. But, we did not do it.

DR. R. L. JACKSON (*University of Cincinnati, Cincinnati, Ohio*): I have two questions. The first is, in your *in vitro* system containing VLDL, HDL$_3$, albumin, and lipase, did you have any LCAT activity present?

DR. EISENBERG: Well, to judge from the chemical analyses, if there was any LCAT present, it was minimal because there was no enrichment of cholesteryl esters in the whole system.

DR. JACKSON: You said it was minimal. Minimal activity?

DR. EISENBERG: I would say almost no activity, simply because we did not generate cholesteryl esters. If you look at one set of data that we published, there is a very small increment of cholesteryl esters in the HDL and we really do not know whether this is true or not.

I tried to measure the LCAT activity in the whole system and I could not detect it. LCAT will not act on a lipolytic system where there is a tremendous generation of fatty acids. My friends tell me that LCAT is inhibited by fatty acids. Moreover, we did carry out the incubations in the presence of LCAT inhibitors and we observed exactly the same transformation.

DR. JACKSON: The second question is, what are the techniques that you use to show this transformation from HDL$_3$ to HDL$_2$ besides the zonal rotor.

DR. EISENBERG: We use the zonal rotor as our basic procedure. Changes are also observed by agarose columns and by analytical ultracentrifugation.

DR. JACKSON: Would you care to comment on the mechanism of interconversion caused by bacterial lipase and lipoprotein lipase? Since they have different specificity I was surprised that both enzymes produced the same kind of disc.

DR. EISENBERG: Let me point out that, as I mentioned, I did not have time to present those comparative studies. We actually did use four different lipases during the last six months or so. It is the bacterial lipase which we have studied intensively, a lipase isolated from the tongue, the lingual lipase, and the triglyceride lipase of hepatic origin.

As for the bacterial lipase, the enzyme has a very potent triglyceridease activity and hydrolyzes triglycerides in lipoproteins. It has almost no phospholipase activity. Practically, in the experiment that we carried out, there was zero phospholipase activity. You may remember that with lipoprotein lipase, the phospholipase activity is quite marked. It does not have any cholesterol esterase or any cholesterol hydrolase activity, neither does it have protease activity. The experimental condition is the simplest we can think about; we take VLDL and the enzyme, and incubate them together with a fatty acid receptor. The enzyme does not even need fatty acid acceptors.

DR. B. SHEN (*University of Chicago, Chicago, Ill.*): So, you are suggesting that this special lipase has lipoprotein lipase activity.

DR. EISENBERG: I do not know what lipoprotein lipase is anymore. It is an enzyme that hydrolyzes triglycerides in lipoproteins. Some people object very much to the term "lipoprotein lipase of hepatic origin" because they feel it is not a true lipoprotein lipase. But, obviously, the liver enzyme does not see anything but lipoproteins.

DR. SHEN: Is the activity of the bacterial enzyme stimulated by apoC-II?

DR. EISENBERG: Not that I know of; we do get activity with and without apoC.

EVOLUTION OF THE LDL RECEPTOR CONCEPT— FROM CULTURED CELLS TO INTACT ANIMALS *

Michael S. Brown, Petri T. Kovanen, and Joseph L. Goldstein

*Departments of Molecular Genetics and Internal Medicine
University of Texas Health Science Center at Dallas
Dallas, Texas 75235*

In 1973 a new mechanism was described for the regulation of cholesterol metabolism. Cultured human skin fibroblasts were shown to derive membrane cholesterol from plasma low-density lipoprotein (LDL), but not from high-density lipoprotein (HDL).[1, 2] This was the first clue that extrahepatic cells might have a specific mechanism for extracting cholesterol from specific lipoproteins. In the months that followed, it was shown that fibroblasts and other cells derive cholesterol from LDL by binding the lipoprotein to a cell surface receptor, which was named the LDL receptor.[3, 4] But binding of the lipoprotein was not sufficient for cholesterol delivery. The cells had to internalize the bound LDL and take it apart to extract its cholesterol.[3-6] This internalization and degradation involved the concerted interaction of several cellular organelles in a sequence that was called the LDL receptor pathway.[7]

LDL Receptor Pathway in Cultured Cells

FIGURE 1 shows the sequence of steps in the LDL receptor pathway as it eventually emerged from the studies in cultured fibroblasts. To deliver cholesterol, LDL first binds to its receptor, which is localized in specialized regions of the plasma membrane called coated pits.[8] The coated pits have one important property: they rapidly invaginate into the cell and pinch off to form coated endocytic vesicles that contain the receptor-bound LDL. The coated vesicles then migrate through the cytoplasm until they fuse with cellular lysosomes.[9] Within the lysosome, the protein of LDL is hydrolyzed to amino acids, and the cholesteryl esters in the core of LDL are hydrolyzed, liberating free cholesterol that is used by the cell for membrane synthesis.[5-7] This cholesterol also regulates three events in cellular cholesterol metabolism. First, it suppresses the activity of 3-hydroxy-3-methylglutaryl coenzyme A reductase (HMG CoA reductase), the rate-controlling enzyme in cholesterol biosynthesis, thereby suppressing cholesterol synthesis by the cell. Second, it activates an acyl-CoA: cholesterol acyltransferase (ACAT), which re-esterifies some of the incoming cholesterol for storage as cholesteryl ester droplets in the cytoplasm. Third, cholesterol derived from LDL suppresses the synthesis of LDL receptors, allowing the cell to control the rate of entry of LDL by regulating the number of LDL receptors (reviewed in References 7 & 10). Under the usual conditions of cell culture, human and animal cells do not synthesize their own cholesterol, but rather they use the LDL receptor pathway to derive cholesterol from LDL.

The LDL pathway was elucidated entirely through studies of cultured human

* Supported by Grant HL-20948 from the National Institutes of Health.

skin fibroblasts. This was a departure from the traditional way in which metabolic pathways are delineated. Usually, these pathways are worked out through
studies of living animals or of organ slices excised from living animals. The
LDL pathway, however, was worked out in a much more artificial environment:
It was observed in cells that had been propagated for many generations in tissue
culture. And this raised a crucial question: Does this LDL pathway also
operate in the body of living humans and animals? After all, cells in tissue
culture might express functions that are encoded in the genes but that might
not be expressed *in vivo*.

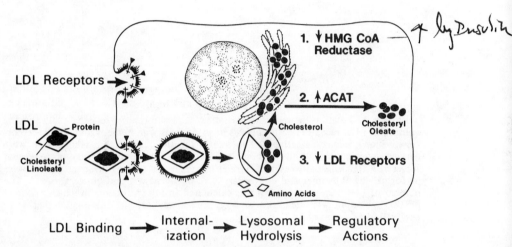

FIGURE 1. Sequential steps in the LDL pathway in cultured human fibroblasts. LDL
denotes low-density lipoprotein; HMG CoA reductase denotes 3-hydroxy-3-methyl-
glutaryl coenzyme A reductase; and ACAT denotes acyl-CoA:cholesterol acyltran-
ferase.

GENETIC EVIDENCE FOR LDL RECEPTORS *in Vivo*

We were encouraged at the outset to believe that the LDL receptor is expressed *in vivo* because of certain genetic considerations. Early in our studies,
we observed that fibroblasts cultured from patients with the homozygous form
of familial hypercholesterolemia (FH) failed to express LDL receptors.[2-4] As a
result of their receptor defect, these mutant FH homozygote cells were unable
to take up and degrade LDL.

The inability of FH homozygote cells to degrade LDL was consistent with
the known abnormality of LDL degradation in the body of FH patients. Studies
of the plasma turnover of ^{125}I-labeled LDL by a number of investigators, including Langer and Levy,[11] Myant and co-workers,[12, 13] Bilheimer and co-
workers,[14, 15] and Packard and Shepherd,[16] have shown that the elevated LDL
level in FH was due primarily to a reduction in the fractional catabolic rate
for circulating LDL. These *in vivo* results correlated with the levels of LDL
receptors measured *in vitro*.[10] Thus, as shown in FIGURE 2, normal subjects
whose cultured fibroblasts expressed a normal number of receptors catabolized

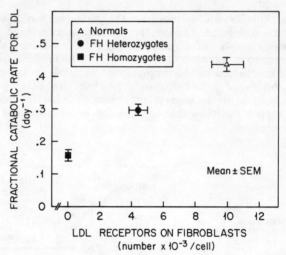

FIGURE 2. Relation between the fractional catabolic rate for plasma LDL and the number of LDL receptors on fibroblasts in 11 patients with homozygous FH (receptor-negative or receptor-defective). The values for the fractional catabolic rate were derived from studies of the turnover of [125I]apo-LDL in the plasma of 6 normal subjects, 6 FH heterozygotes, and 11 FH homozygotes. These turnover studies were performed by Bilheimer and co-workers [14, 15] and by Myant and co-workers.[12, 13] The number of LDL receptors per cell was calculated from experiments in which maximal [125I]LDL binding was measured at 4° C in actively growing fibroblasts that were deprived of LDL for 48 hr.[43]

about 45% of their circulating LDL pool per day. FH heterozygotes whose cells expressed half the normal number of receptors catabolized only 30% of their LDL pool per day, and FH homozygotes whose cultured fibroblasts expressed no receptors catabolized only 15% of their plasma LDL pool per day.

The correlation between the decreased number of LDL receptors on fibroblasts in tissue culture and the defect in plasma LDL catabolism in patients with FH gave us confidence that the LDL receptor must be working constantly *in vivo* and that it must play a major role in degrading plasma LDL. These findings led us to propose a model for LDL catabolism in man.[17] This model is illustrated in FIGURE 3. We postulated that in normal man two-thirds of the LDL that is catabolized daily goes through the receptor pathway and one-third goes through an LDL receptor-*independent* pathway, which we called the scavenger cell pathway. In FH homozygotes the LDL receptor pathway is absent and all LDL is degraded through the less efficient scavenger pathway.

Evidence in support of this model has come from studies of a human fetus of 20 weeks gestation in whom the earliest expression of the FH mutation was observed.[18] The L. family from Leuven, Belgium consists of a married couple, both of whom are FH heterozygotes. Their first son had the homozygous form of FH and died of a myocardial infarction at age 8. Soon after his death, the mother became pregnant. Because her genetic risk of producing another homozygote was 1 in 4, the family physician asked that we attempt a prenatal diagnosis. Accordingly, a sample of amniotic fluid was removed from the uterus at the 16th week of pregnancy. Fetal cells were cultured from the amniotic fluid and sent to our laboratory for analysis. Assays of [^{125}I]LDL binding on the cultured amniotic fluid cells from the fetus at risk, which is called the L. fetus, showed an absence of LDL receptor activity. All of the functional consequences of LDL binding to the receptor were also shown to be markedly reduced in the cells of the L. fetus; that is, there was no suppression of HMG CoA reductase and no stimulation of cholesteryl ester formation when these cells were incubated with LDL.[18]

Based on these biochemical findings, we predicted that the L. fetus was a FH homozygote, and a therapeutic abortion was performed at the 20th week of gestation. The serum cholesterol level in the aborted L. fetus was 279 mg/dl, a value that is 9-fold higher than the mean value observed in other fetuses of similar gestational age. More than 85% of the total cholesterol in the plasma of the L. fetus was in the LDL fraction, confirming that the L. fetus had indeed been affected with homozygous FH. Again the lack of LDL receptors measured *in vitro* was associated with an accumulation of LDL in the plasma *in vivo*.

These genetic results strongly suggest that LDL receptors are normally expressed in some tissues in the body. However, they do not tell us which tissues express LDL receptors and what conditions promote this expression.

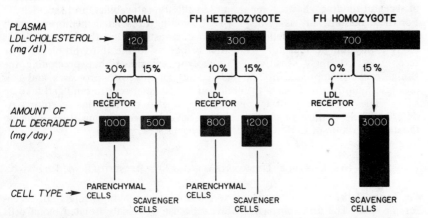

FIGURE 3. Proposed model for the clearance of plasma LDL-cholesterol. The quantitative estimates are based on studies of the turnover of [^{125}I]apo-LDL in the plasma of human subjects that have been performed by Langer *et al.*,[11] Bilheimer *et al.*,[14, 15] Simons *et al.*,[12] and Packard *et al.*[16] In general, these studies show that in normal subjects a total of about 45% of the plasma LDL pool is removed from the plasma daily, whereas in FH heterozygotes this value is about 25% and in homozygotes it is about 15%. In using these data to develop the above model, we have made two assumptions: (1) that the 15% clearance in the FH homozygote represents LDL cleared by LDL receptor-independent pathways (i.e., in "scavenger cells"); and (2) that this same 15% clearance through the scavenger cell pathway occurs in all subjects and is independent of the plasma level of LDL.[10, 13, 14] The daily degradation of LDL-cholesterol (i.e., the sum of the absolute values for the clearance through the LDL receptor and scavenger cell pathways) is highest in the FH homozygote (3000 mg cholesterol), intermediate in the FH heterozygote (2000 mg cholesterol), and lowest in the normal subjects (1500 mg cholesterol). These numbers are within the range of the respective synthetic rates for apo-LDL as measured in steady-state turnover studies. (From Goldstein & Brown.[17] By permission of *Metabolism*.)

To answer these questions, we have set up methods to measure directly LDL receptor activity in tissues removed from living man and experimental animals.

EXPERIMENTAL APPROACHES TO THE STUDY OF LDL RECEPTORS *in Vivo*: POTENTIAL PITFALLS

As we began our *in vivo* studies, we realized that the task would not be simple. The fibroblast studies warned us of many pitfalls, some of which are listed in TABLE 1. First, the tissue culture studies demonstrated that the LDL receptor is expressed in relatively small amounts in nondividing cells and is expressed in much larger amounts in rapidly dividing cells.[4, 10] Moreover, the receptor is tightly regulated. In nondividing cells, LDL receptor activity is just high enough to replace the cholesterol that the cells lose as a result of membrane turnover. The number of receptors can be markedly enhanced by temporarily depriving the cells of LDL so that they develop a deficit of cholesterol.[19-21] The demonstration of LDL receptors *in vivo* would be easier if we could find a way to deprive cells of cholesterol while they are still in the body. Second, [125I]-labeled LDL is a sticky ligand; it adheres to many surfaces. In fact, it can even bind to glass beads in such a way that it mimics most of the characteristics of receptor binding, showing apparent high affinity, saturability, and specificity.[22] For these reasons, any assay of [125I]LDL binding to isolated membranes must be validated by some functional assay to demonstrate that the binding site is really a physiologic receptor. And that brings us to the third problem: The receptor is extremely sensitive to proteolytic enzymes,[4] thus precluding the straightforward approach of first dissociating organs with proteases and collagenases and then measuring the ability of the isolated cells to bind and take up LDL. The proteases used to dissociate cells also destroy the receptor. As described below, most of these problems have been overcome, thus allowing the demonstration of LDL receptors in body cells.

FOUR SYSTEMS FOR DEMONSTRATING LDL RECEPTORS *in Vivo*

TABLE 2 lists four systems that have been used to demonstrate LDL receptors *in vivo*. The first approach involves the use of freshly isolated blood cells from humans. Either normal lymphocytes or malignant leukemia cells express

TABLE 1

FACTORS TO CONSIDER WHEN STUDYING THE LDL RECEPTOR *in Vivo*

1. LDL receptor is tightly regulated, its expression in a given cell type depending on the cell's cholesterol requirements. In general, the receptor is expressed in small amounts in nondividing cells and in larger amounts in rapidly dividing cells.

2. [125I]LDL is a "sticky" ligand. Assays of [125I]LDL binding must be accompanied by functional assays.

3. Receptor is extremely sensitive to proteolytic enzymes, precluding use of protease-isolated cells.

TABLE 2

FOUR SYSTEMS FOR DEMONSTRATING LDL RECEPTORS *in Vivo*

1. Freshly Isolated Blood Cells from Humans
2. Binding of LDL to Membranes from Bovine and Human Organs
3. Uptake of LDL by Organs of Lipoprotein-Deficient Animals
   A. 4-Aminopyrazolopyrimidine (4-APP)
   B. 17α-Ethinyl Estradiol
4. Use of Chemical Modifications to Demonstrate Delayed Plasma Clearance of Modified LDL That Can No Longer Bind to Receptors

functional LDL receptors that regulate cholesterol metabolism via the entire LDL pathway.[21, 23-25] Second, we can demonstrate specific [^{125}I]LDL binding to membranes isolated from homogenates of fresh bovine and human organs.[26-28] Third, high affinity uptake of LDL can be demonstrated *in vivo* in organs of animals that have been rendered lipoprotein-deficient by two different techniques.[28-31] Fourth, chemical modifications can be used to demonstrate delayed plasma clearance of modified LDL particles that can no longer bind to receptors.[32, 33] Each of these systems is discussed below.

LDL Pathway in Freshly Isolated Human Blood Cells

When mononuclear cells from normal individuals are isolated and incubated immediately thereafter with [^{125}I]LDL, they degrade the lipoprotein by a process that is competitively inhibited by an excess of unlabeled LDL, indicating that a specific surface receptor is involved.[24] When this degradation assay is used to measure the number of receptors on freshly isolated cells, normal subjects have easily detectable LDL receptor activity, cells from FH heterozygotes have a half-normal number of receptors, and cells from FH homozygotes have no detectable LDL receptor activity.[24] Thus, normal unstimulated mononuclear cells, which are freshly isolated from the human bloodstream, express functional LDL receptors on their surfaces at the time they are isolated. Moreover, the number of receptors is proportional to the number of functional genes at the receptor locus.

Lymphocytes are nondividing cells that have been exposed to plasma LDL all their life. The studies with fibroblasts predict that if lymphocytes are deprived of lipoproteins, they should develop a cholesterol deficit and an enhanced LDL receptor activity. This prediction was verified experimentally in the following way. When freshly isolated lymphocytes from normal subjects were incubated in the absence of LDL, the number of lipoprotein receptors increased markedly.[21] Under the same conditions of receptor induction, the receptors remained undetectable in FH homozygotes, and the lymphocytes from FH heterozygotes continued to express half the normal number of LDL receptors.[24]

Are the LDL receptors on lymphocytes functional in a physiologic sense, i.e., do they deliver cholesterol to the cells and allow suppression of cholesterol synthesis? The answer is yes. When fresh lymphocytes are incubated for 72 hours in the absence of LDL, they develop a maximal number of LDL receptors and a high rate of cholesterol synthesis. If, at this time, increasing amounts of LDL are added back to the cells, the lipoprotein completely suppresses cholesterol synthesis in cells from normal subjects. In cells from FH homozygotes, however, the lack of LDL receptors completely prevents LDL from suppressing cholesterol synthesis. In cells from FH heterozygotes, a 2.5-fold higher concentration of LDL is required to produce the same degree of suppression as in normal cells.[23, 24] This pattern of response is the same as in cultured fibroblasts.

Recall that rapidly dividing cells in culture express more LDL receptors than nondividing cells. To determine whether this phenomenon also occurs *in vivo*, we screened peripheral blood cells from patients with hematologic malignancies.[25] FIGURE 4 shows the number of LDL receptors on freshly isolated mononuclear cells. The column on the left shows the receptor activity in cells freshly isolated from 18 normal subjects. The column on the right shows the receptor activity in mononuclear cells isolated from seven patients with acute myelogenous leukemia (AML). The LDL receptor activity in these malignant cells ranged from 3- to 100-fold above normal.[25]

The human blood cell studies can be summarized as follows: In all respects so far studied, the LDL receptor in human mononuclear blood cells isolated directly from the body faithfully reflects the properties of the LDL receptor in cultured fibroblasts.

Binding of [^{125}I]LDL to Membranes from Bovine and Human Organs

A second approach to the demonstration of LDL receptor *in vivo* involves the use of membrane binding assays. For this purpose, human or animal organs are homogenized, the membranes are isolated, and their ability to bind [^{125}I]LDL is assayed. Dr. Sandip Basu in our laboratory validated this binding assay by comparing the binding activity of intact fibroblasts with those of membranes isolated from the same cells.[26] Under the conditions of this assay, the receptor that binds [^{125}I]LDL in isolated membranes is the same as the one that functions physiologically to carry LDL into cells.[26] This assay has recently been used to survey LDL receptor activity in membranes prepared from homogenates of 16 tissues of the cow.[27] The results of this survey are shown in FIGURE 5. Membranes from nearly all of these fresh tissues showed detectable LDL binding activity. The number of [^{125}I]LDL binding sites was highest in the membranes of the adrenal cortex and the ovarian corpus luteum, the two tissues that secrete steroids and thus have the highest requirements for cholesterol. In contrast, the adrenal medulla and the ovarian interstitium, which do not produce large amounts of steroid, showed much lower [^{125}I]LDL binding activity. High affinity binding was also detected in many other tissues including adipose tissue, myocardium, skeletal muscle, and so forth. No high affinity binding of [^{125}I]LDL was detected in mature red cells.[27]

It is not surprising that the number of LDL receptors *in vivo* is highest in tissues that actively secrete steroids. We had earlier demonstrated that cultured mouse and bovine adrenal cells have large numbers of LDL receptors.[35, 36] The finding in FIGURE 5 of such a characteristic distribution of receptors in the tissues of the cow reinforces the notion that these receptors are functional *in vivo*. In a survey of human fetal tissues, we have also found that the adrenal gland and gonads express the highest level of high affinity [^{125}I]LDL binding activity.[28]

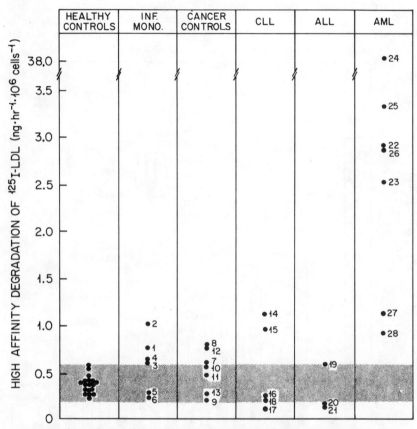

FIGURE 4. High affinity degradation of [^{125}I]LDL in freshly isolated mononuclear cells from 18 healthy subjects (left panel) and 7 patients with acute myelogenous leukemia (AML) (right panel). The middle four panels show control values obtained on 6 patients with infectious mononucleosis (inf. mono.), 7 patients with nonhematologic malignancies (cancer patients), 5 patients with chronic lymphocytic leukemia (CLL), and 3 patients with acute lymphocytic leukemia (ALL). Approximately 4×10^6 freshly isolated mononuclear cells were incubated in 1 ml of medium with 30% lipoprotein-deficient serum and 25 μg protein/ml of [^{125}I]LDL (200 to 496 cpm/ng) in the absence or presence of 500 μg protein/ml of unlabeled LDL. After incubation for 4 to 6 hr at 37°, the content of ^{125}I-labeled acid-soluble (noniodide) material formed by the cells and released into the medium was determined. High affinity (i.e., receptor-mediated) degradation of [^{125}I]LDL was calculated as the difference between values obtained in the absence and presence of unlabeled LDL. Each data point represents the mean of triplicate incubations performed on cells from a single subject. (From Ho *et al*.[25] By permission of Blood.)

Uptake of LDL by Organs of Lipoprotein-Deficient Animals

The third model system for demonstrating lipoprotein receptors *in vivo* is the lipoprotein-deficient animal. The rationale for these studies lay in the observation that when human fibroblasts are grown in the presence of LDL

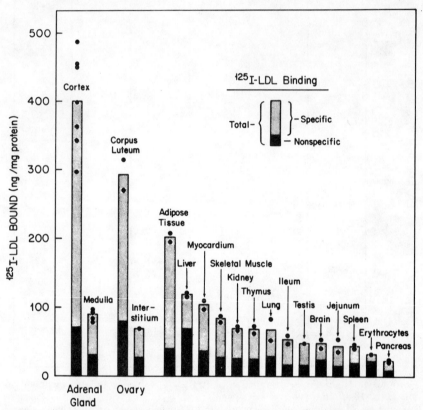

FIGURE 5. Comparison of [^{125}I]LDL binding activity to membranes prepared from different bovine tissues. Fresh tissues were homogenized, the 8000g to 100,000g membrane pellets were isolated, and [^{125}I]LDL binding assays were performed at 4° C as previously described.[27] Total binding represents the amount of [^{125}I]LDL bound to the membranes in the absence of excess unlabeled LDL. Specific (high affinity) binding and nonspecific binding are those components of the total binding that were, respectively, inhibited and not inhibited competitively by the presence of the excess unlabeled LDL. Each point represents the average of duplicated assays performed in the membranes obtained from one animal. (After Kovanen *et al.*[27])

they derive their cholesterol from LDL and hence keep their cholesterol synthesis suppressed.[1, 2] When LDL is removed from the culture medium, fibroblasts continue to grow because they increase their cholesterol synthesis. When LDL is subsequently added back, the lipoprotein binds to the LDL receptor, delivers cholesterol to the cells, and again suppresses cholesterol synthesis.

At the time we began these studies, circumstantial evidence indicated that a similar suppression of cholesterol synthesis also operates in extrahepatic tissues *in vivo*. From studies of cholesterol metabolism in the rat, it had long been known that the rate of cholesterol synthesis is low in most extrahepatic tissues.[37] Based on the LDL receptor hypothesis, we predicted that this low rate prevailed because extrahepatic cells normally derive their cholesterol from plasma lipoproteins.[7] If we could find a way to deprive tissues of lipoproteins *in vivo*, their rates of cholesterol synthesis should rise. An approach to this problem grew out of a discussion that we had in 1975 with Richard J. Havel, who told us of an early observation by Howard Eder.

4-APP-Treated Rat and Mouse

In 1971 Schiff, Roheim, and Eder showed that the drug 4-aminopyrazolo-pyrimidine (4-APP) blocked the secretion of lipoproteins from the liver of rats and that this, in turn, led to a profound drop in the plasma cholesterol level.[38] If we could reproduce this finding, it would give us the opportunity to deprive extrahepatic tissues of plasma lipoproteins *in vivo* and to ask whether the cholesterol synthesis in these tissues would increase.

When 4-APP was given to rats, the plasma level of lipoprotein-cholesterol declined dramatically. This was accompanied by a marked increase in the activity of HMG CoA reductase in the kidney and the lung.[29] The increase in the activity of this rate-limiting enzyme was accompanied by the expected increase in cholesterol biosynthesis in tissue slices as measured from [^{14}C] acetate.

The tissue that showed the most dramatic changes in cholesterol metabolism when the plasma cholesterol level was lowered by 4-APP was the adrenal gland.[28, 30] The drop in plasma cholesterol was accompanied by a drastic fall in the content of stored cholesteryl esters within the adrenal gland. At the same time, there was a rise in the adrenal HMG CoA reductase activity.[30] If these changes were due to a deprivation of plasma lipoproteins, then they should be reversed by the subsequent infusion of lipoproteins. Accordingly, we treated rats with 4-APP until the plasma cholesterol level had dropped, the adrenal cholesteryl ester content had fallen, and the adrenal HMG CoA reductase had risen. We then infused the animals with increasing amounts of human LDL. When increasing amounts of LDL were given to the 4-APP-treated rat, all of the above changes were reversed. The plasma cholesterol level rose, the level of adrenal cholesteryl esters was restored, and adrenal HMG CoA reductase became suppressed.[30] We also found that the infusion of human HDL could similarly reverse all of the changes in the adrenal gland of the 4-APP-treated rat.[30] Andersen and Dietschy have also performed extensive experiments along these same lines and have obtained similar results.[39, 40]

We have recently repeated these 4-APP experiments in another species, the mouse. Using ^{125}I-labeled LDL, we have gone on to show that the uptake of LDL-cholesterol is due to the binding of the lipoprotein by the adrenal gland to a saturable and specific receptor that resembles in all respects the LDL receptor originally demonstrated *in vitro*.[31] We have also observed that the adrenal glands from the mouse have a separate set of receptors that recognize HDL. Thus, the adrenal of the mouse is able to use cholesterol derived from either HDL or LDL.[31]

The important physiologic point to emerge from these 4-APP studies is that the adrenal gland in the rat and in the mouse normally obtains its cholesterol from plasma lipoproteins through lipoprotein receptors and that removal of lipoproteins causes the gland to synthesize its own cholesterol—just as in cultured fibroblasts.

Rats Treated with 17α-Ethinyl Estradiol

We have recently used a different technique to lower plasma lipoprotein levels in the rat and observed the same results that were originally obtained with 4-APP. FIGURE 6 shows an experiment in which rats were treated with 17α-ethinyl estradiol, a compound that profoundly lowers the plasma lipoprotein level,[41] but is not as toxic to the animal as 4-APP. As with 4-APP,

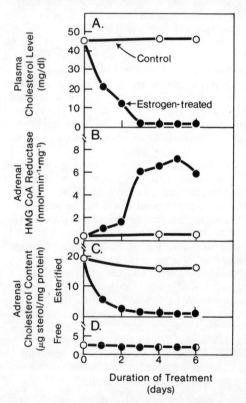

FIGURE 6. Plasma cholesterol levels (A), adrenal HMG CoA reductase activity (B), and adrenal content of free (D) and esterified (C) cholesterol as a function of duration of administration of 17α-ethinyl estradiol to rats. Ethinyl estradiol was administered subcutaneously (5 mg/kg body weight per day) to 6 groups of male rats (●) as previously described.[44] Three control groups of male rats received daily subcutaneous injections of propylene glycol (○). All the animals were killed on the same day 2 hr after the last dose, and the indicated measurements were made by previously described methods.[30] Each point represents the average of values obtained from 2 to 4 rats.

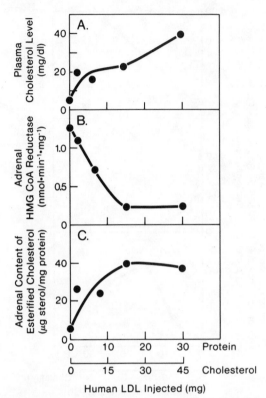

FIGURE 7. Effect of human LDL on the plasma cholesterol level (A), adrenal HMG CoA reductase activity (B), and adrenal esterified cholesterol content (C) of rats previously treated with 17α-ethinyl estradiol. Five groups of male rats were treated subcutaneously with ethinyl estradiol (5 mg/kg body weight per day) as previously described.[44] On day 10 of treatment, 4 groups of rats received the indicated amount of human LDL (*d*, 1.019 to 1.063 g/ml) intravenously as a bolus. The control groups received an intravenous injection of 0.15 M NaCl. All of the animals were killed 12 hr after the intravenous injections, and the indicated measurements were made as previously described.[30] Each point represents the average of values obtained from 2 to 4 rats.

when the plasma cholesterol level dropped (FIGURE 6A), the adrenal gland became depleted of cholesteryl esters (FIGURE 6C), and the activity of HMG CoA reductase rose (FIGURE 6B). And again, as with the 4-APP-treated rat, these changes in adrenal cholesterol metabolism due to 17α-ethinyl estradiol treatment could be reversed by infusing either human LDL (FIGURE 7) or human HDL (FIGURE 8).

*Use of Chemical Modifications to Demonstrate Delayed Plasma
Clearance of Modified LDL That Can No Longer Bind to Receptors*

The fourth system for demonstrating LDL receptors *in vivo* involves the use of modified lipoproteins. Studies by Mahley and co-workers have demon-

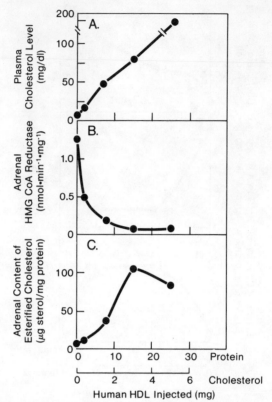

FIGURE 8. Effect of human HDL on the plasma cholesterol level (A), adrenal HMG CoA reductase activity (B), and adrenal esterified cholesterol content (C) of rats previously treated with 17α-ethinyl estradiol. Five groups of male rats were treated subcutaneously with ethinyl estradiol (5 mg/kg body weight per day) as previously described.[44] On day 10 of treatment, 4 groups of rats received the indicated amount of human HDL₃ (d, 1.125 to 1.215 g/ml) intravenously as a bolus. The control group received an intravenous injection of 0.15 M NaCl. All of the animals were killed 12 hr after the intravenous injections, and the indicated measurements were made as previously described.[30] Each point represents the average of values obtained from 2 to 4 rats.

strated that LDL can be modified in certain specific ways so as to block its ability to bind to the LDL receptor.[32] Mahley has shown that one way to accomplish this is to methylate the lysine residues of LDL.[32, 33] We have confirmed Mahley's observations as shown by the data of FIGURE 9, which compare the binding and degradation of [¹²⁵I]LDL and [¹²⁵I]methyl-LDL by monolayers of human fibroblasts. The [¹²⁵I]methyl-LDL has lost its ability to bind to the LDL receptor (FIGURE 9A) and to be degraded by the cells (FIGURE 9B).

The ability to prevent the in vitro receptor-mediated uptake of LDL by methylation of the lipoprotein provides a powerful way to determine whether LDL is being metabolized through the receptor site in vivo. If [¹²⁵I]methyl-LDL were administered intravenously and its decay followed, one would predict that the methylated lipoprotein would disappear from the plasma at a slower rate than unmodified [125I]LDL. And if the original hypothesis were correct that about two-thirds of LDL clearance in man *in vivo* was due to the receptor,[17] then the clearance of [125I]methyl-LDL should be reduced by two-thirds.

Mahley *et al*. have recently compared the simultaneous turnover of [125I] methyl-LDL and normal [131I]LDL in the rhesus monkey.[33] The clearance of the [125I]methyl-LDL was markedly retarded. The calculated fractional catabolic rate was reduced by slightly more than 50%, a value that is in reasonable agreement with the 66% reduction predicted for man. Mahley has made similar findings in the rat.[33] These important experiments provide strong support for the role of the LDL receptor in clearing LDL from the plasma in these two species.

Building on Mahley's experience, we have compared the uptake of normal [125I]LDL and [125I]methyl-LDL by adrenal glands of intact rats treated with 17α-ethinyl estradiol (FIGURE 10A) and intact mice treated with 4-APP (FIGURE 10B). These results show that large amounts of intravenously administered normal [125I]LDL were rapidly taken up by the adrenal glands of such animals, whereas only small amounts of the [125I]methyl-LDL were taken up. Again, these results support the view that LDL receptors operate in the intact rat and the intact mouse.

The most dramatic experiments using modified lipoproteins have been performed in man by Shepherd and Packard.[42] These workers took advantage of

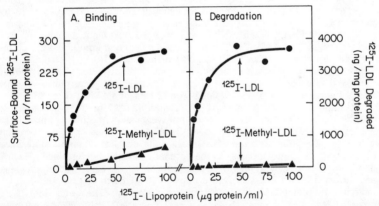

FIGURE 9. Comparison of the cell surface binding (A) and proteolytic degradation (B) of native [125I]LDL (●) and [125I]methyl-LDL (▲) by monolayers of cultured human fibroblasts. Monolayers of normal fibroblasts were prepared as previously described.[43] After incubation for 48 hr in 10% human lipoprotein-deficient serum, the actively growing cells were incubated with the indicated concentration of either [125I]LDL (56 cpm/ng protein) (●) or [125I]methyl-LDL (48 cpm/ng) (▲). After incubation for 5 hr at 37° C, the amount of surface-bound [125I]lipoprotein (i.e., [125I]lipoprotein released by dextran sulfate) and the amount of [125I]LDL degraded (i.e., trichloroacetic-acid-soluble [noniodide] 152I-radioactivity formed by the cells and excreted into the culture medium) were determined as described.[4, 43] Each value represents the average of duplicate incubations. Methyl-LDL was prepared by treatment of LDL with formaldehyde and sodium borohydride [32] and was radiolabeled with 125I as described for native LDL.[3]

Mahley's observation that modification of the arginine residues in LDL by reaction with cyclohexanedione blocked the ability of the lipoprotein to bind to the LDL receptor.[32] Shepherd and Packard administered simultaneously normal [^{125}I]LDL and cyclohexanedione-modified [^{131}I]LDL to four normal subjects and four patients with heterozygous FH. Assuming that the cyclohexanedione-treated [^{131}I]LDL was cleared from the plasma only through

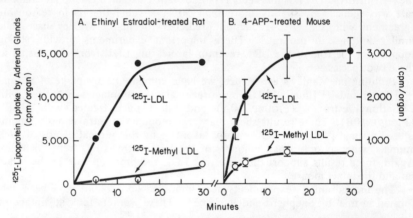

FIGURE 10. Time course of uptake of human [^{125}I]LDL (●) and human [^{125}I]methyl LDL (○) by adrenal glands of lipoprotein-deficient animals. (A) Rats were treated subcutaneously for 7 days with 17α-ethinyl estradiol (5 mg/kg body weight per day) as previously described.[44] Each rat was then injected intravenously with 0.2 ml of a solution containing 0.15 M NaCl, 20 mg/ml bovine serum albumin, and 2.8 μg protein (1×10^6 cpm) of either human [^{125}I]LDL (●) or human [^{125}I]methyl-LDL (○). After the indicated time intervals, whole-body perfusions were carried out, the adrenal glands were removed, and their total content of ^{125}I-radioactivity was determined. Each point represents the average of values obtained from 2 rats. (B) Mice received 5 doses of 4-APP (20 μg/g body weight) and ACTH (2 units) at 12 hr intervals as previously described.[31] Each mouse was then injected intravenously with either human [^{125}I]LDL (●) or human [^{125}I]methyl LDL (○) (1×10^6 cpm, 2.8 μg protein) as described above in (A). The animals were killed at the indicated time interval after injection, and the content of ^{125}I-radioactivity in the adrenal glands was determined. Each point represents the average of values obtained from 3 mice. The brackets represent 1 standard error. In (A) and (B), more than 95% of the total tissue content of ^{125}I-radioactivity was precipitable by 10% trichloroacetic acid. The wet weights for pairs of adrenal glands for the rats (A) and mice (B) were 72±6 mg and 4.9±0.1 mg (mean ±1 SE), respectively. Methyl-LDL was prepared by treatment of LDL with formaldehyde and sodium borohydride[32] and was radio-labeled with ^{125}I as described for native LDL.[3]

receptor-independent pathways, the data indicated that in normal man one-third of the daily clearance of LDL is via the receptor pathway and two-thirds by receptor-independent routes. In normal man the calculated fractional catabolic rate for LDL through the receptor pathway was 0.110 per day. In FH heterozygotes this value was reduced to 0.032 per day. Thompson *et al.* have carried these studies one step further.[45] Applying the same technique to an FH homozygote, they showed that the fractional catabolic rate through the receptor pathway was even further reduced, to 0.019 per day. Taken together, these pioneering studies provide strong evidence for the existence of an LDL receptor pathway in normal man and for its disruption in familial hypercholesterolemia.

SUMMARY

The initial observations in cultured fibroblasts made six years ago allowed the formulation of a series of hypotheses concerning LDL metabolism in tissues of animals and man. The most important of these hypotheses was that a large fraction of LDL was removed from plasma by a specific receptor-mediated uptake mechanism whose function was to supply cholesterol to extrahepatic cells. This hypothesis is strongly supported by genetic observations in patients with familial hypercholesterolemia and by studies of the four model systems discussed above. These studies by no means solve all of the important questions about LDL metabolism. We still need to know which tissues take up the most LDL; we need to know how much LDL is cleared by the liver and whether this clearance involves the same LDL receptor that operates in extrahepatic cells; we need to know the mechanism for the clearance of the one-half to two-thirds of LDL that leaves the plasma by receptor-independent pathways; and finally we need to know how an abnormal accumulation of LDL in the plasma leads to the deposition of cholesterol in scavenger cells and produces atherosclerosis.

REFERENCES

1. BROWN, M. S., S. E. DANA & J. L. GOLDSTEIN. 1973. Regulation of 3-hydroxy-3-methylglutaryl coenzyme A reductase activity in human fibroblasts by lipoproteins. Proc. Natl. Acad. Sci. USA **70:**2162–2166.
2. GOLDSTEIN, J. L. & M. S. BROWN. 1973. Familial hypercholesterolemia: Identification of a defect in the regulation of 3 hydroxy-3-methylglutaryl coenzyme A reductase activity associated with overproduction of cholesterol. Proc. Natl. Acad. Sci. USA **70:**2804–2808.
3. BROWN, M. S. & J. L. GOLDSTEIN. 1974. Familial hypercholesterolemia: Defective binding of lipoproteins to cultured fibroblasts associated with impaired regulation of 3-hydroxy-3-methylglutaryl coenzyme A reductase activity. Proc. Natl. Acad. Sci. USA **71:**788–792.
4. GOLDSTEIN, J. L. & M. S. BROWN. 1974. Binding and degradation of low density lipoproteins by cultured human fibroblasts: Comparison of cells from a normal subject and from a patient with homozygous familial hypercholesterolemia. J. Biol. Chem. **249:**5153–5162.
5. BROWN, M. S., S. E. DANA & J. L. GOLDSTEIN. 1975. Receptor-dependent hydrolysis of cholesteryl esters contained in plasma low density lipoprotein. Proc. Natl. Acad. Sci. USA **72:**2925–2929.
6. GOLDSTEIN, J. L., G. Y. BRUNSCHEDE & M. S. BROWN. 1975. Inhibition of the proteolytic degradation of low density lipoprotein in human fibroblasts by chloroquine, concanavalin A, and Triton WR 1339. J. Biol. Chem. **250:**7854–7862.
7. BROWN, M. S. & J. L. GOLDSTEIN. 1976. Receptor-mediated control of cholesterol metabolism. Science **191:**150–154.
8. ANDERSON, R. G. W., J. L. GOLDSTEIN & M. S. BROWN. 1976. Localization of low density lipoprotein receptors on plasma membrane of normal human

fibroblasts and their absence in cells from a familial hypercholesterolemia homozygote. Proc. Natl. Acad. Sci. USA **73:**2434–2438.

9. ANDERSON, R. G. W., M. S. BROWN & J. L. GOLDSTEIN. 1977. Role of the coated endocytic vesicle in the uptake of receptor-bound low density lipoprotein in human fibroblasts. Cell **10:**351–364.

10. GOLDSTEIN, J. L. & M. S. BROWN. 1977. The low-density lipoprotein pathway and its relation to atherosclerosis. Ann. Rev. Biochem. **46:**897–930.

11. LANGER, T., W. STROBER & R. I. LEVY. 1972. The metabolism of low density lipoprotein in familial type II hyperlipoproteinemia. J. Clin. Invest. **51:**1528–1536.

12. SIMONS, L. A., D. REICHL, N. B. MYANT & M. MANCINI. 1975. The metabolism of the apoprotein of plasma low density lipoprotein in familial hyperbetalipoproteinaemia in the homozygous form. *Atherosclerosis* **21:**283–298.

13. THOMPSON, G. R., T. SPINKS, A. RANICAR & N. B. MYANT. 1977. Non-steady-state studies of low-density-lipoprotein turnover in familial hypercholesterolaemia. Clin. Sci. Mol. Med. **52:**361–369.

14. BILHEIMER, D. W., J. L. GOLDSTEIN, S. M. GRUNDY & M. S. BROWN. 1975. Reduction in cholesterol and low density lipoprotein synthesis after portacaval shunt surgery in a patient with homozygous familial hypercholesterolemia. J. Clin. Invest. **56:**1420–1430.

15. BILHEIMER, D. W., N. J. STONE & S. M. GRUNDY. 1979. Metabolic studies in familial hypercholesterolemia: Evidence for a gene-dosage effect *in vivo*. J. Clin. Invest. **64:**524–533.

16. PACKARD, C. J., J. L. H. C. THIRD, J. SHEPHERD, A. R. LORIMER, H. G. MORGAN & T. D. V. LAWRIE. 1976. Low density lipoprotein metabolism in a family of familial hypercholesterolemic patients. Metabolism **25:**995–1006.

17. GOLDSTEIN, J. L. & M. S. BROWN. 1977. Atherosclerosis: The low-density lipoprotein receptor hypothesis. Metabolism **26:**1257–1275.

18. BROWN, M. S., P. T. KOVANEN, J. L. GOLDSTEIN, R. EECKELS, K. VANDENBERGHE, H. V. D. BERGHE, J. P. FRYNS & J. J. CASSIMAN. 1978. Prenatal diagnosis of homozygous familial hypercholesterolaemia: Expression of a genetic receptor disease *in utero*. Lancet (1):526–529.

19. BROWN, M. S. & J. L. GOLDSTEIN. 1975. Regulation of the activity of the low density lipoprotein receptor in human fibroblasts. Cell **6:**307–316.

20. GOLDSTEIN, J. L., M. K. SOBHANI, J. R. FAUST & M. S. BROWN. 1976. Heterozygous familial hypercholesterolemia: Failure of normal allele to compensate for mutant allele at a regulated genetic locus. Cell **9:**195–203.

21. HO, Y. K., M. S. BROWN, D. W. BILHEIMER & J. L. GOLDSTEIN. 1976. Regulation of low density lipoprotein receptor activity in freshly isolated human lymphocytes. J. Clin. Invest. **58:**1465–1474.

22. DANA, S. E., M. S. BROWN & J. L. GOLDSTEIN. 1977. Specific, saturable, and high affinity binding of ^{125}I-low density lipoprotein to glass beads. Biochem. Biophys. Res. Comm. **74:**1369–1376.

23. HO, Y. K., J. R. FAUST, D. W. BILHEIMER, M. S. BROWN & J. L. GOLDSTEIN. 1977. Regulation of cholesterol synthesis by low density lipoprotein in isolated human lymphocytes. J. Exp. Med. **145:**1531–1549.

24. BILHEIMER, D. W., Y. K. HO, M. S. BROWN, R. G. W. ANDERSON & J. L. GOLDSTEIN. 1978. Genetics of the low density lipoprotein receptor: Diminished receptor activity in lymphocytes from heterozygotes with familial hypercholesterolemia. J. Clin. Invest. **61:**678–696.

25. HO, Y. K., R. G. SMITH, M. S. BROWN & J. L. GOLDSTEIN. 1978. Low-density lipoprotein (LDL) receptor activity in human acute myelogenous leukemia cells. Blood **52:**1099–1114.

26. BASU, S. K., J. L. GOLDSTEIN & M. S. BROWN. 1978. Characterization of the low density lipoprotein receptor in membranes prepared from human fibroblasts. J. Biol. Chem. **253:**3852–3856.

27. KOVANEN, P. T., S. K. BASU, J. L. GOLDSTEIN & M. S. BROWN. 1979. Low

density lipoprotein receptors in bovine adrenal cortex. II. Low density lipoprotein binding to membranes prepared from fresh tissue. Endocrinology **104:** 610–616.

28. BROWN, M. S., P. T. KOVANEN & J. L. GOLDSTEIN. 1979. Receptor-mediated uptake of lipoprotein-cholesterol and its utilization for steroid synthesis in the adrenal cortex. Recent Prog. Hormone Res. **35:**215–257.

29. BALASUBRAMANIAM, S., J. L. GOLDSTEIN, J. R. FAUST & M. S. BROWN. 1976. Evidence for regulation of 3-hydroxy-3-methylglutaryl coenzyme A reductase activity and cholesterol synthesis in nonhepatic tissues of rat. Proc. Natl. Acad. Sci. USA **73:**2564–2568.

30. BALASUBRAMANIAM, S., J. L. GOLDSTEIN, J. R. FAUST, G. Y. BRUNSCHEDE & M. S. BROWN. 1977. Lipoprotein-mediated regulation of 3-hydroxy-3-methylglutaryl coenzyme A reductase activity and cholesteryl ester metabolism in the adrenal gland of the rat. J. Biol. Chem. **252:**1771–1779.

31. KOVANEN, P. T., W. J. SCHNEIDER, G. M. HILLMAN, J. L. GOLDSTEIN & M. S. BROWN. 1979. Separate mechanisms for the uptake of high and low density lipoproteins by mouse adrenal gland *in vivo*. J. Biol. Chem. **254:**5498–5505.

32. WEISGRABER, K. H., T. L. INNERARITY & R. W. MAHLEY. 1978. Role of the lysine residues of plasma lipoproteins in high affinity binding to cell surface receptors on human fibroblasts. J. Biol. Chem. **253:**9053–9062.

33. MAHLEY, R. W., K. H. WEISGRABER, G. W. MELCHIOR, T. L. INNERARITY & K. S. HOLCOMBE. 1979. Inhibition of receptor-mediated clearance of lysine- and arginine-modified lipoproteins from the plasma of rats and monkeys. Proc. Natl. Acad. Sci. USA. **77:**225–229.

34. BROWN, M. S. & J. L. GOLDSTEIN. 1979. Familial hypercholesterolemia: Model for genetic receptor disease. Harvey Lectures **73:**163–201.

35. FAUST, J. R., J. L. GOLDSTEIN & M. S. BROWN. 1977. Receptor-mediated uptake of low density lipoprotein and utilization of its cholesterol for steroid synthesis in cultured mouse adrenal cells. J. Biol. Chem. **252:**4861–4871.

36. KOVANEN, P. T., J. R. FAUST, M. S. BROWN & J. L. GOLDSTEIN. 1979. Low density lipoprotein receptors in bovine adrenal cortex. I. Receptor-mediated uptake of low density lipoprotein and utilization of its cholesterol for steroid synthesis in cultured adrenocortical cells. Endocrinology **104:**599–609.

37. DIETSCHY, J. M. & J. D. WILSON. 1970. Regulation of cholesterol metabolism. N. Engl. J. Med. **282:**1241–1249.

38. SHIFF, T. S., P. S. ROHEIM & H. A. EDER. 1971. Effects of high sucrose diets and 4-aminopyrazolopyrimidine on serum lipids and lipoproteins in the rat. J. Lipid Res. **12:**596–603.

39. ANDERSEN, J. M. & J. M. DIETSCHY. 1977. Regulation of sterol synthesis in 15 tissues of rat. II. Role of rat and human high and low density plasma lipoproteins and of rat chylomicron remnants. J. Biol. Chem. **252:**3652–3659.

40. ANDERSEN, J. M. & J. M. DIETSCHY. 1978. Relative importance of high and low density lipoproteins in the regulation of cholesterol synthesis in the adrenal gland, ovary, and testis of the rat. J. Biol. Chem. **253:**9024–9032.

41. DAVIS, R. A. & P. S. ROHEIM. 1978. Pharmacologically induced hypolipidemia: The ethinyl estradiol-treated rat. Atherosclerosis **30:**293–299.

42. SHEPHERD, J., S. BICKER, A. R. LORIMER & C. J. PACKARD. 1979. Receptor mediated low density lipoprotein catabolism in man. J. Lipid Res. **20:**999–1006.

43. GOLDSTEIN, J. L., S. K. BASU, G. Y. BRUNSCHEDE & M. S. BROWN. 1976. Release of low density lipoprotein from its cell surface receptor by sulfated glycosaminoglycans. Cell **7:**85–95.

44. KOVANEN, P. T., M. S. BROWN & J. L. GOLDSTEIN. 1979. Increased binding of low density lipoprotein to liver membranes from rats treated with 17α-ethinyl estradiol. J. Biol. Chem. **253:**5126–5132.

45. THOMPSON, G. R., A. K. SOUTAR, B. L. KNIGHT, S. GAVIGAN, N. B. MYANT & J. SHEPHERD. 1980. Evidence for defect of receptor-mediated low density

lipoprotein catabolism in familial hypercholesterolemia *in vivo*. Clin. Sci. **58**: 2p–3p.

DISCUSSION OF THE PAPER

DR. H. L. SEGAL (*SUNY, Buffalo, N.Y.*): Dr. Brown, it was not clear to me whether you think that the methyl derivative and the cyclohexanedione derivative of LDL is taken up by a specific receptor and, if so, is this the same as the acetylated LDL receptor?

DR. M. S. BROWN: As Robert Mahley has shown, either modification of the lysine residues of LDL by reductive methylation or modification of the arginine residues by cyclohexanedione blocks the binding of LDL to these specific receptor sites.

In the case of the methylated LDL, it does not bind *in vitro* to the site in macrophages that binds acetyl LDL for the probable reason that the methylated LDL has not undergone a change in charge. In other words, the methylated LDL still has the same net charge that it had before it was methylated.

Now, when the methylated LDL is injected into the animals, its decay is retarded because it fails to bind to the receptor so it cannot escape from the plasma through the receptor route. The amount of methylated LDL that does escape from the plasma presumably reflects nonspecific pathways or scavenger cell pathways, so that one can make the assumption that the difference between the clearance of native LDL and the clearance of the methylated LDL reflects the amount that is normally being cleared through the receptor pathway. From the studies in the various species, it comes out that about ⅓ to ½ of the LDL are being metabolized through the receptor dependent pathway and the rest through receptor independent pathways.

DR. SEGAL: As you showed, there is a specific receptor in fixed and circulating macrophages for the acetylated LDL. Is there a specific receptor in those same cells for methylated LDL?

DR. BROWN: No. Not for the methylated LDL. We have not studied the cyclohexanedione system. I think that Dr. Mahley has some data on this subject. But, the methylated LDL does not bind to macrophages and is not taken up and degraded by macrophages; that is what allows you to use clearance of this modified particle to reflect a nonspecific receptor independent pathway.

DR. R. W. MAHLEY (*University of California, San Francisco, Calif*): Just a comment on that last response. The cyclohexanedione-modified lipoprotein is also not recognized by the macrophage. But, and as Dr. Brown said, the methylated is also not. The acetylated is, however.

DR. A. M. GOTTO, JR.: Is there any evidence whether the LDL that is taken up by the scavenger pathway regulates cholesterol synthesis in the body?

DR. BROWN: No, there is no evidence one way or the other in that regard.

DR. E. T. KAISER (*University of Chicago, Chicago, Ill.*): The converse to the experiment regarding a modified lipoprotein would be to try to irreversibly inactivate the receptor. It would be possible then to look at the clearance of the LDL itself. Do you consider experiments along such lines feasible?

DR. BROWN: Well, I think that nature has inactivated a receptor for us in the FH homozygotes. But, in terms of chemical manipulation of the receptor itself, experiments to purify the receptor are now making substantial progress. Dr. Wolfgang Schneider in our laboratory has been able to solubilize the receptor and to purify it about 40-fold from bovine adrenal cortex. We are just beginning to do some modification studies to find out how we can specifically block the binding. We know that the receptor is pronase sensitive but the question of whether one can do the analagous chemical modifications of the receptor that one does with LDL would be of interest. It still would not help you in the whole body. We do not know of a good way to block LDL binding in the body. High levels of things like heparin will block LDL interaction with a receptor in the body but I do not know that one could get high enough levels *in vivo* to perform these types of experiments.

DR. P. LAGGNER (*Austrian Academy of Sciences, Graz, Austria*): There have been suggestions that the physical state of the lipids in LDL has an effect on its catabolic fate. From your experiments, do you have any evidence, positive or negative, whether the receptor is sensitive to the physical state of the lipids?

DR. BROWN: Dr. Monty Krieger in Dallas has been able to extract the core cholesteryl esters from LDL and to reconstitute the lipoprotein with a variety of exogenous lipids so that he can have the lipoprotein in a state in which the core, say, at 10° is either liquid or solid. If one carries out binding studies at this temperature no difference is observed in the binding to the receptor of intact fibroblasts, which may be interpreted to mean that the binding of the lipoprotein to the fibroblast receptor is not affected by the physical state of the lipid core in LDL.

DR. GOTTO: In regard to the experiments that you and also Drs. Mahley, Shepherd and Packard have carried out in which the lysine or arginine residues are modified, have there been any experiments done with other proteins to see whether or not modification of the charge on the protein, would alter their distribution in the plasma?

DR. BROWN: Shepherd and Packard did cyclohexanedione treatment of HDL and found no effect on plasma clearance of HDL. I do not know whether Bob has done any other proteins. But, let me say that, as far as I am aware, these studies by Mahley and by Shepherd and Packard are landmark studies, not only in lipoprotein metabolism but in protein catabolism in general. Except for certain very isolated systems like the Ashwell asialoglycoprotein receptor system, I am not aware of modifications that one can make to plasma proteins that retard their clearance. In other words, we do not know how to modify albumin or gamma globulins to prevent them from being removed from plasma. The recognition markers for removal from plasma are generally not very well understood, although generally a modified protein is expected to be removed instantaneously from the circulation. So, the idea that one can modify a protein specifically and retard its clearance means that you are preventing the interaction with some specific receptor mechanism and this opens the way to start looking at other plasma proteins to see whether receptors are involved in their clearance. I am not aware of any extensive studies on these lines.

Dr. Gotto: Did you say whether or not Sheperd and Packard did their experiments also with patients with FH?

Dr. Brown: They conducted them in heterozygotes with FH and observed that the proportion of LDL that they calculated to be leaving the plasma by the receptor-dependent route, i.e., the proportion that was affected by cyclohexanedione treatment, was reduced by about 50%. The amount of LDL going out through the scavenger cell pathway was increased and the proportion of LDL going out through the receptor pathway was decreased fairly much in proportion to the values that we predicted based on the receptor studies. In other words, a 50% reduction in receptors seems to produce a 50% reduction in the proportion of LDL that exits from the plasma via the receptor pathway.

GENERAL DISCUSSION

A. M. Gotto, Jr., *Moderator*

Baylor College of Medicine
Houston, Texas 77030
The Methodist Hospital
Houston, Texas 77030

DR. A. M. GOTTO, JR.: I wanted to ask Dr. Lindgren and Dr. Eisenberg if they would make a comment about reports of a series of LDLs isolated from patients with hyperlipidemia of different molecular weight, this primarily by Fisher *et al.*

DR. F. T. LINDGREN: I do not quite recall whether Waldo gave actual patterns and flotation characteristics, but I do know that even in the normal there are LDL species in a range from about 2 to 4 million molecular weight, all having different properties.

DR. S. EISENBERG: This is an interesting point. As far as I know, regardless of the methods used to separate LDL subfractions, there is one consistent observation and this relates to the constant amount of protein presumably apoB per particle. If one looks at the population of particles that Frank and Waldo separated, one observes that as the particles become smaller, or the molecular weight decreases, the percent contribution of the protein increases resulting in the same amount of apoB per particle. It is true that in some cases, it is possible to find as much as 20% difference in apoB per particle; but these data may reflect problems in methodology.

DR. LINDGREN: I think that there might be some real interest in relating the catabolic products of the subfractions of VLDL to different LDL. Since these different LDL are related to differences in the distribution of HDL all this, again, suggests that we are dealing with a population of relatively different atherogenic particles.

DR. A. M. SCANU: Dr. Fless in our laboratory has been looking at the problem of LDL atherogenicity and relate it to LDL subclasses. By using a combination of rate zonal and density gradient ultracentrifugation, at least three LDL subfractions are isolated from normolipidemic rhesus monkey serum. In these particles, although we recognize the difficulty of assessing the actual mass in each lipoprotein, we do not encounter a constancy in the amount of apoB per particle. An interesting thing about this observation is that if the same animals are analyzed after several months on the same diet they will have exactly the same LDL profile.

More recently, in collaboration with Dr. Wissler we have been examining these various LDL for their proliferative effect on primary cultures of smooth muscle cells. We find that only certain LDLs are able to exhibit a proliferative effect.

It is apparent, therefore, that there is a close structure–function relationship, which we recently found to also apply to human LDL.

DR. R. J. HAVEL: In considering the heterogeneity of the particles isolated

69

in the LDL density interval, I think that we must keep very carefully in mind functional as well as structural differences.

Functionally, from our liver perfusion studies, I would tend to define LDL as a particle which the normal liver takes up very slowly. Now, there may be particles in that density interval that the liver takes up avidly. For example, in functionally hepatectomized rats it is not difficult to see particles produced in the LDL density interval. These particles contain a fair amount of the arginine-rich protein or apoE. Such particles we would predict would be avidly taken up by the liver and therefore, we would classify them as remnants.

I think I have a little difficulty in calling LDL a remnant just because it is obviously some kind of a product of VLDL metabolism, which differs tremendously in the protein components that it has on the surface. So, I would like to say that an LDL particle, functionally, is probably a particle that has only apoB as its protein component. If we have other particles, whether we produce them *in vitro* or under any other conditions, I think that to call them LDL is fine—that is the operational definition Dr. Lindgren has been emphasizing—but, it is the functional heterogeneity that we must keep very uppermost in our minds in considering the metabolic properties of these lipoprotein particles.

DR. K. W. A. WIRTZ (*University of Utrecht, Utrecht, The Netherlands*): I have a question for Dr. Havel with respect to the transfer of cholesteryl ester from HDL to the other lipoproteins. Is there any evidence that apoD transfers the cholesteryl ester to the remnant particle or does apoD just shuttle between particles?

DR. HAVEL: There is certainly no published evidence. I really should not speak for Dr. Fielding authoritatively here, but I think to date there is no conclusive evidence that apoD goes with the cholesteryl ester. I think the exact mechanism of shuttling is not clear. What is very exciting and what Dr. Fielding talked about at the Gordon Conference was that apoD forms a complex with LCAT and that the particle that contains apoD in native plasma probably comprises a very tiny fraction of the total HDL spectrum, and that is where the action is—probably in a particle the concentration of which is very low but which is turning over very rapidly. The cholesterol ester would be formed in that complex. In a paper, which is due to appear fairly soon, he has data on the properties of that complex, which I do not think I should comment on at this time.

DR. WIRTZ: Would you suggest that the apoD operates through the cholesteryl esters at the surface of the particle?

DR. HAVEL: I do not think I am the person to ask about that. I think all we know is what is seen in a functional sense. The evidence that we have at present is not sufficient to comment further.

DR. D. STEINBERG: My comments are directed at the sites of degradation of LDL, and I shall present tomorrow some data from our lab that deal with this issue directly. But right now I wanted to comment on the question raised by the findings of Brown and Goldstein on the scavenger pathway. They have presented some very intriguing work on the macrophage that has quite a different receptor mechanism and proposed the interesting idea that maybe the scavenger pathway is one that involves different cells from those containing the high-affinity receptor pathway, which is certainly possible.

I would like to point out though that in the case of the low-affinity process of LDL uptake, one that is shared with the high-affinity process, the uptake could account for at least part of what is called the low-affinity or scavenger pathway, and I would like to hear what Dr. Brown thinks about that. Even in fibroblasts, if you run the simple experiment of degradation as a function of LDL concentration, you find a biphasic curve in which degradation first increases rapidly and then more slowly and does reach, in our hands, an absolute plateau indicating that there is a low-affinity process. We have done studies comparing fluid pynocytosis measured with [^{14}C]sucrose and actually observed LDL degradation. In the homozygous cells, fluid pynocytosis would not account for the observed degradation. So, we feel that the low-affinity process may be one that goes on in all cells and not just in a different set of cells such as RE cells, and I would like to ask Dr. Brown his thoughts on this point.

DR. M. S. BROWN: Well, I would certainly agree that it is possible that a nonspecific uptake mechanism in a variety of cells accounts for the LDL degradation observed in FH homozygotes. The problem that we have is that it is difficult to study because of the very nature of these nonspecific processes. So we have no clear answers at this time.

DR. N. PAPADOPOULOS: I would like to comment on the methodology. All the studies that have been mentioned were carried out by ultracentrifugation. I would like to comment on the high-resolution agarose gel electrophoresis where we see two β lipoproteins that are associated with LDL, four pre-β lipoproteins, which by ultracentrifugation are named VLDL, and two α lipoproteins. It is possible that all these lipoproteins are not seen in each individual, but become apparent in the analysis of different subjects.

The other comment is that the agarose system is very rapid and is likely to represent more accurately the circulating lipoproteins since they are analyzed immediately after their removal from the blood, within 2 minutes, and the electrophoresis is accomplished in about 10 minutes. The electrophoresis itself is the closest to the ideal liquid electrophoresis since it is 99.5% buffer liquids and only 0.5% agarose, so that a minimum alteration of the lipoproteins is expected.

In regard to HDL, if the plasma is analyzed immediately, we find only one HDL with traces of a second band; after the plasma remains at room temperature for hours or in the refrigerator overnight, other HDLs appear. So, all HDL heterogeneity remains a puzzle, and one must establish how much was there to start with and how much was created artificially.

DR. SCANU: I wish to direct a question to Dr. Brown. You mentioned modifying your LDL core for instance by changing the physical state of the cholesteryl esters from solid to liquid; then you stated that in all of these conditions the binding is similar. What is the fate of these lipoproteins once they are internalized?

DR. BROWN: In order to make a liquid core, in the most common case that we have studied, we put in methylelnoleate, the methyl ester of linoleic acid. Now, in that case if we have the protein labeled, the lipoprotein is taken up by the cells, the protein is hydrolyzed, but the HMG CoA reductase is not suppressed because we have extracted all the cholesterol from the lipoprotein. We really have not studied the fate of the methyl esters and whether they get hydrolyzed or not.

DR. LINDGREN: A last comment which I should have made a moment ago: Alex Nichols has been doing some of the gel studies that Dr. Papadopoulos described and is getting these kinds of multiplicity of compents, which he is relating to their corresponding centrifugal components. But there are some problems with this procedure. It is not that simple at least in Dr. Nichols' hands in that there are problems and changes occur very shortly after the material is dyed. However, ideally the method may become very useful, inexpensive, and quick. But, it has some limitations at the moment.

DR. A. R. TALL: I just wanted to make a comment about Peter Laggner's earlier question about how the state of the core cholesteryl esters in LDL might affect the binding to the surface receptor. In studies that I did in Don Small's lab with Robert Mahley, we looked at hypercholestermic swine LDL in the calorimeter and found that the order–disorder transition of cholesteryl esters was well above body temperature so that their LDL was circulating in an ordered state.

In earlier studies that Dr. Mahley had done with Brown and Goldstein using the same LDL from the same animals, it was shown to bind normally, i.e., in the same way that normal human LDL binds to human fibroblasts. So, even though they were not done simultaneously, those back-to-back findings indicate that the more ordered core of cholesteryl esters in that system does not affect the binding of the LDL to human fibroblast.

DR. J. D. MORRISETT: In that regard, we recently completed some experiments with the cholesterol-fed rabbit in which the transition that Dr. Tall was talking about is much higher than the physiological temperature, and while we have not done the binding studies, we have done reductase suppression and found that those particles are much more suppressive than they are in their normal counterpart.

DR. S. R. BATES (*University of Chicago, Chicago, Ill.*): We have done some studies with rhesus monkeys fed 25% peanut oil and 2% cholesterol and determined that the binding of normal LDL was greater than that of hyperlipidemic LDL. In competition experiments we determined that when you compete normal LDL with hyperlipidemic LDL, the latter competes better than the former. So, we found definite differences in the binding and uptake of normal versus hyperlipidemic LDL.

DR. BROWN: Just as a point of information, has anyone conducted LDL turnover studies in these hyperlipidemic animals? Are the LDLs homogenous enough to label? It would be interesting to know what the turnover rate in the plasma of these particles is. Can anybody answer this question?

DR. STEINBERG: In connection with the issue of whether modification of the lipid interferes with or changes in any way the interaction of LDL with the receptor, it seems that there is a great deal of evidence suggesting that the core is unimportant. The studies that were done by Dr. Weinstein and Dr. Nestel in our laboratory showed that you could take out all of the nonpolar lipids by extraction and still get perfectly normal interaction with the receptor. So, whether you have no core lipid, normal core lipid or core lipid that has been converted into cholesterol linoleate, it seems that no change in binding occurs. But, this might be expected since the configuration of apoB would be influenced by phospholipids and free cholesterol that are in the shell with the apoproteins. Thus, I see no incompatibility between the preliminary results that Sandra Bates mentioned and the negative results with regard to the core lipid.

DR. GOTTO: Yes, the cholesterol feeding experiments might certainly be expected to change the apoprotein composition, which could in turn affect the binding to the receptor.

DR. R. W. MAHLEY: You just took my response, Dr. Gotto. This goes back to a comment by Dr. Havel a few minutes ago. We really ought to define what we mean by apoLDL because so many of the hyperlipidemic LDLs also contain a significant amount of the E apoprotein, and, as we know, that is going to change the binding activity and the metabolism of those particles significantly.

DR. GOTTO: I wonder if I could briefly raise another subject, that which was touched on by Dr. Havel and Dr. Brown: the experiments with ethinyl-estradiol. Are these effects sex-dependent or dosage-dependent, and how do they relate with other experiments, for instance with the cockerel in which hypolipidemia is induced?

DR. BROWN: Based on my own knowledge, the ethinylestradiol effect is restricted to the rat. You do not get the same response in other animals. You can practically turn the mouse into a crystal of estrogen and you do not change its plasma lipids. As it was early described—Dr. Getz probably knows the history better than I since he was one of the early people who worked with this—this is clearly a pharmacologic effect; i.e., it requires massive doses of the estrogen in the range of milligrams per kilogram, and does not occur at doses below 1 milligram per kilogram. As I mentioned, unfortunately, this effect is restricted to the rat and the mechanism, as postulated early, appears to be due to the increased catabolism of the lipoproteins causing a reduction in their level in the plasma.

DR. HAVEL: I also would like to stress that it is a pharmacological effect, and I think nobody should leave here thinking this is the difference between boys and girls. In fact, in perfused livers from female rats, we see very little difference from male rats in the uptake in catabolism with LDL.

DR. BROWN: Let me just add one thing, that the estrogen effect occurs in females as well as in males. All of our experiments, I think Dr. Havel's too, and all the ones in the literature have been done with male rats for some reason but, in fact, if you give female rats the same doses similar things happen.

DR. GOTTO: What about extrapolating the estrogen findings to the clearing of LDL or remnants by the liver since in such an artificial system one is dealing with a highly abnormal physiological situation?

DR. BROWN: Well, if I can speculate, I think that what estrogens do is to unmask a binding site in the liver, namely, a receptor very similar in its characteristics to the LDL receptor that we can study in cultured human fibroblasts. This unmasked receptor, according to Dr. Havel's study, seems to catalyze the uptake and degradation of a variety of lipoproteins that contain apoB and apoE.

Now, the question is why we cannot normally see such a receptor? We have a difficulty in detecting a receptor in the untreated animal and yet we know that there must be some way of getting these remnants into the liver even in an untreated animal. Then, the question arises, are we causing the appearance of a new receptor or are we simply unmasking or enhancing the activity of a receptor that is already there? I do not think that we can answer this question right now.

COMMENT: Dr. Gotto, you referred to studies in the cockerel and I would like to mention some observations we made in that system. When we give the animal a pharmacological dose of estrogen before the synthesis of VLDL is stimulated, we actually see a decreased level of those lipoproteins. This probably reflects a stimulation of the degradative pathway of the VLDL remnants. Also, if you look at the half-life of VLDL after prolonged administration of estrogens, the half-life is considerably shorter than you would expect as compared with a physiological situation. This is probably an indication of increased degradation, as well as increased synthesis. In the rat system, Dr. Havel mentioned that there is some preliminary evidence suggesting that the synthesis of lipoproteins is increased after pharmocological doses of estrogen. So it seems that when you look at plasma levels of lipoproteins alone, you are really looking at two factors: increase in the rate of lipoprotein synthesis and also increased rate of degradation. If you do the same experiments in ovariectomized rats, and place them on physiological doses of the hormone, then the main thing you see is the effect on the rate of lipoprotein synthesis so that you can restore their plasma levels back to normal.

DR. M. STEINBERG (Schering Corp., Bloomfield, N.J.): To continue with estrogens in the rat, I only wish someone else would pick up on the following observation because we ourselves are not working with it. Not only is it not a pharmacological effect, but it is not even due to the estrogen itself. If you remove the pituitary gland you completely eliminate the effect of the estrogen; pituitary homogenates can replace the activity but not individual pituitary hormones. There is apparently a hormone in the pituitary which in some way mediates the effects of estrogen on cholesterol. It is apparently present in very high levels in commercially available growth hormone and is either an impurity or is in some way related to the hormone. Some of this work was published quite some time ago and there has been really very little done on the endocrine influences on lipid and lipoprotein metabolism.

DR. HAVEL: I just want to enlarge a bit on the estrogen effect. The data we have in the liver perfusate from estrogen-treated rats on the secretion of triglycerides and of certain apoproteins such as apoA-I is unaltered, but when we put the apoproteins back in the system they are taken up more rapidly. So, the inference from these studies is that probably the total secretion rate has increased. For example, we see very little accumulation of apoE in these perfusates. We put back apoE in and the uptake goes up so rapidly that it is very difficult to use the accumulation as a reflection of secretion rate. So, I think, as with the cockerels and other situations, even with these pharmacological doses, there is an increased lipoprotein production as well as an altered catabolic state.

DR. GOTTO: Did you measure the hepatic lipase?

DR. HAVEL: No, we have not. This has been done, of course, with estrogens and other situations, and the hepatic lipase has been found to be depressed. But, we have not measured it in our rats.

APOLIPOPROTEINS A AND C:
INTERACTION WITH LIPID MONOLAYERS *

R. L. Jackson

*Departments of Pharmacology and Cell Biophysics, Biological
Chemistry, and Medicine
University of Cincinnati College of Medicine
Cincinnati, Ohio 45267*

F. Pattus,† G. de Haas, and R. A. Demel

*The Biochemical Laboratory
State University of Utrecht
Padualaan 8 Utrecht, The Netherlands*

INTRODUCTION

Plasma lipoproteins function to transport lipids in a water-soluble form. The majority of plasma triglycerides are transported by chylomicrons and very-low-density lipoproteins (VLDL). Low-density lipoproteins (LDL) and high-density lipoproteins (HDL) are the primary vehicles for the transport of cholesteryl esters. It is generally accepted that the neutral lipids, triglycerides and cholesteryl esters, occupy the central core of the lipoprotein particles, whereas the more polar lipids, phospholipids and cholesterol, are in a surface film. In addition to lipids, each lipoprotein class contains specific apoproteins, which also occupy the surface. These apoproteins interact with lipids and, as such, make the lipoprotein particle water-soluble. The apoproteins function not only to transport lipids but also play an important role in lipoprotein metabolism.[1, 2] Apolipoprotein C-II (apoC-II), an apoprotein of VLDL and HDL, is required for maximal activity of lipoprotein lipase.[3] ApoA-I, a major apoprotein of HDL, is required for maximal activity of lecithin cholesterol acyltransferase (LCAT).[4] The other apoC proteins (apoC-I and apoC-III), and apoA-II and apoE also function to transport lipid. However, their specific roles in the regulation of lipoprotein metabolism are unknown. Since all of the apoproteins have been isolated and are well characterized, there have been many studies on the association of the apoproteins with lipids.[5] In most of these studies, purified apoproteins have been added to phospholipid vesicles. As a result of interaction there are marked structural changes in both the proteins and lipids. These types of studies using bilayer phospholipid structures have given much insight into the mechanism of lipid–protein interaction in the plasma lipoproteins and have led to a theory [6] that accounts for the lipid-binding properties of these proteins. Since it is generally thought that the apoproteins in an

* This work was supported in part by the Netherlands Foundation for Chemical Research (SON) and with the financial aid from the Netherlands Organization for the Advancement of Pure Research, by U.S. Public Health Service Grants HL-22619 and HL-23019, by the American Heart Association, by the Lipid Research Clinic Program of the National Heart, Lung, and Blood Institute (NIH NHLBI 72–2914), and by General Clinical Research Center Grant RR-00068–15.

† Present address: Centre National de la Recherche Scientifique, Marseille, France.

75

intact lipoprotein particle are associated at the surface and bind to a monolayer of phospholipids, we have begun to investigate the interaction of specific apoproteins using monolayer techniques. Three representative plasma apoproteins have been used in these studies and include apoC-II and apoC-III from human VLDL, and apoA-I from human HDL. In addition to studying the effects of these apoproteins on monolayer lipids, we have also studied their interaction with specific lipoproteins at a lipid interface. The rationale for this aspect of the study is related to the fact that the apoC proteins exchange between VLDL and HDL, whereas apoA-I remains with HDL. It seemed reasonable to assume that monolayer studies at a phospholipid interface could give some insight as to why the apoC's transfer between VLDL and HDL, while apoA-I does not. In addition, the studies were designed to understand the mechanism by which apoC-II activates lipoprotein lipase. The results of these studies show that all three apoproteins interact with the phospholipid monolayer, but only apoC-II and apoC-III are capable of removing phospholipid from an interface. ApoC-II has two effects on lipoprotein lipase activity: (1) it prevents surface denaturation of the enzyme, and (2) it stimulates product formation. ApoC-III and apoA-I also affect lipoprotein lipase activity. However, with these apoproteins, the effect is not specific and is only observed at low surface pressures.

Materials and Methods

Preparation of Apoproteins, Lipids, and Lipoprotein Lipase

VLDL and HDL were isolated from normal fasting subjects by ultracentrifugation between $d < 1.006$ and 1.063–1.210 g/ml, respectively. ApoC-II and apoC-III were isolated from VLDL obtained from plasma of fasting subjects with type IV hyperlipoproteinemia as described previously.[7] Human apoA-I was prepared from HDL.[8] Each of the purified apoproteins contained less than 0.02 mol% phospholipid as determined by the method of Bartlett.[9] Phosphatidylcholine was isolated from egg yolk and purified with silicic acid chromatography. 1,2-Didecanoyl glycerol was kindly supplied by Dr. R. Verger (Marseille). Lipoprotein lipase was isolated from fresh skimmed bovine milk by affinity chromatography on heparin-Sepharose as described by Kinnunen.[10]

Interfacial Measurements

Monolayer studies were performed in a 15 ml Teflon trough (5.4 × 5.9 × 0.5 cm).[11] The trough was filled with 0.05 M Tris-HCl, pH 7.4. Surface pressure and surface radioactivity were monitored as described previously. Lipid films were spread from a chloroform/10%-methanol solution until the desired interfacial pressure was reached. Apoproteins were dissolved in 0.05 M Tris-HCl, pH 7.4, containing 6 M guanidine-HCl to give 1 mg/ml and were incubated at 22° C for 2 hr prior to injection underneath the monolayer. Reaction rates for lipoprotein lipase were determined at $25 \pm 0.5°$ C in a zero-order Teflon trough as described by Verger and de Haas.[12] The compartment containing the enzyme had a total volume of 210 ml and a total surface area of 91 cm². Reaction rates were determined graphically using the maximal slope of the kinetic curves. In all assays the aqueous subphase contained 10 mM Tris-acetate-0.1 M NaCl, pH 7.4.

RESULTS

Interaction of Apoprotein with Phospholipid Monolayers

In the absence of a lipid monolayer, apoC-II, apoC-III, and apoA-I were all surface active and collected at the air–water interface to a final surface pressure of approximately 18 dyne/cm; the time for maximal changes in surface pressure was inversely proportional to the amount of apoprotein added to the subphase. When a lipid monolayer was first formed at 20 dyne/cm and then the apoproteins were added underneath the monolayer, there was a further increase in surface pressure to 30 dyne/cm. The increase in surface pressure observed by adding the apoproteins to the subphase was not specific for the lipid in the monolayer. At an initial surface pressure of 20 dyne/cm, increases were found for egg yolk phosphatidylcholine, cholesterol, phosphatidylinositol, 1,2-dimyris-toyl-*sn*-glycero-3-phosphatidylcholine, 1,2-dimyristoyl-*sn*-glycero-3-phosphatidyl-glycerol, 1,2-diethermyristoyl-*sn*-glycero-3-phospatidylcholine, and ergosterol. The injection of apoC-II or apoC-III underneath a monolayer of ^{14}C-labeled egg phosphatidylcholine at 20 dyne/cm not only caused an increase in surface pressure but, as seen in FIGURE 1A, after the maximal attainment of surface pressure, there was a decrease in surface radioactivity, indicating a loss of radio-labeled phosphatidylcholine from the interface to the subphase. At an initial surface pressure of 20 dyne/cm, the rate of surface radioactivity decrease was proportional to the amount of apoC-II or apoC-III injected into the subphase and was maximal with 3 nmol apoprotein. Although there was an increase in surface pressure with the addition of apoA-I, the surface radioactivity did not decrease. Using ^{125}I-labeled apoC-II, apoC-III, and apoA-I, we found that all of the apoproteins collected at the lipid interface. With apoA-I the amount that collected was constant after the surface pressure reached 30 dyne/cm and corresponded to approximately 3% of the injected apoprotein. With apoC-II and apoC-III, the decrease in surface radioactivity, viz., loss of phospholipid from the monolayer, correlated inversely with the accumulation of apoC at the interface, suggesting that apoproteins were replacing the lipid that was removed and, thus, maintaining a constant surface pressure. Although not all lipids were tested, apoC-II and apoC-III did not cause a decrease in surface radioactivity using monolayers of [^{14}C]cholesterol or phosphatidyl [^{14}C]inositol, suggesting that the interaction of the apoC peptides was specific for phosphatidylcholine.

It is well known that both the apoA and apoC proteins interact with phospholipid vesicles and as a result there are structural changes in both the lipid and protein.[5] Therefore, it was of interest to determine if the addition of phospholipid vesicles to the subphase affected the removal of apoprotein and phospholipid from the interface. As shown in FIGURE 1, the addition of vesicles to a subphase, to which apoproteins had been previously added, greatly facilitated the removal of phosphatidylcholine from the interface to which apoC-II or apoC-III were previously added. However, the addition of vesicles to a subphase containing apoA-I had no effect on surface radioactivity or pressure.

Since it is well known [1] that both VLDL and HDL contain the apoC proteins and that HDL are the physiologic acceptors for the apoC proteins during

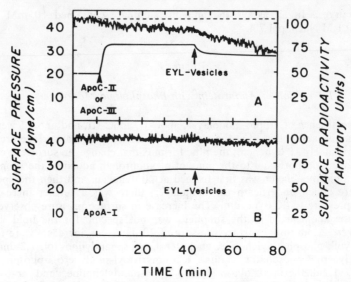

FIGURE 1. Interaction of (A) apoC-II and apoC-III, and (B) apoA-I with egg phosphatidylcholine monolayer. The monolayers consisted of egg phosphatidyl [Me-^{14}C]choline (6 nmol) at an initial surface pressure of 20 dyne/cm. The subphase contained 15 ml of 0.05 M Tris-HCl, pH 7.4. At the indicated time (↑), the apoproteins (25 μg) were added to the subphase and the changes in surface pressure and surface radioactivity were recorded. At 45 min, egg phosphatidylcholine vesicles (1 μmol) containing 2 mol% phosphatidic acid were added to the subphase.

lipolysis, it was of interest to determine the effects of these lipoproteins on the rate of decrease of surface radioactivity. As shown in FIGURE 2, the injection of either VLDL or HDL underneath a monolayer of ^{14}C-labeled egg phosphatidylcholine caused an increase in the rate of decrease of surface radioactivity by apoC-II. Using ^{125}I-labeled apoC-II, we found by ultracentrifugation that the apoC-II was associated with both VLDL and HDL. Injection of VLDL or HDL alone without apoC-II first being added to the trough caused no decrease in surface radioactivity. Thus, we conclude from the results shown in FIGURES 2A and B that VLDL and HDL interact with apoC-II in a monolayer of ^{14}C-labeled egg phosphatidylcholine and enhance the rate of apoprotein-phospholipid removal from the interface.

To further determine the specificity of the interaction between lipoproteins and apoprotein–phospholipid interfaces, LDL was injected under the monolayer (FIGURE 2C). As seen in FIGURE 2C, injection of LDL underneath a monolayer of egg [^{14}C]phosphatidylcholine did not enhance the rate of decrease of surface radioactivity by apoC-II. Since there was also a slight decrease in surface pressure with the addition of LDL to the subphase, we conclude that the decrease in radioactivity observed with VLDL and HDL was not caused by the decrease in surface pressure but was due to a specific interaction between the lipoproteins and the apoC-II–phospholipid complex.

Interaction of Apolipoproteins with Diglyceride Monolayers:
Effects on Lipoprotein Lipase Activity

In general, the surface pressure changes observed with apoC-II, apoC-III, and apoA-I when injected underneath a film of diglyceride were similar to those observed with phospholipids in the monolayer. Since it is known that apoC-II potentiates the activity of lipoprotein lipase,[1] it was of interest to study the mechanism of activation of the enzyme. In FIGURES 3A and B are shown the kinetics of hydrolysis by lipoprotein lipase (0.5 µg) of 1,2-didecanoyl glycerol films at 15 dyne/cm and 25 dyne/cm in the absence and presence of apoC-II. At 15 dyne/cm the kinetics of hydrolysis gave a sigmoidal curve with an initial lag period indicative of a presteady state condition, a steady-state condition, and then the reaction progressively slowed down suggesting enzyme inactivation. The addition of apoC-II (50 µg) to the subphase had a three-fold effect on the kinetics of hydrolysis at 15 dyne/cm (FIGURE 3A): the apoprotein (1) made the kinetics more linear, (2) decreased the pre-steady-state condition, and (3) increased lipase activity. The effects were observed either when apoC-II was added first to the subphase and then lipase added, or when apoC-II and

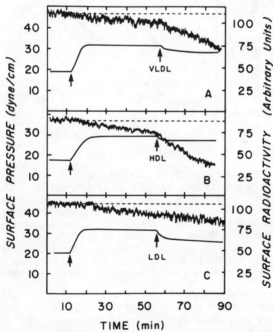

FIGURE 2. Effects of human VLDL, HDL, and LDL on the interaction of apoC-II with egg phosphatidylcholine (PC) monolayers. As indicated (↑), apoC-II (25 µg) was injected under a monolayer of ^{14}C-labeled egg PC (6 nmol) at 20 dyne/cm as in FIGURE 1. After 1 hr lipoproteins were then injected under the monolayer: (A) VLDL (0.3 mg protein, 1.0 µmol phospholipid), (B) HDL (1.0 mg protein, 0.8 µmol phospholipid), (C) LDL (1.0 mg protein, 1.5 µmol phospholipid).

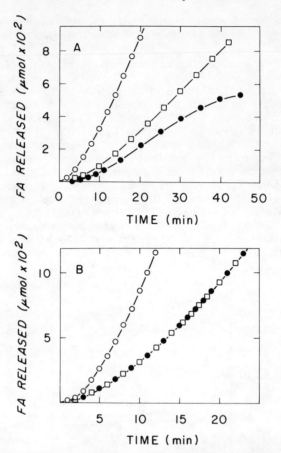

FIGURE 3. Kinetics of hydrolysis of 1,2-didecanoyl-glycerol monolayers by bovine milk lipoprotein lipase at 15 dyne/cm (A), or 25 dyne/cm (B). The kinetics were performed at 25° C in a 210 ml zero-order trough at constant surface pressure. The reaction mixtures contained bovine milk lipoprotein lipase (0.5 μg) in 0.01 M Tris-acetate buffer containing 0.1 M NaCl, pH 7.4. The kinetics of hydrolysis for enzyme alone are shown in curve ●—●. In addition, 50 μg of the following were added to the trough 10 min prior to the addition of lipase; zero time corresponds to the addition of lipase: apoC-III, apoA-I, or BSA (□—□), and apoC-II (○—○). The reaction rates were determined graphically using the maximal slope of the kinetic curves.

lipase were premixed and then added to the subphase. At the concentration (0.24 μg/ml) of apoprotein used in these experiments, apoC-II alone gave a surface pressure increase of only 0.5 dyne/cm. In the studies described above with the interaction of apoC-II with phospholipid monolayers, the concentration of apoC-II was 3.3 μg/ml. Thus, the increased kinetics of hydrolysis of substrate by lipase in the presence of apoC-II was not due to changes in surface pressure. At 25 dyne/cm (FIGURE 3B) the kinetics of hydrolysis after the initial lag period was linear both in the absence and presence of apoC-II. The addition of apoC-II to the subphase enhanced product formation and reduced the lag time. Furthermore, the rates of hydrolysis at 25 dyne/cm in either the absence or presence of apoC-II were greater than that at 15 dyne/cm. The addition of apoC-II increased the apparent reaction velocity at all surface pressures. At the lower surface pressures, the lipase was active in the presence of apoC-II. The activation factor was >10. At higher surface pressures the activation factor was approximately 2. With either substrate the induction or lag time (τ) observed during pre-steady-state conditions was independent of surface pressure but did decrease when apoC-II was added to the subphase. With 1,2-didecanoyl-glycerol, the lag time was 7.2 min in the absence and 3.0 min in the presence of apoC-II. In FIGURE 3 are also shown the effects of apoC-III, apoA-I, and bovine serum albumin (BSA) on the kinetics of lipid hydrolysis. At 15 dyne/cm, the addition of each apoprotein or BSA to the subphase made the kinetics more linear and increased the rate of hydrolysis without changing the lag time. Although the apparent reaction velocity was 1.5-fold greater than that observed with lipase alone, apoC-III, apoA-I, and BSA were not as effective as apoC-II in enhancing lipase activity or decreasing the lag time. At 25 dyne/cm, each of the apoproteins and BSA had no effect on the kinetics of hydrolysis (FIGURE 3B); at this pressure the addition of apoC-II gave a 1.6-fold increase in activity. The effects of each protein on the apparent activity are summarized in TABLE 1. At 15 dyne/cm, apoproteins and BSA accumulate at the interface and presumably protect the enzyme from surface denaturation. At higher surface pressures, the enzyme is not denatured at the lipid–air interface and, thus, the proteins (at the concentrations used) have no effect on activity. However, at higher concentrations, the proteins do affect the activity of the enzyme, as shown below.

Effects of ApoC-III and ApoA-I on the Kinetics of Activation by ApoC-II

In FIGURE 4 is shown the effect of apoC-III and apoA-I on the activation of lipoprotein lipase by apoC-II. In these experiments, apoC-II (50 μg) was added

TABLE 1

EFFECT OF VARIOUS PROTEINS ON THE KINETICS OF LIPOPROTEIN LIPASE HYDROLYSIS
OF 1,2-DIDECANOYL GLYCEROL MONOLAYERS *

	Activity	
Addition	15 dyne/cm	25 dyne/cm
None	3.5 (1.0)	12.2 (1.0)
ApoC-II	12.2 (3.5)	20.2 (1.6)
ApoC-III	5.9 (1.7)	12.9 (1.0)
ApoC-I	5.2 (1.5)	13.5 (1.1)
BSA	5.5 (1.6)	13.9 (1.1)

* Kinetics were performed in a zero-order trough containing a reaction compartment of 91 cm² (210 ml). After the film of lipid was formed at either 15 or 25 dyne/cm, the various proteins (50 μg each) were added underneath the monolayer. After 10 min, lipoprotein lipase (0.5 μg) was added and the kinetics recorded. Activity is expressed as μmol free fatty acid released/min per mg lipase injected into the subphase. The numbers in parentheses are the relative activities.

to the subphase of a trough containing a monolayer of 1,2-didecanoyl glycerol at 25 dyne/cm. The surface pressure was then monitored as shown in the solid line (FIGURE 4). Twelve minutes after the addition of apoprotein, the surface pressure increased 0.5 dyne/cm to a constant value of 25.5 dyne/cm. After 50 min, lipoprotein lipase (0.5 μg) was added. When the pressure decreased to 25 dyne/cm, the pressure was maintained constant at 25 dyne/cm and the kinetics of lipid hydrolysis were recorded (open circles). The curve obtained when lipase alone was added at zero time is shown for comparison. In the next experiment, apoC-III (50 μg) or apoA-I (50 μg) was added to the trough 10 min after the addition of apoC-II (50 μg). As shown in FIGURE 4 (Exp. 2), the addition of apoprotein caused a marked increase in surface pressure to approximately 30.2 dyne/cm (solid line). After constant pressure was maintained, lipase (0.5 μg) was added to the trough. After 2 min, there was a precipitous drop in surface pressure. When the surface pressure reached 25 dyne/cm, the pressure was again maintained constant and the kinetics of hydrolysis recorded. Because of the surface pressure changes after the addition of lipase, it was not possible to measure the kinetics of hydrolysis during this period; viz., activity is dependent on surface pressure.[13] However, after the surface pressure reached 25 dyne/cm and the pressure maintained constant, the kinetics of hydrolysis was remarkably different from that found for lipase alone or lipase plus apoC-II; the rate of hydrolysis was linear but interestingly was considerably less than lipase alone or with apoC-II (50 μg). From these results, we conclude that the inhibition of apoC-II stimulated bovine milk lipoprotein lipase activity by other apolipoproteins is not specific. In fact, the effects on enzyme activity observed by these proteins at high concentrations is not possible to interpret since they have such profound tensioactive properties;

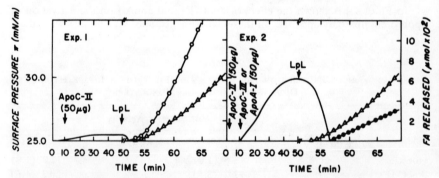

FIGURE 4. Effects of apoC-II, apoC-III, and apoA-I on the kinetics of lipid hydrolysis by lipoprotein lipase (LpL). In experiment 1, apoC-II (50 μg) was injected underneath a monolayer of 1,2-didecanoyl glycerol at an initial pressure of 25 dyne/cm. Surface pressure was recorded (———). After 50 min LpL was injected, and when the pressure reached 25 dyne/cm, it was held constant and the kinetics of lipid hydrolysis recorded (O—O). The curve (△—△) represents the kinetics of lipid hydrolysis for lipase alone at 25 dyne/cm. In experiment 2, apoC-II (50 μg) was injected and then 10 min later apoC-III (50 μg) or apoA-I (50 μg) was injected. Surface pressure was recorded (———). At 50 min LpL was added, and when the surface pressure reached 25 dyne/cm, the kinetics of hydrolysis were again recorded at a constant pressure: apoC-III (●—●), apoA-I (△—△).

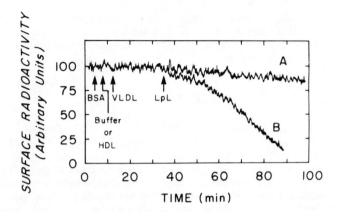

FIGURE 5. Effects of *in vitro* lipolysis of VLDL by lipoprotein lipase on the removal of egg phosphatidylcholine from a monolayer. The monolayer consisted of ^{14}C-labeled egg PC (6 nmol) at an initial surface pressure of 20 dyne/cm. As indicated, fatty-acid-free BSA (75 mg), human plasma VLDL (85 μg protein, 1.0 μmol triacylglycerol), buffer or HDL (5 mg protein) and bovine milk lipoprotein lipase (LpL) were injected under the monolayer: A, buffer; B, HDL.

when 100 μg of apoC-II (vs 50 μg) was added to the subphase, it too was inhibitory.

Effects of Apoproteins Released During Lipolysis of VLDL on the Removal of Monolayer Phospholipid

It is well known that during lipolysis of VLDL the apoC proteins are released from the surface of VLDL.[1] We reasoned that during lipolysis the apoproteins would be free to interact with a monolayer of egg [^{14}C]phosphatidylcholine and cause a decrease in surface radioactivity. Furthermore, the addition of HDL (the acceptor for apoC proteins) would be expected to bind the apoC proteins and, thus, decrease the removal of phospholipid. As a prerequisite to these studies, a number of experiments were necessary to establish the monolayer system. In separate studies [14] we have shown that (1) the addition of BSA to a final concentration of 5 mg/ml (75 mg total) was the optimal concentration required to bind fatty acids produced during lipolysis; (2) BSA had no effect on the surface radioactivity when the initial surface pressure was 20 dyne/cm; (3) VLDL or HDL did not affect surface radioactivity by themselves; (4) milk lipoprotein lipase did not hydrolyze the phospholipid monolayer at high (>20 dyne/cm) surface pressure to cause hydrolysis of the lipid. FIGURE 5 shows the decrease in surface radioactivity of a phospholipid film when lipoprotein lipase was added to a subphase containing VLDL. The rate of decrease of surface radioactivity was significantly greater than that observed when HDL were added to the subphase after apoC-II or apoC-III were previously added (FIGURE 2B). The addition of a physiologic amount of HDL (HDL to VLDL protein ratio of 5) to the subphase caused a decrease in the rate of surface radioactivity leaving the surface. Thus, we conclude that HDL serves as an acceptor of the apoC proteins during lipolysis of VLDL. In other studies [14] we have fractionated the HDL after lipolysis and have demonstrated that the apoC peptides that were released during lipolysis were indeed associated with HDL.

DISCUSSION

Using monolayer methods as a technique to study lipid–protein interaction, we have shown that apoC-II, apoC-III, and apoA-I are all surface active, even in the absence of a lipid interface. When a surface film of lipid was first formed and then the apoproteins injected underneath a monolayer of lipid, then there was a further increase in surface pressure beyond that found for the lipid alone. The increase in pressure was not specific for apoproteins at low surface pressures since bovine serum albumin also caused a further increase. However, at pressures greater than 18 dyne/cm, bovine serum albumin had no further effect on the surface pressure of the lipid. It seems unlikely that all of the increase in surface pressure observed with the injections of apolipoproteins underneath a lipid monolayer was due to specific interaction between the apoproteins and lipids, since all lipids tested showed this increase in surface pressure. There was, however, specificity with respect to the type of lipid removed from the interface and the apoproteins which facilitated the removal. A significant new finding in these studies was that only apoC-II and apoC-III caused a decrease in the surface radioactivity of phosphatidylcholine. ApoA-I, on the other hand, caused an increase in surface pressure, but there was no removal of phospholipid from the interface. While a complete understanding of these differences between the two classes of apoproteins is still unknown, the importance of these findings to the known role of the apoproteins in lipoprotein metabolism may be of some significance. It is known that the apoC proteins transfer between HDL and VLDL.[1] On the other hand, apoA-I remains with HDL and does not transfer between VLDL and HDL. Based on the present studies, we suggest that the reason the apoC proteins transfer between lipoproteins is because of their ability to interact with phospholipid monolayers and to remove phospholipid from an interface. This speculation may also be of some importance in lipoprotein metabolism when we consider that there is a reciprocal relationship between plasma concentrations of HDL, particularly HDL_2, and VLDL triglycerides. Patsch et al.[15] have demonstrated in an in vitro study that concomitant with lipolysis of VLDL, apoC proteins, phospholipids, and cholesterol are transferred to HDL_3, giving rise to a less dense lipoprotein particle, which the authors have designated HDL_2. In the transfer of apoproteins from VLDL to HDL during lipolysis, the question remains as to whether the phospholipid transfers in a complex associated with the apoC proteins or not. The present studies using monolayer techniques suggest that the phospholipids are complexed with apoC's, and move as a unit. The studies also show that apoC-II becomes associated with HDL during in vitro lipolysis of VLDL and confirm the earlier work of Glangeaud et al.[16]

Although there were differences between the lipid binding properties of apoA-I and the apoC proteins, the data presented in FIGURE 3 indicate that all of the apolipoproteins appear to activate lipoprotein lipase when the surface pressure of the lipid film is maintained at 15 dyne/cm. At this surface pressure, even bovine serum albumin appeared to activate the enzyme. One possible mechanism that might account for the stimulation of lipase activity at low surface pressures by surface active proteins is that any tensioactive protein protects the enzyme from surface denaturation at the lipid interface. The unfolding and denaturation of lipolytic enzymes at lipid–water interfaces is a well-known phenomenon. For example, Momsen and Brockman [17] have shown that taurodeoxylate protects against surface inactivation of pancreatic lipase when added to glass beads covered with tripropionin. Verger *et al.*[18] have also shown that at low surface pressures colipase and bovine serum albumin protect pancreatic lipase from being denatured. The activation of the lipase by these tensioactive peptides at low surface pressures was not seen at high surface pressures. At all surface pressures tested, apoC-II showed a stimulatory effect. This stimulatory effect was dependent upon protein concentration. At high protein concentrations, apoC-II, apoC-III, and apoA-I inhibited lipase activity. While we are not completely certain as to the mechanism of this inhibition, it is evident from the data presented in FIGURE 4 that the increase in surface pressure due to the larger amount of apoprotein added to the monolayer system could explain the decreased activity. At the higher surface pressures, we suggest that the apoproteins modify the properties of the substrate itself, which accounts for lipase inhibition at high apoprotein concentrations. Ostlund-Lindqvist and Iverius,[19] using a triglyceride–phospholipid emulsion as substrate, have also shown that high concentrations of apoC-II inhibit the lipase.

In summary, we have shown that all of the apolipoproteins are surface active and interact with either phospholipids or diglycerides to affect surface pressure. ApoC-II and apoC-III remove phospholipids from a monolayer. ApoC-II has a specific effect on the activity of lipoprotein lipase.

ACKNOWLEDGMENTS

We acknowledge the assistance of Ms. Gwen Kraft in preparing the figures, and of Ms. Janet Boynton in preparing the manuscript for publication.

REFERENCES

1. SMITH, L. C., H. J. POWNALL & A. M. GOTTO. 1978. Ann. Rev. Biochem. **47:** 751–777.
2. SCHAEFER, E. J., S. EISENBERG & R. I. LEVY. 1978. J. Lipid Res. **19:**667–687.
3. FIELDING, C. J. & R. L. HAVEL. 1977. Arch. Pathol. Lab. Med. **101:**225–229.
4. FIELDING, C. J., V. G. SHORE & P. E. FIELDING. 1972. Biochem. Biophys. Res. Commun. **46:**1493–1498.
5. MORRISETT, J. D., R. L. JACKSON & A. M. GOTTO. 1977. Biochim. Biophys. Acta **472:**93–133.
6. SEGREST, J. P., R. L. JACKSON, J. D. MORRISETT & A. M. GOTTO. 1974. FEBS Lett. **38:**247–253.
7. JACKSON, R. L., H. N. BAKER, E. B. GILLIAM & A. M. GOTTO. 1977. Proc. Natl. Acad. Sci. USA **74:**1942–1945.
8. BAKER, H. N., R. L. JACKSON & A. M. GOTTO. 1973. Biochemistry **12:**3866–3871.
9. BARTLETT, G. R. 1959. J. Biol. Chem. **234:**466–468.
10. KINNUNEN, P. K. J. 1977. Med. Biol. **55:**187–191.
11. DEMEL, R. A., R. KALSBEEK, K. W. A. WIRTZ & L. L. M. VAN DEENEN. 1977. Biochim. Biophys. Acta **466:**10–12.
12. VERGER, R. & G. H. DE HAAS. 1973. Chem. Phys. Lipids **10:**127–136.

13. JACKSON, R. L., F. PATTUS & G. DE HAAS. 1980. Biochemistry **19:**373–378.
14. JACKSON, R. L. & R. A. DEMEL. 1979. Biochim. Biophys. Acta **556:**369–387.
15. PATSCH, J. R., A. M. GOTTO, T. OLIVECRONA & S. EISENBERG. 1978. Proc. Natl. Acad. Sci. USA **75:**4519–4523.
16. GLANGEAUD, M. C., S. EISENBERG & T. OLIVECRONA. 1977. Biochim. Biophys. Acta **586:**23–35.
17. MOMSEN, W. E. & H. L. BROCKMAN. 1976. J. Biol. Chem. **251:**384–388.
18. VERGER, R., J. RIETSCH & P. DESNUELLE. 1977. J. Biol. Chem. **252:**4319–4325.
19. OSTLUND-LINDQVIST, A. M. & P. H. IVERIUS. 1975. Biochem. Biophys. Res. Commun. **65:**1447–1455.

DISCUSSION OF THE PAPER

DR. D. M. SMALL (*Boston University, Boston, Mass.*): What do you think the surface pressure is in your substrate *in vivo?*

DR. R. L. JACKSON: That is a hard question to answer. In the literature the values range from around 15 to 17 dynes but we do not know what it is because in most of the systems where the value has been calculated proteins were not present.

DR. B. SHEN: In your constant pressure measurement, regarding milk lipoprotein lipase, this enzyme is probably surface active. Is that possible that you are measuring enzyme absorption together with substrate hydrolysis? If so, the two processes compensate each other. At low pressure there is hydrolysis but you cannot measure it.

DR. JACKSON: The amount of lipase that we add to the system when a film of lipid is formed is very, very small, 0.5 μg per 210 ml. At this concentration the enzyme has no effect on the surface pressure. In order to do the surface pressure studies with LpL, one has to add enzyme in the order of micrograms, for instance, 50 μg. The same holds true for apoCs and apoA-I.

DR. SHEN: Did you ever measure the surface pressure in the presence of an inert substrate?

DR. JACKSON: Yes, by using a substrate that is not hydrolyzed the surface pressure does not increase at least at the concentration of 0.5 μg per 210 ml.

STUDIES ON THE PRIMARY STRUCTURE
OF APOLIPOPROTEIN B *

W. A. Bradley,† M. F. Rohde, and A. M. Gotto, Jr.

Department of Medicine
Baylor College of Medicine
Texas Medical Center
Houston, Texas 77030

INTRODUCTION AND OVERVIEW

Recent years have seen considerable accumulation of physical-chemical and functional data concerning the low-density lipoproteins (LDL). Elegant studies designed to demonstrate core regions of cholesteryl esters which perform cooperative phase transitions have been well-documented.[1-3] Low angle x-ray [4, 5] and neutron scattering [6] experiments suggest a quasispherical structure with protein and polar lipids surrounding a nonpolar lipid core. Functionally LDL interacts with a variety of cells by a high-affinity receptor, presumably to the protein, which initiates a series of events all aimed at cellular control of cholesterol synthesis.[7] Such intensity of interest about the LDL particle has been justified by the epidemiological suggestion that it is directly involved in the atherogenic process.[8] In spite of all that has been documented concerning the structure and function of low-density lipoproteins, the characterization of perhaps its most important component, that of the apoprotein, remains uniquely obscure. Handling of the apoprotein has proven a test (of abilities and patience) to anyone who has attempted it. If one has not worked with the apoprotein of LDL, it is difficult to understand all the fuss over it. That this protein presents a unique chemical problem is apparent by the fact that, although for many years apolipoprotein B (apoB) has been an intensely studied moiety, and large quantities are readily available, very little is confidently known about the apolipoprotein. In our attempts to obtain primary sequence data on the apoprotein, we have continually struggled with the solubility and aggregation problems associated not only with the protein but also with fragments of apoB. Some of the problems with the cyanogen bromide peptides have been discussed by us [9] and others.[10, 11] In the following report, we outline our recent approaches to obtaining chemical and sequence information on apoB. Because of the difficulties involved in working with both the apoprotein and its fragments, we emphasize some of the problems that we have encountered in the hope that our experiences will be of aid to others. The bulk of data presented here will concern the initial attempts to isolate, purify, and characterize the peptides generated from intact LDL by tryptic digestion. We will demonstrate that enumerable purification steps were often necessary, leading to overall low yields. We also suggest that several peptides are from partial cleavages, probably leading

* This work was supported by National Heart and Blood Vessel Research and Demonstration Center Grant HL 17269.

† Address correspondence to: Dr. W. A. Bradley, The Methodist Hospital, 6516 Bertner Blvd., Mail Station A601, Houston, Tex. 77030.

to the complexity of the peptide mixture released from the surface. Finally, we briefly discuss additional approaches that have begun to yield chemical and sequence information about the water-insoluble apoB.

MATERIALS AND METHODS

LDL lipoproteins were isolated by either sequential ultracentrifugation with KBr in the density range 1.025–1.050 g/ml or by rate zonal ultracentrifugation as described by Patsch et al.[12] On occasion when large volumes of plasma (>5 liters) were worked up, sodium phosphotungstate precipitations were used to concentrate the low-density lipoproteins. The precipitates were redissolved as described by Burstein et al.,[13] returned by dialysis to plasma densities, and then isolated by sequential ultracentrifugation.

Lipoproteins were stored at 4° C in the presence of PMSF and 0.02% sodium azide.

Organic delipidation with ether:ethanol (3:1) was performed as described earlier.[14] Ethanol:acetone (1:1, vol/vol) delipidations were carried out at —20° C by injection of LDL (14–35 mg/ml) solutions into 10 volumes of organic solvent. Detergent delipidations (sodium dodecylsulfate and sodium deoxycholate) were essentially the procedures described by Simon and Helenius.[15]

Trypsin was purified by affinity chromatography on 6-aminocaproyl-p-aminobenzamidine-Sepharose 4B.[16]

Tryptic Digestion and Removal. Tryptic digestion of intact LDL was carried out in 0.1 M NH_4HCO_3, pH 8.0. One hundred mg of protein (475 mg LDL) in 15–30 ml buffer was digested. To this solution, 20 mg of trypsin was added. After a 30–45 min incubation at 25°, the trypsin was removed by passage over a 1.5×5 cm column of 6-aminocaproyl-p-aminobenzamidine-Sepharose 4B. The unbound material was pooled and applied to a 2.6×200 cm G-50 column.

PCase Method. The procedure of Podell and Abraham[17] was used for the treatment of apoB with pyroglutamate amino carboxylase: 10 mg of apoB in 10 ml of pH 8.0, 0.1 M phosphate buffer, 5 mM DTT, 10 mM EDTA, 5% glycine was incubated for 9 hr at 4° with 0.5 mg Boehringer Mannheim PCase. Another 0.5 mg was added and incubated overnight at 37°. The solution was desalted on a G-10 column equilibrated with 0.05 M HOAc and lyophilized.

Gel filtration chromatography and ion-exchange procedures have been described previously.[9, 18]

Concanavalin A (ConA) Sepharose was equilibrated with a buffer containing 10 mM Tris-HCl (pH 8.1), 1 mM $CaCl_2$, 1 mM $MnCl_2$, and 1 M NaCl. The tryptic peptides were introduced onto the column at 0.5 ml/min. The column was washed with 2 bed volumes of the equilibration buffer. The bound peptides were eluted with the equilibration buffer containing 0.2 M α-D-mannoside. The α-D-mannoside was removed by desalting on P-2 BioGel in 0.1 M NH_4HCO_3.

Thiopropyl-Sepharose chromatography relies on the formation of disulfide linkages between the covalently linked Sepharose ligand and the cysteinyl residue of the peptide.[19] In order to ensure free sulfhydryls in the peptide(s), β-mercaptoethanol or dithiothreitol was added in excess in the presence of 6 M guanidine·HCl. Just prior to application to thiopropyl-Sepharose, the peptides were desalted over a short G-50 Sephadex column to remove the reducing reagent. Binding of peptides to the thiopropyl column was monitored at 343 nm by release of 2-thiopyridone. The covalently attached peptides were in turn released by addition of β-mercaptoethanol (0.2 M).

Two-dimensional paper chromatography was accomplished on Whatman No. 1 paper with the high voltage electrophoresis conducted at pH 3.7 and 2.5 kV (<100 mA) for 1.5 hr. The second dimension was performed on the equilibrated paper at 90° to the electrophoresis with butanol, water, acetic acid, and pyridine (BWAP) (60:48:12:40). Fluorescamine spraying was used to detect peptides.

Peptides were hydrolyzed in 6 N HCl containing 0.1% phenol at >50 millitorr in a 110° heating block for 18–22 hr.

Amino acid analyses were carried out on an amino acid analyzer (Beckman, Model 119).

Automated Edman degradations were done on a Backman 290 B (updated) sequencer using the dimethylbenzylamine (DMBA) program described by Hermodsen *et al.*[20] Depending on solubility of the peptides, Sequanal grade sodium dodecylsulfate[21] was occasionally included in the cup. Small tryptic fragments were sequenced either in the presence of apocytochrome C,[22] or introduced after two wash cycles with polybreen and Gly-Gly.[23]

Phenylthiohydantoin (PTH) amino acids were identified by either gas-liquid chromatography (GLC),[24] back hydrolysis with hydriotic acid (HI),[9] or by high-pressure liquid chromatography (HPLC) on a Spectra-Physics Model 8000 utilizing a du Pont Zorbax (5 pm) ODS column at 50° C.

RESULTS

Tryptic Digestion of LDL and Removal of Trypsin. Because of the extreme lack of solubility of the protein in aqueous solutions, the trypsinization of the apoprotein of LDL is not conveniently carried out under conditions that are suitable for optimal activity of the enzyme. Other investigators[25-27] have reported successful digestions up to 25%–30% of the total protein from the water-soluble intact lipoproteins. In addition, such digestions are intended as an initial fractionation of water-soluble and lipid-soluble peptides. We, therefore, chose to employ trypsin at high enzyme substrate ratios for short times (30–45 min, up to 1:5) in order to maximize the release of surface tryptic peptides. Tryptic digestions were quenched by passage of the digestion mixture over aminocaproyl-*p*-aminobenzamidine-Sepharose 4B, which also removed the active enzyme. Tryptic activity of the effluent was monitored using Azacoll and shown to be absent. After passage of 2 bed volumes over the trypsin affinity column, the effluent was pooled, placed on a G-50 Sephadex column (2.6 × 150 cm) and eluted. A typical elution profile of the tryptic digestion is shown in FIGURE 1.

Characterization and Subfractionation of Tryptic Fragments. Four major peaks were usually obtained (plus an occasional post-salt fraction). Pooled regions for subsequent fractionation are designated G-50-A–F. The void volume (pool A) contains the partially digested lipid–protein complex, also called the trypsin LDL core by others.[28] The B pool contains generally small amounts of the released peptide material (<1% by weight) and was not further studied. The amounts of material isolated from each pooled region were determined by amino acid analyses and are shown in TABLE 1. Recoveries were

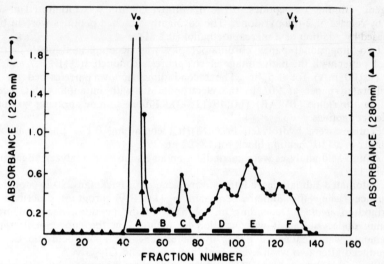

FIGURE 1. Gel filtration profile on G-50 Sephadex of the tryptic digestion products of intact LDL. Absorbance at 280 nm is indicated by the triangles and at 226 nm by the circles. Pooled regions are designated by the bars.

usually greater than 75% with approximately 10%–30% of the protein material released into solution by trypsin. A general flow diagram of the main steps involved in fractionation of each region is shown in FIGURE 2.

G-50-C Region. Pool C, in most cases, contained only one major peptide, with minor amounts of contaminant in different digestions.

Initial amino acid analyses indicated the possible presence of cysteine. This was then confirmed by production of the carboxymethyl cysteine derivative and by oxidation to cysteic acid. The peptide was reduced with 2-mercaptoethanol and applied to thiopropyl-Sepharose 4B. All material escaped binding to this

TABLE 1

G-50 COLUMN REGIONS OF TRYPSIN-DIGESTED LOW-DENSITY LIPOPROTEINS (AMOUNT BY AAA)

Region	mg	%	Size
A	65.5	90 (66)	>30,000
B	0.8	1.1 (0.8)	~14,000
C	0.9	1.2 (0.9)	~7,000
D	3.1	4.2 (3.1)	~2,500
E	3.0	4.1 (3.0)	~1,400
F	<0.2	0.2 (0.2)	
Total	73.3		
Total applied	98.8		
% Recovery	74%		

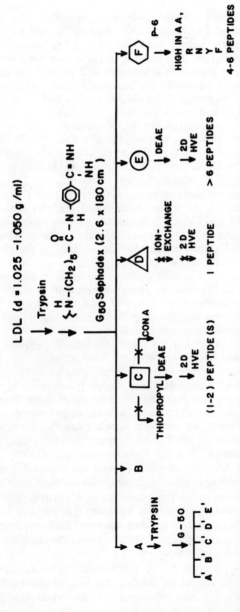

FIGURE 2. Flow diagram of the fractionation steps of the tryptic release peptides of the low-density lipoproteins (LDL).

column. The protein was then reduced in the presence of 6 M guanidine·HCl, which was included in all the reducing steps and in the desalting and thiopropyl-Sepharose columns. Again the peptide remained unbound and still contained cysteine.

Next ion exchange chromatography was attempted. A column of DEAE-cellulose was prepared and equilibrated with 0.05 M NH_4HCO_3. The sample, pool C, (2000 nmoles lysine) was applied and the column washed with 2 volumes of starting buffer, then a linear gradient was run from 0.05 to 1.0 M NH_4HCO_3. The only change in absorbance at 226 nm from start to finish was a linear climb, which paralleled the absorbance expected for the increase in buffer salts. Since recoveries from DEAE in this buffer are somewhat lower than expected, a Tris buffer was used with a gradient of sodium chloride. The absorbance profile of this column (2500 nmoles lysine applied) indicated essentially no fractionation or recovery of peptides. Finally, the column was rerun using the sample size to 5000 nmoles and including 6 M urea in all the buffers to induce the DEAE to break its stronghold on the peptide mixture, but again an absolutely flat chromatogram was obtained.

High voltage paper electrophoresis (HVE) of pool C at pH 3.7 yielded three fluorescamine-staining spots. Amino acid analyses indicated no peptide material in one spot and identical compositions in the other two. The composition of pool C of the average of three separate tryptic digestions is shown in TABLE 2. It is a 14-residue peptide based on 1.0 Lys. We attribute the multiple spots on HVE to partial deamidation.

G-50-D Region. In a similar manner, the G-50-D pool was refractory to all our separation techniques. It again is apparently a single tryptic peptide whose composition is shown in TABLE 2. Interestingly, the G-50-D peptide contains one methionine and should prove useful as an overlap peptide for the alignment of cyanogen bromide peptides.

G-50-E Region. Region E of the G-50 column provided the first set of fragments that could be manipulated by classical methods. A representative profile of the DEAE ion exchange separation is shown in FIGURE 3. The major peak (underlined with a solid bar) was further fractionated by two-dimensional paper chromatography and revealed the presence of seven fluorescamine staining spots (FIGURE 4). By amino acid analysis, all but spot 6 contained peptide material. The compositions of these peptides can be found in TABLE 3. In general, these peptides are small as might be guessed from their elution positions from the G-50 column. Peptide 5 obtained in about 10% yield apparently contains no Lys or Arg. Whether this peptide is a carboxyterminal fragment of apoB must await further studies. Although we have used highly purified trypsin at very short exposure times, the possibility of a chymotryptic clip cannot yet be excluded. It should, in all fairness, be stated that we have on occasion found another peptide, obtained from a separation using cholestyramine resin (Dowex 1-X2-Cl) of the E region at about an 8% yield, whose composition is similar but not identical to this peptide.

G-50-F Region. Region F (or the post-salt fraction) is indeed curious! Fractionation of this region on BioGel P-6 yielded the profile illustrated in FIGURE 5. This column was monitored by absorbance at 226 nm and with fluorescamine. Peaks A, D, E, and F contain little or no peptide material by amino acid analyses. Peaks B and C are rich in hydrophobic and aromatic residue and appear to contain either multiple Lys/Arg regions or remain an

TABLE 2

MAJOR PEPTIDES FOUND IN REGIONS C AND D OF G-50 SEPHADEX COLUMN *

	G-50 C	G-50 D
Asp	1.3 (1)	2.0 (2)
Thr	0.7 (1)	0.9 (1)
Ser	2.2 (2)	1.8 (2)
Glu	1.3 (1)	2.1 (2)
Pro	0.9 (1)	0.9 (1)
Gly	2.4 (2)	1.1 (1)
Ala	1.2 (1)	1.4 (1)
Cys	(1)	
Val	1.3 (1)	1.1 (1)
Met		0.4 (1)
Ile	0.8 (1)	1.1 (1)
Leu	0.9 (1)	1.9 (1)
Tyr		
Phe		
Lys	1.0 (1)	1.0 (1)
His		
Arg		
Total residues	(14)	(15)

* Average from three separate digestions, based on Lys as 1. Amounts less than 0.2 not recorded.

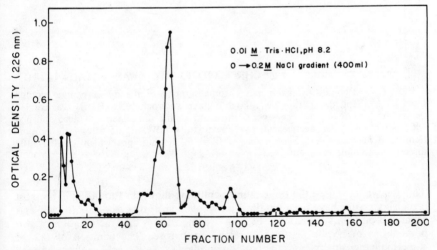

FIGURE 3. DEAE Sephadex profile of the fractionation of the released tryptic peptides of native LDL from the G-50E region of the column described in FIGURE 1. The column was equilibrated with 10 mM Tris-HCl, pH 8.2. A linear gradient from 0 to 0.2 NaCl (400 ml total volume) was initiated at the arrow. The major peak (fractions 60–70) was pooled for further fractionation. The other peaks contained minor amounts of material and varied among digestions.

unresolved mixture. TABLE 3 contains the composition of the peptides isolated from P-6. This work remains in progress.

In addition to our work on surface tryptic mapping, we would like to briefly describe a more general approach we have taken to obtain fragments of whole apoB and to indicate some of our progress.

The general methodology is illustrated in FIGURE 6. Apolipoprotein B is characterized as a peptide with regions of different functionality with regard to the method of fractionation. Once fragmented either by chemical or enzymatic methods, we separate the peptides based on a particular functional separation.

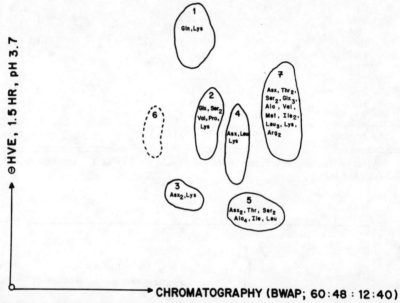

FIGURE 4. Two-dimensional paper chromatography of the major peptide pooled from DEAE Sephadex (FIGURE 3). High voltage electrophoresis (HVE) was carried out in the first direction. The second chromatographic dimension was accomplished with a butanol, water, acetic acid, pyridine mixture (BWAP) at volumetric proportions seen in the figure. Spot 6 was a faint fluorescing spot which yielded little material upon amino acid analyses.

To date, we have used the three affinity columns shown in FIGURE 6. The most promising results have been obtained on whole tryptic digests of apoB itself and separated on ConA-Sepharose. FIGURE 7 demonstrates the fractionation of two populations of tryptic peptides on ConA-Sepharose. The addition of 0.2 M α-methylmannoside releases the bound peptide(s). Amino acid analyses of each population is shown in TABLE 5. The unbound peptides are compositionally very similar to B itself. The bound fraction, on the other hand, is rich in Asx and Ser, and poor in Leu. Although the tryptic digestions are carried out on a water-insoluble precipitate of apoB, we have consistently obtained these results over eight separate experiments. N-terminal and preliminary sequence data

TABLE 3

TRYPTIC FRAGMENTS FROM DEAE-CELLULOSE CHROMATOGRAPHY
SEPARATED BY TWO-DIMENSIONAL PAPER CHROMATOGRAPHY *

Amino Acid	Spot No.							Total Spots
	1	2	3	4	5	6 †	7	
Asp			1.8	1.0	1.7		0.9	6
Thr					0.9		1.9	3
Ser		2.0			1.8		1.7	6
Glu	1.1	1.3			1.0		3.0	6
Pro		1.3						1
Gly								—
Ala					3.4		1.0	4
Val		0.9					1.0	2
Met							1.0	1
Ile					0.5		1.5	3
Leu				0.7	0.7		2.7	5
Tyr								
Phe								
Lys	1.0	1.5	1.0	1.0			1.1	5
His								
Arg							2.0	2
Total residues	2	6	3	3	11		18	44
	Lys	Lys	Lyr	Lys			Lys/Arg	

* Cysteine and tryptophan not determined.
† >0.2 nmole material in analysis.

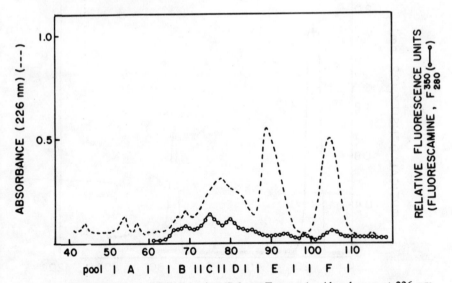

FIGURE 5. BioGel P-6 profile of region F from FIGURE 1. Absorbance at 226 nm is indicated by the dashed lines while fluorescamine fluorescence (F_{280}^{350}) is indicated by the open circles.

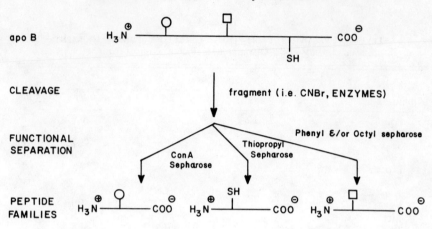

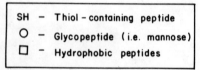

FIGURE 6. Schematic illustration of the general separation scheme for apolipoprotein B fragments.

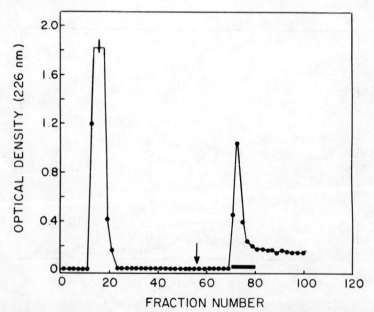

FIGURE 7. Elution profile of tryptic fragments of apolipoprotein B on ConA-Sepharose. 0.2 M α-D-mannoside was added to the column at the elution volume indicated by the arrow.

TABLE 4

AMINO ACID COMPOSITIONS OF G-50-F REGION PEPTIDES
FRACTIONATED ON BIOGEL P-6

Amino Acid	Peak	
	B *	C †
Asp	1.4	0.8
Thr	0.9	0.8
Ser	1.3	1.3
Glu	2.3	0.9
Gly	1.4	0.8
Ala	0.9	0.7
Val	0.4	—
Ile	1.1	—
Leu	1.3	1.1
Tyr	0.3	1.1
Phe	1.1	—
Lys	2.0	1.0
His	0.8	0.8
Arg	1.2	2.3
Trp	—	(1)

* Based on 2.0 Lys.
† Based on 1.0 Lys.

TABLE 5

COMPARISON OF THE AMINO ACID COMPOSITIONS OF TRYPTIC
FRAGMENT(S) FRACTIONATED BY CONCANAVALIN A-SEPHAROSE

	Residues/1,000		
	ApoB	ConA-Unbound	ConA-Bound *
Asp	105	115	139
Thr	63	67	82
Ser	78	82	116
Glu	118	119	99
Pro	38	42	36
Gly	47	63	68
Ala	75	74	72
Half Cys	— †	— †	1
Val	17	19	6
Ile	58	57	37
Leu	117	119	85
Tyr	32	22	39
Phe	49	49	82 ‡
Lys	78	76	41
His	25	20	17
Arg	35	30	15

* Average of eight separate experiments.
† Not determined.
‡ Glucosamine and phenylalanine coelute in this system.

indicate one major peptide obtained by this method. The N-terminal is Phe and the first eight amino acid residue(s) are: Phe-Val-Glu-Ser-Leu-Glu-Val-Leu. . . .

The use of thiopropyl-Sepharose also appears promising and yields peptides that bind covalently. It is necessary to insure that the peptide be in the reduced form. We, therefore, treat the tryptic mixture with a reducing agent in 6 M guanidine·HCl before applying the sample to the thiopropyl-Sepharose. Binding is monitored by the release of a chromophore 2-thiopyridone. Release of the peptide is accomplished by addition of a suitable reductant to the column.

FIGURE 8 shows such an experiment with the tryptic fragments of whole apoB derived in the same manner as in the ConA experiment. Binding is

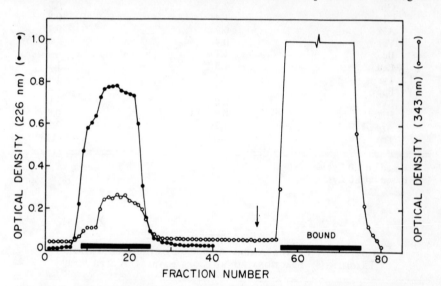

FIGURE 8. Elution pattern of the tryptic peptides generated from approximately 50 mg of apolipoprotein B and fractionated on thiopropyl-Sepharose. The covalent binding of free thiol-containing peptides to the thiopropyl-Sepharose is indicated by the initial release of 2-thiopyrilone monitored at 343 nm. The covalently bound peptides are released from the column upon addition of 0.2 M β-mercaptoethanol indicated by the arrow. The thiopropyl-Sepharose-bound peptides fractionated into two pools on G-75 Sephadex (not shown).

achieved as indicated by the release of 2-thiopyridone and peptide(s) are recovered after addition of the reductant. The reproducibility of this experiment is more in keeping with the expected results of enzymatic digestions of an insoluble protein; that is, it has been variable. However, such methods allow us to extract specific regions of the protein and we are continuing work to develop reproducible tryptic digestion of the insoluble and detergent solubilized apoprotein.

DISCUSSION AND CONCLUSION

Although all of the peptides from the surface of LDL have *not* been completely resolved and characterized, one gets the general impression that the peptides released in each digestion are relatively similar. We find some differences between digestions when fractionation is complete. This might have been expected considering the complexity of the surface and the many parameters involved in such digestions. However, we are left with the fact that at least 12–15 tryptic peptides are released with possibly some multiple basic partially digested peptides. This suggests strongly from the primary structure alone that apoB has clustering of basic charge near or at the surface of the lipoprotein, a finding which is consistent with the protein modification studies of the lipoprotein [33] controlling its interaction with the LDL receptor.

In summary, then, we have shown: (1) that tryptic surface mapping of the low-density lipoproteins yields a peptide mixture, which, although complex, can be fractionated to yield peptides that are suitable for sequence analysis; (2) that the released tryptic fragments from LDL are composed of intermediate (10–20 residues) and small peptides (<10 residues) along with partially digested fragments suggesting a clustering of basic residues at or near the surface of the lipoprotein; (3) and finally we have shown a methodology for the separation of fragments generated from whole apoB, which has allowed the initiation of sequence information.

We recognize that such studies as described here seem primitive compared with modern peptide separations and protein sequence analyses. However, fractionation of this protein and/or its fragments has not been forthcoming even with the utilization of a variety of techniques by a number of investigators.[9–11, 26, 34] ApoB has proven itself to be a singularly difficult protein to characterize by conventional methods for soluble or membrane proteins. Perhaps a whole new methodology is necessary. Recently, a number of novel techniques for its solubilization have been reported by Lee [29] and Camejo.[30] Although in both reports this protein is water-soluble, it remains in a highly heterogeneous and aggregated state. This ability to aggregate under seemingly all conditions and in the presence of detergents and denaturants [31, 32] is at the crux of understanding the chemistry of apolipoprotein B. We maintain that even though the peptides of apoB are extremely difficult to isolate reproducibly, that this approach remains a viable method to the eventual elucidation of the chemistry and primary amino acid sequence.

ACKNOWLEDGMENTS

The authors are indebted to Ms. Alice Lin for her patience and excellent technical assistance, to Ms. Debbie Mason for her excellent preparation of the manuscript, and to Ms. Kaye Shewmaker for the preparation of the figures. We wish to acknowledge the helpful discussions and positive criticisms of our colleagues, Drs. Louis C. Smith, James T. Sparrow, Henry J. Pownall, Joel D. Morrisett, and Josef R. Patsch. In addition, Dr. William Hancock provided both insight and encouragement in the development of the HPLC techniques.

REFERENCES

1. DECKELBAUM, R. J., G. G. SHIPLEY, D. M. SMALL, R. S. LEES & P. K. GEORGE. 1975. Thermal transitions in human plasma low density lipoproteins. Science **190:**392–394.

2. ATKINSON, D., R. J. DECKELBAUM, D. M. SMALL & G. G. SHIPLEY. 1977. Structure of human plasma low-density lipoproteins: Molecular organization of the central core. Proc. Natl. Acad. Sci. USA **74**:1042–1046.

3. DECKELBAUM, R. J., G. G. SHIPLEY & D. M. SMALL. 1977. Structure and interactions of lipids in human plasma low density lipoproteins. J. Biol. Chem. **252**:744–754.

4. LAGGNER, P., K. MÜLLER, O. KRATKY, G. KOSTNER & A. HOLASEK. 1976. X-ray small angle scattering on human plasma lipoproteins. J. Colloid Interface Sci. **55**:102–108.

5. TARDIEU, A., L. MATEU, C. SARDET, B. WEISS, V. LUZZATI, L. AGGERBECK & A. M. SCANU. 1976. Structure of human serum lipoprotein in solution. II. Small angle x-ray scattering of HDL$_3$ and LDL. J. Mol. Biol. **101**:129–153.

6. LUZZATI, V., A. TARDIEU, L. MATEU, C. SARDET, H. B. STUHRMANN, L. AGGERBECK & A. M. SCANU. 1975. Neutron scattering for the analysis of biological structures. Brookhaven Symposia in Biology, No. 27.

7. BROWN, M. S. & J. L. GOLDSTEIN. 1974. Familial hypercholesterolemia: Defective binding of lipoproteins to cultured fibroblasts associated with impaired regulation of 3-hydroxy-3-methylglutaryl coenzyme A reductase activity. Proc. Natl. Acad. Sci. USA **71**:788–792.

8. GOFMAN, J. W., F. GLAZIER, A. TAMPLIN, B. STRISOWER & O. DeLALLA. 1954. Lipoproteins, coronary heart disease, and atherosclerosis. Physiol. Rev. **34**: 589–607.

9. BRADLEY, W. A., M. F. ROHDE, A. M. GOTTO, JR. & R. L. JACKSON. 1978. The cyanogen bromide peptides of the apoprotein of low density lipoprotein (apoB): Its molecular weight from a chemical view. Biochem. Biophys. Res. Commun. **81**:928–935.

10. DEUTSCH, D. G., R. L. HEINRIKSON, J. FORMAN & A. M. SCANU. 1978. Studies of the cyanogen bromide fragments of the apoprotein of human serum low density lipoproteins. Biochim. Biophys. Acta **529**:342–350.

11. KUEHL, D. S., L. E. RAMM & R. G. LANGDON. 1977. Chemical evidence for subunit structure of low density lipoprotein. Fed. Proc. **36**:828, 2941 Abstr.

12. PATSCH, J. R., S. SAILER, G. KOSTNER, F. SANDHOFER, A. HOLASEK & H. BRAUNSTEINER. 1974. Separation of the main lipoprotein density classes from human plasma by rate-zonal ultracentrifugation. J. Lipid Res. **15**:356–366.

13. BURSTEIN, M. & H. R. SCHOLNICK. 1973. Lipoprotein-polyanion-metal interactions. Adv. Lipid Res. **11**:68–105.

14. BROWN, W. V., R. I. LEVY & D. S. FREDRICKSON. 1969. Studies of the proteins in human plasma very low density lipoproteins. J. Biol. Chem. **244**:5687–5694.

15. HELENIUS, A. & K. SIMONS. 1971. Removal of lipids from human plasma low-density lipoprotein by detergents. Biochemistry **10**:2542–2547.

16. JANY, K. D., W. KEIL, H. MEYER & H. H. KILTZ. 1976. Preparation of a highly purified bovine trypsin for use in protein sequence analysis. Biochim. Biophys. Acta **453**:62–66.

17. PODELL, D. N. & G. N. ABRAHAM. 1978. A technique for the removal of pyroglutamic acid from the amino terminus of proteins using calf liver pyroglutamate amino peptidase. Biochem. Biophys. Res. Commun. **81**:176–185.

18. BRADLEY, W. A. & G. A. SOMKUTI. 1979. The primary structure of sillicin, an antimicrobial peptide from *Mucor pusillus*. FEBS Lett. **97**:81–83.

19. BROCKLEHURST, K., J. CARLSSON, M. P. J. KIERSTAN & E. M. CROOK. 1973. Covalent chromatography. Preparation of fully active papain from dried papaya latex. Biochem. J. **133**:573–584.

20. HERMODSEN, M. A., L. H. ERICSSON, K. TITANI, H. NEURATH & K. A. WALSH. 1972. Application of sequenator analyses to the study of proteins. Biochemistry **11**:4493–4502.

21. BAILEY, G. S., D. GILLETT, D. F. HILL & G. B. PETERSEN. 1977. Automated sequencing of insoluble peptides using detergent. Bacteriophage fl coat protein. J. Biol. Chem. **252**:2218–2225.

22. BONICEL, J., M. BRUSCHI, P. COUCHOUD & G. BOVIER-LAPIERRE. 1977. Improvement of peptide sequencing by the use of apocytochrome C as a protecting protein. Biochimie **59:**111–113.

23. HUNKAPILLER, M. W. & L. E. HOOD. 1978. Direct microsequencing analysis of polypeptides using an improved sequenator, a nonprotein carrier (polybrene), and high pressure liquid chromatography. Biochemistry **17:**2124–2133.

24. PISANO, J. J., T. J. BRONZERT & H. B. BREWER, JR. 1972. Advances in the gas chromatographic analysis of amino acid phenyl- and methylthiohydantoins. Anal. Biochem. **45:**43–59.

25. TRIPLETT, R. B. & W. R. FISHER. 1978. Proteolytic digestion in the elucidation of the structure of low density lipoprotein. J. Lipid Res. **19:**478–488.

26. CHAPMAN, M. J., S. GOLDSTEIN & G. L. MILLS. 1978. Limited tryptic digestion of human serum low-density lipoprotein: Isolation and characterisation of the protein-deficient particle and of its apoprotein. Eur. J. Biochem. **87:**475–488.

27. S. MARGOLIS & R. G. LANGDON. 1966. Studies on human serum β_1-lipoprotein. III. Enzymatic modifications. J. Biol. Chem. **241:**485–493.

28. LAGGNER, P., M. J. CHAPMAN & S. GOLDSTEIN. 1978. An x-ray small-angle-scattering study of the structure of trypsin treated low density lipoprotein from human serum. Biochem. Biophys. Res. Commun. **82:**1332–1339.

29. HUANG, S. S. & D. M. LEE. 1979. A novel method for converting apolipoprotein B, the major protein moiety of human plasma low density lipoproteins, into a water-soluble protein. Biochim. Biophys. Acta **577:**424–441.

30. SOCORRO, L. & G. CAMEJO. 1979. Preparation and properties of soluble, immunoreactive apoLDL. J. Lipid Res. **20:**631–638.

31. CHEN, C.-H. & F. ALADJEM. 1978. Further studies on the subunit structure of human serum low density lipoproteins. Biochem. Med. **19:**178–187.

32. STEELE, J. C., JR. & J. A. REYNOLDS. 1979. Molecular weight and hydrodynamic properties of apolipoprotein B in guanidine hydrochloride and sodium dodecyl sulfate solutions. J. Biol. Chem. **254:**1639–1643.

33. WEISGRABER, K. H.., T. L. INNERARITY & R. W. MAHLEY. 1978. Role of the lysine residues of plasma lipoproteins in high affinity binding to cell surface receptors on human fibroblasts. J. Biol. Chem. **253:**9053–9062.

34. HEINRIKSON, R. L., J. J. KOZIARZ & S. C. MEREDITH. 1980. Solubilization and enzymatic degradation of the apoprotein from human serum low-density lipoproteins. Ann. N.Y. Acad. Sci. This volume.

<hr/>

DISCUSSION OF THE PAPER

DR. P. LAGGNER: I have two questions. One is, what was the molecular weight of your trypsinized apoB and that of the untrypsinized material? The second question is, on the basis of your cleavage patterns, would it care to comment on the possibility or impossibility of the proteins being arranged in four discrete patches on the surface of LDL as proposed by the Luzzati group?

DR. W. A. BRADLEY: It never fails that when you talk on apoB, whether or not the chemistry of the peptides is involved, the only question that appears of importance is the size of the apoprotein. I would prefer taking this question up during the general discussion, although my data does not permit me to answer your question. But, I would like to say that both the fragments that comprise the C and D pools apparently consist of one major peptide. From the data on the cyanogen bromide digestion the molecular weight of apoB is around 30,000.

DR. A. M. SCANU: Thank you, Dr. Bradley. We will devote about 15–20 minutes to the molecular weight of apoB in the General Discussion.

DR. BRADLEY: I think that it is important that those working on the subject get together and examine the difficulties encountered in the study of the chemistry of apoB.

As to the other question by Dr. Laggner, I do not think my data allow an interpretation of whether or not apoB is arranged on the surface of LDL in a tetrahedral symmetry.

DR. R. L. JACKSON: In your experiment with the Con-A column, was the material still coming through the column represented by glycopeptides.

DR. BRADLEY: Well, part of it.

DR. JACKSON: What percentage of the total carbohydrate containing tryptic peptides were actually sticking to the Con-A column?

DR. BRADLEY: The quantity was somewhat variable, although the amino acid composition was the same. However, about 30% was bound.

DR. R. L. HEINRIKSON (*University of Chicago, Chicago, Ill.*): Dr. Bradley, your original fractionation gave peaks A through F; from the relative compositions that you presented, about 65 mg was in A. Am I correct?

DR. BRADLEY: Yes, at least in that particular digestion. We can actually shift that pattern to get more material released.

DR. HEINRIKSON: So, you think that what is in A is undigested material?

DR. BRADLEY: Yes. That particular pool can be redigested and you get essentially the same pattern as the other fractions.

DR. HEINRIKSON: So, you would conclude that apoB is really comprised of the kind of peptides that you are getting in those low molecular weight ranges if trypsin has a chance to do its job?

DR. BRADLEY: Right.

DR. JACKSON: I agree with Dr. Bradley on that. In our hands we can degrade apoB completely with trypsin so that there is almost nothing in the void volume and have a very similar pattern to that of Dr. Bradley on a G 50 column in ammonium bicarbonate.

DR. SCANU: I suppose that your data do not allow you to address yourself to the question of the potential heterogeneity of apoB.

DR. BRADLEY: Heterogeneity in terms of the peptides? No, not yet. The data on that particular aspect of the problem as you probably are well aware, are also quite controversial. Depending on who does it, everyone gets a different answer as to the number of carboxyl terminals. The results appear to be dependent upon how this apoprotein is handled. One may see Lys, Leu, and Ser in the various carboxypeptidase experiments. However, the quantitation is always somewhat lacking. So, it is very difficult right now to say how many peptide chains are present in apoB.

DR. SCANU: So much has been said on the effects of the history of the sample, the potential effect of proteolytic enzymes, bacterial contamination, and so on. How do you deal with your LDL preparation before chemical analysis?

DR. BRADLEY: Well, we are very careful. We do put in protease inhibitors although we have never seen a breakdown of apoB by the production of end terminals, which, I think, is one of the more valid ways to be sure that there is, in fact, proteolysis going on. We use this criterion for assessing whether breakdown of the polypeptide chain has occurred.

DR. SCANU: We will come back to this subject in the General Discussion.

SOLUTION PROPERTIES OF THE
PLASMA APOLIPOPROTEINS

James C. Osborne, Jr. and H. Bryan Brewer, Jr.

Molecular Disease Branch
National Heart, Lung, and Blood Institute
National Institutes of Health
Bethesda, Maryland 20205

The solution properties of apolipoproteins have been investigated extensively by several laboratories over the past few years [1-7] and reviewed recently.[8] In the present report we shall summarize briefly the unique molecular properties of these proteins. The *intra*molecular and *inter*molecular interactions of apolipoproteins respond dramatically to mild perturbations in their environment and thus an analysis of their structure has yielded valuable insight into the forces responsible for the stability of macromolecules in aqueous solution. It should be stressed that although the molecular properties of apolipoproteins are complex, they are quite reproducible and in many cases predictable. In this review we shall emphasize three major features of the molecular properties of apolipoproteins:

1. The self-association of human apolipoproteins in aqueous solution.
2. Changes in the structure of apolipoproteins as a function of environment, solvent composition, temperature, and protein concentration.
3. Heterologous interactions of apolipoproteins with the formation of specific mixed oligomeric species.

Finally, we shall comment on possible mechanisms for the transfer and/or exchange of apolipoproteins between plasma lipoproteins and on the important role the apolipoproteins play in the metabolism of plasma lipoproteins.

SELF-ASSOCIATION OF HUMAN PLASMA APOLIPOPROTEINS

Self-association is defined as the reversible intermolecular interaction between two identical protomeric species, which may or may not be monomers, to form specific oligomeric complexes, i.e., dimers, trimers, and so forth. This interaction is governed by the laws of mass action and can be characterized thermodynamically by appropriate equilibrium constants.

The first major consequence of self-associating systems is that in nondissociating solvents their molecular properties depend upon the concentration of protein in solution. This feature is illustrated in the elution profile from gel permeation columns, which can change dramatically with initial (loading) protein concentrations. This effect is especially evident with apoA-I where monomers, dimers, tetramers, and octamers exist in equilibrium (FIGURE 1).[9] With increasing initial concentrations of protein the elution volume of the faster migrating component decreases significantly; thus, the elution volume for self-associating systems cannot be related easily to the size and shape of the species in solution. Similar effects are found with other techniques that depend

104

upon size and rates of migration such as gel electrophoresis and sedimentation velocity and flotation measurements.

An excellent method for evaluating quantitatively self-associating systems is sedimentation equilibrium. This technique does not depend on shape or rate processes and the results can be evaluated easily in terms of equilibrium constants. From the profile of concentration versus distance from the center of rotation (FIGURE 2) one can obtain the corresponding weight average molecular weight versus concentration profile by classical methods (inset, FIGURE 2). These data can then be analyzed statistically in terms of various modes of association. However, as indicated below, the modes of interaction for apolipo-

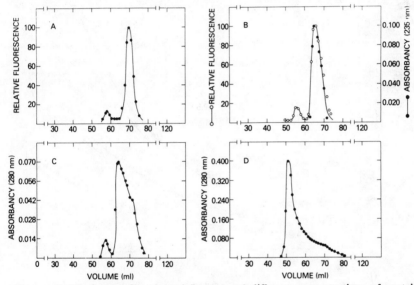

FIGURE 1. Elution profile of apoA-I at several different concentrations of protein, from a Sephadex G-150 superfine column in 0.01 M Tris, 0.1 M potassium chloride, 0.001 M sodium azide, pH 7.4 buffer (25° C). Initial apoA-I volumes and concentrations were: (A) 1.5 ml of apoA-I at 0.05 mg/ml; (B) 1.5 ml of apoA-I at 0.20 mg/ml; (C) 1.5 ml of apoA-I at 0.50 mg/ml; (D) 1.5 ml of apoA-I at 2.0 mg/ml.

proteins are best analyzed by an examination of the primary data, i.e., the concentration versus radius profile.[3]

CHANGES IN THE MOLECULAR STRUCTURE OF APOLIPOPROTEINS
AS A FUNCTION OF ENVIRONMENT

The observation that apolipoproteins self-associate in aqueous solution is not unexpected since many, if not the majority, of proteins self-associate. The most striking observations with the apolipoproteins are the major changes in secondary structure, determined by circular dichroic measurements in the UV, which accompany this self-association. The mean residue ellipticity at 220 nm

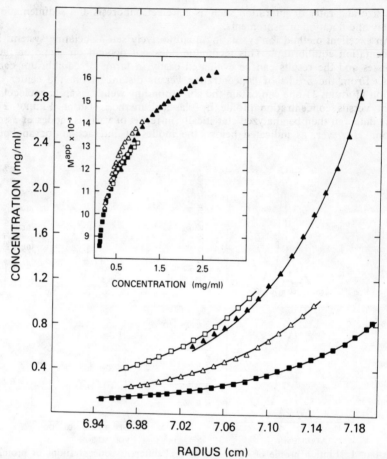

FIGURE 2. Results of sedimentation equilibrium experiments plotted as the concentration of apoC-I versus distance from the center of rotation. The rotor speed was 30,000 rpm and the buffer used was 0.1 M potassium chloride, 0.001 M sodium azide, 0.01 M potassium phosphate, pH 7.4 (25° C). Initial concentrations of protein were: 1.34 mg/ml (▲, □); 0.67 mg/ml (△); and 0.34 mg/ml (■). Inset: Plot of the apparent weight average molecular weight of apoC-I as a function of protein concentration. The symbols correspond to those used in the concentration versus radius profile.

for apoA-I, apoC-I, and apoA-II as a function of protein concentration are shown in FIGURE 3. For each of these apolipoproteins the mean residue ellipticity decreases with decreasing protein concentration. The shape of the circular dichroic spectra also changes from that characteristic of an α helix at high concentrations of protein to a more random configuration with decreasing protein concentration. These results are consistent with a molecular unfolding with dissociation. Also illustrated in FIGURE 3 is the mean residue ellipticity of apoC-III$_2$. In contrast to apoA-I, apoC-I, and apoA-II, the secondary structure of apoC-III$_2$ is relatively independent of protein concentration.

The conformation of apolipoproteins is also quite sensitive to solvent composition. To illustrate this feature, the anisotropy, fluorescence intensity, and mean residue ellipticity of apoA-II as a function of increasing concentration of guanidinum chloride (GdmCl) are given in FIGURE 4. Each of these parameters decreases with increasing concentration of GdmCl, reaching a minimum by 1.5 M in added perturbant. Each of these parameters decreases even at the lowest concentration of GdmCl employed in these studies, which is in contrast to data obtained with globular proteins where an initial plateau region at low GdmCl concentrations is usually found. The inset gives the anisotropy of apoA-II as a function of protein concentration in 0.6 M GdmCl. Thus, apoA-II also self-associates even in the presence of GdmCl; the main effect of this perturbant is to decrease the corresponding dimerization constant.[10]

Large changes in the secondary structure of apolipoproteins occur also with the addition of other perturbants, including salts such as inorganic phosphate. The mean residue ellipticity of apoC-III$_2$ increases dramatically with increasing inorganic phosphate (FIGURE 5). The shape of the spectra also changes, from that characteristic of a protein with a random configuration to that expected for a protein with a high α-helical content. It should be noted that the secondary structure of apoC-III$_2$ was found to be independent of protein concentration (FIGURE 3).

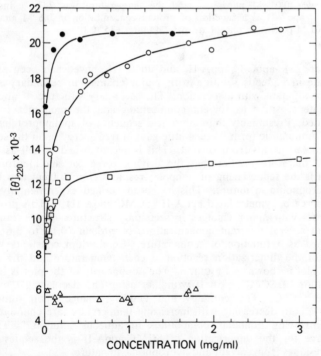

FIGURE 3. The mean residue ellipticity at 220 nm of apoA-I (●), apoC-I (○), apoA-II (□), and apoC-III$_2$ (△), as a function of protein concentration. The buffer was 0.01 Tris, 0.1 M potassium chloride, 0.001 M sodium azide, pH 7.4, and the temperature was maintained at 25° C.

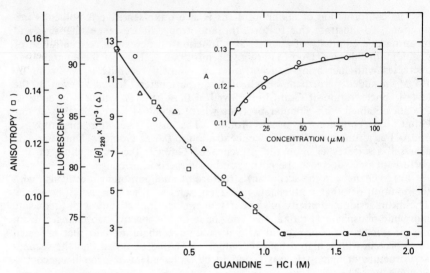

FIGURE 4. The anisotropy, fluorescence intensity, and mean residue ellipticity of apoA-II (0.5 mg/ml) as a function of the concentration of guanidinium chloride. The buffer was 0.01 M phosphate and the temperature was 24° C. Inset: The anisotropy of apoA-II as a function of protein concentration in 0.6 M guanidinium chloride, 0.01 M potassium phosphate, pH 7.4 buffer (25° C).

Thus, apoA-I, apoC-I, apoA-II, and apoC-III$_2$ have each been shown to self-associate in aqueous solution with major changes in secondary structure that are concomitant with association. The secondary structure of apolipoproteins is quite sensitive to solvent composition and the monomer forms are loosely folded. Presumably the amino acid sequence of apolipoproteins is such that in the monomeric form there is little gain in free energy upon the sequestering of nonpolar groups from solvent. This is accomplished by self-association. One would therefore predict that the driving force for apolipoprotein self-association is the sequestering of nonpolar residues from solvent and thus primarily hydrophobic in nature. This has been verified experimentally for the reduced and carboxymethylated apoA-II (SCMC-apoA-II).[11] This protein also self-associates with major changes in secondary structure. The mean residue ellipticity at several different concentrations of protein (0.14 to 3.6 mg/ml) was obtained as a function of temperature. Equilibrium constants were determined for the dimerization reaction at each temperature and the resulting van't Hoff plot is shown in FIGURE 6. The nonlinearity of the plot is indicative of dissociation of SCMC-apoA-II with increasing and decreasing temperature from about 30° C. The enthalpy and entropy change upon dimerization (FIGURE 7), both decreasing with increasing temperature, are characteristic of reactions involving nonpolar compounds in aqueous solution.[12] Thus, the driving force for the dimerization of SCMC-apoA-II is the sequestering of nonpolar residues from solvent and hydrophobic in nature.

A large decrease in the degree of exposure of nonpolar residues to solvent with oligomer formation would be predicted to result in an increase in the partial specific volume of the apolipoprotein. This is presumably due to the ordering of water molecules around nonpolar solutes in aqueous solution. Shielding of nonpolar residues from solvent is associated with a decrease in the amount of "ordered water," and the nonpolar solute is allowed to expand.[13] Such changes in partial specific volume would be predicted to have significant effects on the behavior of oligomeric species in the ultracentrifuge. At the high pressures generated in the ultracentrifuge, those apolipoprotein species with the smaller partial specific volume would be favored and the corresponding oligomers would dissociate with increasing rotor speed. These effects have been observed experimentally with the apoA-I system.[9]

The weight average molecular weight of apoA-I at any given concentration of protein decreases with increasing rotor speed as illustrated in FIGURE 8. With an ideal self-associating system, in the absence of volume changes, the weight average molecular weight at a given concentration of protein would be independent of rotor speed; in other words, the curves in FIGURE 8 would overlap one another. Similar effects of pressure are observed experimentally when data obtained with different column heights at the same rotor speed are compared. As illustrated in the inset to FIGURE 9, the weight average molecular weight at a given concentration of protein decreases with increasing column height (i.e., with increasing pressure). The extreme sensitivity of the weight average molecular weight of apoA-I to rotor speed and column height account for the divergent

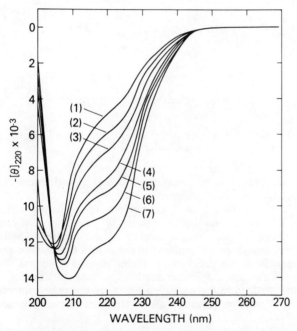

FIGURE 5. The mean residue ellipticity of apoC-III$_2$ as a function of wavelength in 0.01 Tris, 0.001 sodium azide 0.1 M KCl, pH 7.4 buffer at several different concentrations of inorganic phosphate. The concentrations of protein and potassium phosphate were, respectively: (1) 0.225 mg/ml, 0.01 M; (2) 0.210 mg/ml, 0.21 M; (3) 0.197 mg/ml, 0.38 M; (4) 0.175 mg/ml, 0.67 M; (5) 0.137 mg/ml, 0.91 M; (6) 0.119 mg/ml, 1.18 M; and (7) 0.098 mg/ml, 1.50 M.

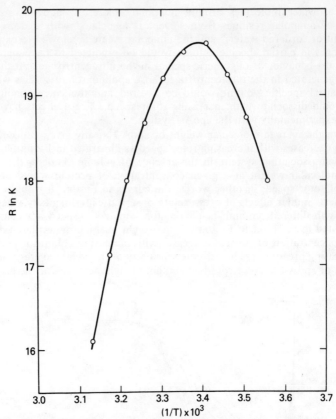

FIGURE 6. van't Hoff plot for the dimerization of reduced and carboxymethylated apoA-II in 0.01 M potassium phosphate buffer (pH 7.4).

sedimentation equilibrium data reported previously by other laboratories.[1, 4, 7] (For a detailed discussion, see Reference 9.)

The routinely employed numerical methods of analyzing self-associating systems by sedimentation equilibrium cannot be employed easily to evaluate systems where large volume changes occur upon interaction. The distribution of apolipoprotein species at atmospheric pressure can however be predicted by appropriate analysis of the data,[14] and for the apoA-I system is illustrated in FIGURE 10. It is emphasized that this distribution of species applies only to the specific conditions stated in the figure legend. Changes in solvent composition, temperature or pressure will result in a redistribution of the oligomeric species.

HETEROLOGOUS INTERACTIONS OF APOLIPOPROTEINS WITH THE FORMATION OF SPECIFIC MIXED OLIGOMERIC SPECIES

Of major importance in our understanding of the structure and function of plasma lipoproteins is the nature and specificity of the interactions between different apolipoproteins. These mixed interactions are much more difficult to analyze quantitatively; for instance, in a mixture of apoA-I and apoA-II there are at least six species in solution; monomers, dimers, tetramers, and octamers of apoA-I, and monomers and dimers of apoA-II plus any mixed oligomeric species. Fortunately, for this system, i.e., apoA-I and apoA-II, the presence of mixed oligomers is demonstrated readily.[15] Since apoA-II contains eight tyrosine and no tryptophan residues and apoA-I contains four tryptophan residues per mole of protein, mixed oligomer formation should result in an increase in the intensity of tryptophanyl fluorescence due to electronic energy transfer from tyrosine. This effect is illustrated in FIGURE 11. The observed fluorescence intensity for the admixture of apoA-I and apoA-II is much higher than that predicted from the spectra of the isolated apolipoproteins, apoA-I and apoA-II. This energy transfer is a saturable phenomenon, as indicated by the increases observed when apoA-II is titrated with apoA-I (FIGURE 12) However, as expected, for the mixed interaction between two self-associating systems, the distribution of apolipoprotein species is quite sensitive to the total concentration of each apolipoprotein as well as their corresponding weight ratio. This latter point is apparent by dilution of the final sample (1:1 ratio of apoA-I to

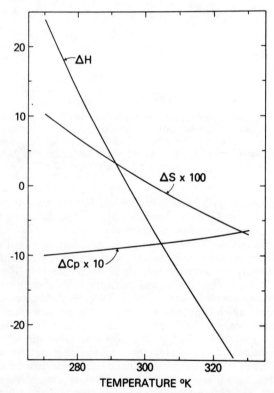

FIGURE 7. The enthalpy (kcal/mol), entropy (kcal/mol deg) and heat capacity (kcal/mol deg) for the dimerization of reduced and carboxymethylated apoA-II in 0.01 M potassium phosphate buffer, pH 7.4 as a function of temperature.

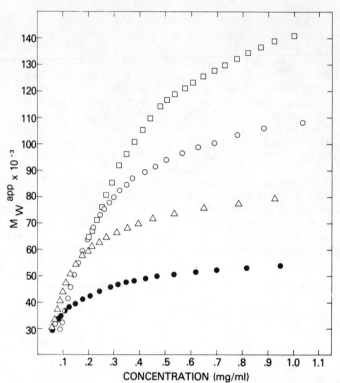

FIGURE 8. The apparent weight average molecular weight of apoA-I as a function of protein concentration obtained from sedimentation equilibrium measurements at several different rotor speeds. The buffer used was 0.01 M Tris, 0.001 M sodium azide, 0.1 M potassium chloride, pH 7.4, and the temperature was 21° C. The rotor speeds were: ($\square$) 10,000, ($\bigcirc$) 15,000, ($\triangle$) 20,000, and ($\bullet$) 22,000 rpm.

apoA-II) in FIGURE 12 with buffer. With dilution there is a substantial increase in fluorescence intensity. This is indicative of the dissociation of homogeneous oligomers prior to the dissociation of mixed oligomers.

These changes in fluorescence are useful for detecting mixed oligomer formation, but cannot be used easily to obtain stoichiometry or equilibrium constants. The analysis of mixed interactions would be simplified greatly by modifying one of the apolipoproteins so that complexes containing this apolipoprotein could be monitored independently. We have modified apoA-II with tetranitromethane, which produces a "red shift" in the absorption spectrum of tyrosine residues. Since apoA-I does not absorb in the visible range, data obtained by absorbancy at 381 nm, the isosbestic point for nitrated tyrosine, will contain contributions from only those species that contain apoA-II. The molecular properties of the modified protein must of course be evaluated and compared to the native species. Nitrated apoA-II closely resembles native apoA-II in that: (1) both apolipoproteins self-associate according to a monomer–dimer scheme; (2) both undergo major conformational changes with association, their secondary structure decreasing with decreasing protein concentration; (3) both interact with antibodies prepared against native apoA-II; and (4) both interact with apoA-I in aqueous solution.[15]

The results of sedimentation equilibrium measurements on nitrated apoA-II in the presence and absence of apoA-I are illustrated in FIGURE 13. The profile of concentration versus radius is shifted to the bottom of the cell in the presence of apoA-I and results in an increase in the apparent weight average molecular weight of nitrated apoA-II (inset, FIGURE 13). These data, when analyzed statistically, are most consistent with mixed oligomers containing an equimolar composition of apoA-I and apoA-II.[19]

The interaction between apoA-II and apoC-I has also been investigated using similar techniques. In these studies the best least squares fit to the data was obtained with a model containing a single mixed oligomer with four molecules of apoC-I and two molecules of apoA-II.[16]

As was found with self-association, mixed interactions between apolipoproteins also result in major changes in secondary structure. The mean residue ellipticity for a mixture of apoC-I and apoA-II is much higher than that pre-

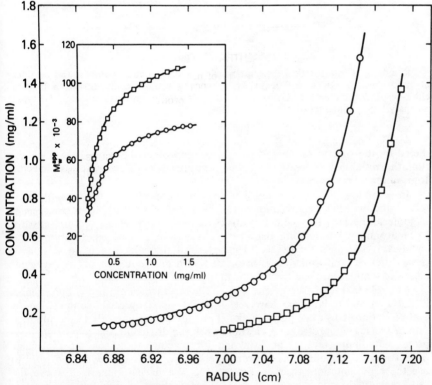

FIGURE 9. The concentration versus distance from the center of rotation profile of apoA-I obtained at equilibrium (15,000 rpm at 21° C) with two different column heights: (●) 11.45 mm; (□) 2.8 mm. The buffer used was 0.01 M Tris, 0.001 M sodium azide, 0.1 M potassium chloride, pH 7.4. Inset: The apparent weight of apoA-I as a function of protein concentration obtained from the data in FIGURE 9.

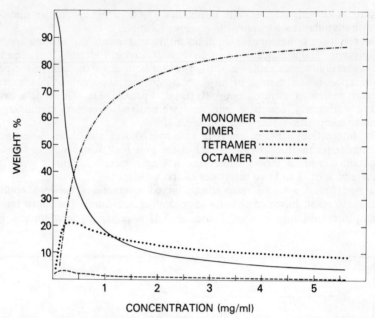

FIGURE 10. The theoretical distribution of monomer, dimer, tetramer, and octamer at atmospheric pressure in 0.01 M Tris, 0.001 M sodium azide, 0.1 M potassium chloride pH 7.4 buffer (25° C) as a function of protein concentration obtained from an analysis of sedimentation equilibrium data.

dicted by the spectra of the individual apolipoproteins (FIGURE 14). In addition, this difference decreases at higher concentrations of protein as is expected for a saturable phenomenon.

In summary, it is now established that apolipoproteins interact with themselves and with other apolipoproteins in aqueous solution to form specific oligomeric species. The secondary structure of apolipoproteins is *quite* sensitive to environment, responding readily to changes in solvent composition. The significant change in the degree of exposure of nonpolar groups to solvent in these different conformations is associated with *dramatic,* but not unexpected, effects of temperature and hydrostatic pressure on these systems.

The role that lipid-free species play in the metabolism of plasma lipoproteins is not known. It is clear, however, that the apolipoprotein composition of plasma lipoproteins must play a major if not the controlling role in the ultimate fate of plasma lipoproteins. As a framework for discussing the role of apolipoproteins in lipoprotein metabolism and for placing studies on the molecular properties of apolipoproteins in proper perspective, we have found it helpful to use the representation given in FIGURE 15. We have summarized above the self (reaction 1) and mixed (reaction 2) interactions of lipid-free apolipoproteins. The overall shape of the monomeric and oligomeric species shown in this diagram emphasizes the loosely folded configuration of the monomeric species and the major increase in secondary structure that is concomitant with association. Each of these apolipoprotein species may bind a few monomeric lipid molecules (reactions 3–5) forming what we have termed "lipoproteins" ("lipidated" apolipoproteins would serve as well) in order to differentiate these species from lipoprotein particles.[8] Apolipoproteins have been shown previously by several laboratories to undergo dramatic increases in their α-helical content in the presence of lipid. (For a recent review, see Reference 17.) These observations, along with the unique sequences of several apolipoproteins, have formed the major framework for current concepts regarding the mode of interaction between lipid and protein to form plasma lipoproteins (i.e., the ability to form amphipathic helices at a lipid–water interface).[18-20] The overall shape of these lipidated species is depicted in FIGURE 15 as being different from the corresponding lipid-free species. A quantitative comparison of the secondary structure of apolipoproteins in different oligomeric forms cannot be made with the present experimental data. Monomeric apolipoproteins are loosely folded and undergo dramatic increases in secondary structure in the presence of ligands, including other apolipoproteins as well as lipids. The effect of apolipo-protein self- and mixed associations on apolipoprotein–lipid interactions is quite

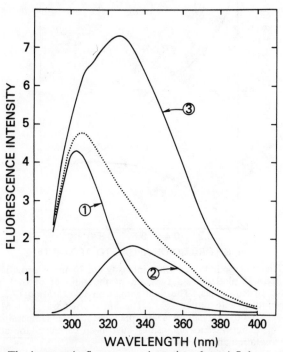

FIGURE 11. The increase in fluorescence intensity of apoA-I due to energy transfer from apoA-II as a function of wavelength at several different apoA-I:apo-II ratios. The buffer used was 0.01 M Tris, 0.1 M potassium chloride, 0.001 M sodium azide, pH 7.4, and the temperature was maintained at 24° C. The excitation wavelength was 280 nm and excitation and emission slit widths were 4 nm. The concentrations of apoA-I and the ratios between apoA-I and apoA-II were, respectively: (1) 0.13 mg/ml, 0.074; (2) 0.057 mg/ml, 0.156; (3) 0.091 mg/ml, 0.320; and (4) 1.13 mg/ml, 0.650. All fluorescence intensities have been corrected for absorption of the excitation and emission beams.

complex.[21-23] The formation of lipoproteins can be viewed as a competition between apolipoprotein–apolipoprotein and apolipoprotein–lipid interactions.

Apolipoproteins and/or lipoproteins may interact with pre-existing lipoprotein particles, reactions 6, 7, and 8 and reactions 9 and 10, respectively. In addition, apolipoproteins may direct the incorporation of many lipid molecules

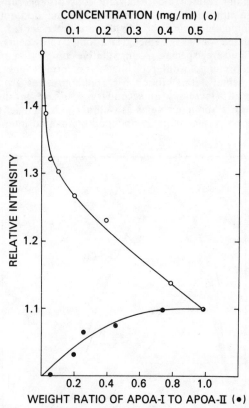

FIGURE 12. The increase in fluorescence intensity at 330 nm of apoA-I due to energy transfer from apoA-II plotted as a function of the ratio of apoA-I to apoA-II is illustrated by the closed circles. The final sample in this titration (AI:AII equal to 0.98) was then diluted with buffer (○). The buffer used was 0.01 M Tris, 0.1 M potassium chloride, 0.001 M sodium azide, pH 7.4, and the temperature was maintained at 24° C. All fluorescence intensities have been corrected for absorption and emission of the excitation and emission beams.

to form a *de novo* lipoprotein particle [24] (reaction 11). Since the conformation of apolipoproteins is quite sensitive to intermolecular interactions, the species depicted in FIGURE 15 (i.e., apolipoprotein and lipoprotein complexes) would be predicted to have different conformations, and thus different affinities for lipoprotein particles. Viewed in these terms, the apolipoprotein composition of plasma lipoproteins is governed through the laws of mass action by the affinity

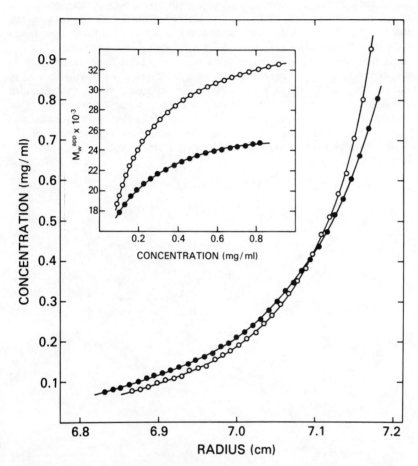

FIGURE 13. Results of sedimentation equilibrium experiments plotted as the concentration of NO_2-apoA-II versus distance from the center of rotation. The buffer used was 0.01 Tris, 0.1 M potassium chloride, 0.001 M sodium azide, pH 7.4, and the temperature was maintained at 21° C. The rotor speed was 20,000 rpm. Data were obtained by determining the absorbancy at 381 nm and thus represents only those species which contain NO_2-apoA-II. The closed circles represent data obtained at equilibrium by centrifuging a solution containing 0.27 mg/ml NO_2-apoA-II in the absence of apoA-I. The open circles represent data obtained at equilibrium (20,000 rpm) by centrifugation of a solution containing 0.27 mg/ml NO_2-apoA-II and 0.27 mg/ml native apoA-I. Inset: Plot of the apparent weight average molecular weight of NO_2-apoA-II in the presence and absence of apoA-I. The symbols correspond to those used in the concentration versus radius profile.

of specific apolipoprotein and/or lipoprotein species for different lipoprotein particles. With metabolism, the lipoprotein particles are modified covalently, changing their affinity for specific apolipoprotein and/or lipoprotein complexes (through reactions 6–11), which results in a redistribution of apolipoproteins. Under the framework of this concept the ultimate fate of a given lipoprotein particle may be governed primarily by its apolipoprotein composition.

This summary of possible interactions between plasma lipoproteins is by no means complete and is presented simply as a framework for discussion and to emphasize the importance of a multidisciplinary approach to the evaluation of the structure and function of plasma lipoproteins. Clearly one of the most important and interesting areas of research in the lipoprotein field over the next few years will be the determination of the quaternary organization of the molecular species involved in plasma lipoprotein metabolism.

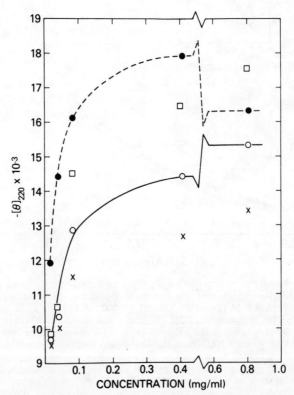

FIGURE 14. The mean residue ellipticity at 220 nm of apoC-I (□), apoA-II (X), and their corresponding admixture (●), as a function of protein concentration. The buffer used was 0.01 M Tris, 0.1 M potassium chloride, 0.001 M sodium azide, pH 7.4 (24° C). The open circles represent the theoretical weight average mean residue ellipticity expected for the admixture of apoC-I and apoA-II at each concentration investigated.

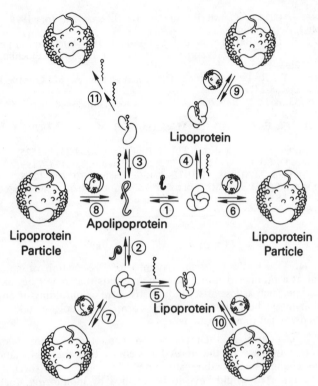

Lipoprotein

Lipoprotein
Particle

Apolipoprotein

Lipoprotein
Particle

Lipoprotein

FIGURE 15. Schematic representation of some of the possible intermolecular interactions between the components of plasma lipoproteins. See text for details.

REFERENCES

1. GWYNNE, J., H. B. BREWER, JR. & H. EDELHOCH. 1974. J. Biol. Chem. **249:** 2411–2416.
2. JONAS, A. 1975. Biochim. Biophys. Acta 393:471–482.
3. OSBORNE, J. C., JR., T. BRONZERT & H. B. BREWER, JR. 1977. J. Biol. Chem. **252:**5756–5760.
4. STONE, W. L. & J. A. REYNOLDS. 1975. J. Biol. Chem. 250:8045–8048.
5. SWANEY, J. B. & K. O'BRIEN. 1978. J. Biol. Chem. 253:7069–7077.
6. TALL, A., G. G. SHIPLEY & D. M. SMALL. 1976. J. Biol. Chem. 251:3749–3755.
7. VITELLO, L. B. & A. M. SCANU. 1976. J. Biol. Chem. 251:1131–1136.
8 OSBORNE, J. C., JR. & H. B. BREWER, JR. 1977. Adv. Protein Chem. 31:253–337.
9. FORMISANO, S., H. B. BREWER, JR. & J. C. OSBORNE, JR. 1978. J. Biol. Chem. **253:**354–360.
10. GWYNNE, J., G. PALUMBO, J. C. OSBORNE, JR., H. B. BREWER, JR. & H. EDELHOCH. 1975. Arch. Biochem. Biophys. 170:204–212.
11. OSBORNE, J. C., JR., G. PALUMBO, H. B. BREWER, JR. & H. EDELHOCH. 1976. Biochemistry 15:317–320.
12. EDELHOCH, H. & J. C. OSBORNE, JR. 1976. Adv. Protein Chem. 30:183–250.
13. NEMETHY, G. & H. A. SCHERAGA. 1962. J. Phys. Chem. 66:1773–1789.
14. OSBORNE, J. C., JR. 1978. J. Biol. Chem. 253:359–360.

15. OSBORNE, J. C., JR., G. M. POWELL & H. B. BREWER, JR. 1979. Biochim. Biophys. Acta. Submitted.
16. SERVILLO, L., H. B. BREWER, JR. & J. C. OSBORNE, JR. Manuscript in preparation.
17. MORRISETT, J. D., R. L. JACKSON & A. M. GOTTO, JR. 1977. Biochim. Biophys. Acta 472:93–133.
18. SEGREST, J. P., R. L. JACKSON, J. D. MORRISETT & A. M. GOTTO, JR. 1974. FEBS Lett. 38:247–253.
19. ASSMANN, G. & H. B. BREWER, JR. 1974. Proc. Natl. Acad. Sci. USA 71:1534–1538.
20. EDELSTEIN, C., F. J. KEZDY, A. M. SCANU & B. W. SHEN. 1979. J. Lipid Res. 20:143–154.
21. RITTER, M. C. & A. M. SCANU. 1979. J. Biol. Chem. 254:2517–2525.
22. JONAS, A. & D. J. KRAJNOVICH. 1977. J. Biol. Chem. 252:2194–2199.
23. RITTER, M. C. & A. M. SCANU. 1977. J. Biol. Chem. 252:1208–1216.
24. HABERLAND, M. E. & J. A. REYNOLDS. 1975. J. Biol. Chem. 250:6636–6639.

DISCUSSION OF THE PAPER

DR. A. R. TALL: Your thermodynamics of dissociation of apoA-II presumably reflect a number of other molecular events that might be taking place at the same time, such as loss of secondary structure or unfolding of any tertiary structure that might be in the monomeric form. How do you take them into account when you get those constants?

DR. J. C. OSBORNE, JR.: Of course, we cannot take them quantitatively into account. Our view of the apoA-I system is that the dissociation has a concomitant change in secondary structure. Of course, the thermodynamics that we have reported would have to be verified by monitoring, for instance, the weight average molecular weight as a function of temperature.

DR. R. L. JACKSON: Dr. Osborne, in the final product or structure that you get when you add apoproteins and lipids together, does it make any difference or not whether the starting material is a monomer, dimer, tetramer, or octamer?

DR. OSBORNE: This is a very difficult question. I have not done those studies myself. I know that Dr. Reynolds has published some of that work as well as Dr. Jonas and Dr. Scanu's laboratories. My only point right now is that the secondary structure of the apolipoproteins is very sensitive to environment. Now, I do not know whether the secondary structure of, for instance, apoA-II in the presence of 1.5 molar phosphate is similar or dissimilar to that obtained in the presence of phosphatidylcholine. I think that those are questions for which we do not have enough quantitative data at this time.

DR. J. A. REYNOLDS (Duke University, Durham, N.C.): This is not a question—but a very quick statement. I do not want anyone to go away from here with a misunderstanding which I am sure Dr. Osborne did not intend to convey, that there have not been other studies on pressure effects. They have been carried out by others but pressure effects were not seen. This discrepancy has not been reconciled. Both Dr. Scanu's lab and my laboratory saw no pressure effects on the association process. Drs. Brewer and Osborne did see a pressure effect. We do not know why. One thing to be concerned about is that the change in partial specific volume that must be postulated if that pressure effect is correct is much larger than has ever been seen in any other associating protein system. Therefore, in trying to sort this out we have to remember that there are very discrepant results, which, if we need to, we can discuss in the general discussion.

DR. OSBORNE: Yes, I think that is one reason why we are here. First of all, the partial specific volume change that we have suggested is larger than that obtained for other self-associating systems, but if you think about it you actually expect it to be much larger. Most associating systems do not have these phenomenal changes in secondary structure when they dissociate. With apoA-I we have a major refolding in the polypeptide chain.

Now, with respect to the differences, in our laboratories we tried to account for those differences in our publication of the pressure effects on apoA-I. I think that one of the things that certainly we have to consider are the conditions under which the data were obtained. Pressure effects will be minimal at low rotor speed and they will be minimal near the meniscus of the cell. So, I agree that there is a controversy and I hope that we can work it out.

DR. G. D. FASMAN (*Brandeis University, Waltham, Mass.*): I would not challenge your statement that hydrophobic interactions are important as you raise the concentration of your various apoproteins, but you showed some data where the secondary structure was higher at an elevated temperature. So, I think, that even though hydrophobic forces are important, there are obviously other forces that are playing an important role here or you would not have that sort of temperature effect.

DR. OSBORNE: I disagree with you. You would expect such temperature effects with hydrophobic interactions.

DR. C. EDELSTEIN (*University of Chicago, Chicago, Ill.*): I was wondering if you ever actually measured the partial specific volume of the associating apoA-I as well as of its monomeric form.

DR. OSBORNE: Unfortunately I do not have the apparatus in my laboratory; so I am looking forward to some interactions with other laboratories. Now, the problem, of course, is that the partial specific volume would be a function of protein concentration, and it would be difficult to differentiate a change in partial specific volume due to protein concentration from a simple nonideality of the apolipoprotein at a higher concentration.

PROPERTIES OF APOLIPOPROTEINS AT THE AIR–WATER INTERFACE *

M. C. Phillips and C. E. Sparks

Department of Physiology and Biochemistry
The Medical College of Pennsylvania
Philadelphia, Pennsylvania 19129

INTRODUCTION

Films of protein adsorbed at fluid interfaces occur in situations that are important in biology and technology so that there has been a long history of studies of protein films at the air–water interface (for reviews, see References 1–3), although there have been no systematic studies on apolipoproteins published. Since apolipoproteins have evolved to perform their biological functions at the surface of lipoproteins, investigations of their intrinsic surface activity and the thermodynamics of their adsorption should provide valuable insights into their *in vivo* behavior.

Protein adsorption and desorption at the air–water interface can be monitored by changes in surface tension and surface radioactivity,[4-6] and these measurements give information about protein surface conformation. Furthermore, addition of an insoluble lipid monolayer prior to protein adsorption gives a model lipid–water interface to mimic the lipoprotein surface. In this paper we compare the surface properties of rat apolipoprotein A-I (apoA-I), rabbit apoE, and bovine serum albumin (BSA). The surface chemistry of BSA has been studied extensively so that the adsorption and surface denaturation of this globular protein make convenient points of reference and contrast for the apoprotein results.

EXPERIMENTAL

Materials

Proteins: Rat Apolipoprotein A-I

High-density lipoprotein (HDL) was isolated ultracentrifugally from rat plasma by flotation at salt densities of 1.06–1.21 g/ml,[7] and was delipidated by treatment with 20 volumes of 2:1 vol/vol chloroform–methanol and 20 volumes of diethyl ether.[8] Apolipoprotein A-I was isolated by subjecting the apoHDL to preparative isoelectric focusing using published procedures [10] except that the Ampholines were in the range pH 5–8. We utilized the front-running (pI 5.80) of the apoA-I bands. The apoA-I fraction gave one band when examined by sodium dodecyl sulfate–polyacrylamide gel electrophoresis (SDS-PAGE) as described previously.[9]

* This work was supported by National Heart, Lung, and Blood Institute Grant PPG HL 22633.

122

Two additional isolation methods were used and the resultant apoA-I gave the same surface properties: (1) The rat HDL was dissolved directly in 30% vol/vol isopropanol–water at room temperature and, after two hours, passed through a 0.22 μm filter. The apoproteins were fractionated in isopropanol by gel filtration on a Sephacryl S-200 (Pharmacia) column. The apoA-I was isolated as a single fraction comprising an aggregate of molecular weight 150,000. The apoA-I isolated by this procedure gave a single band when examined by SDS-PAGE; (2) apoHDL was dissolved in 0.01 M sodium deoxycholate (pH 10, 0.05 M NaCl, 0.05 M Na_2CO_3, 0.02% NaN_3) and the apoproteins separated by gel filtration chromatography on a Sepharose CL-6B (Pharmacia) 200 × 2 cm column at 4° C. The resulting A-I contained about 5% apo C.

Rabbit ApoE

Apolipoprotein E was isolated from the lipoproteins ($d < 1.02$ g/ml) of rabbits that had been fed on rat chow containing 4% cholesterol and 12% corn oil for 5–7 days. The resultant $d < 1.02$ g/ml lipoproteins contained about 30% apoE. The apoproteins were obtained by delipidization with 2:1 vol/vol chloroform–methanol and dissolved in the 0.01 M sodium deoxycholate solution described above and purified by passage through a Sepharose Cl-6B column. Alternatively, the apoproteins were dissolved at 0.5 mg/ml in 0.01 M sodium deoxycholate (pH 8.6, 0.02 M Tris, 0.02% NaN_3) and the apoE isolated by chromatography on a Sephacryl S-300 (Pharmacia) column. The peak of the apoE fraction contained about 0.3 mg protein/ml, and, after pooling, more than 99% of the sodium deoxycholate was removed by exhaustive dialysis as measured with [³H]deoxycholate.

Bovine Serum Albumin (BSA)

Miles fraction V BSA was dissolved in 30% vol/vol isopropanol/water to give a 10% wt/vol solution and passed through a column of Sepharose Cl-6B in the same medium. The albumin fraction was lyophilized and analyzed by SDS-PAGE; applying ten times the standard amount showed that there was a single band of 65–70,000 daltons.

Radioiodination

The apoE was dissolved in 0.01 M sodium deoxycholate to a concentration of about 0.1 mg/ml and treated with ¹²⁵I-labeled ICl.[11] The unreacted ICl and sodium deoxycholate were removed by exhaustive dialysis against saline/EDTA (0.15 M NaCl, 0.002 M EDTA, pH 7.4). The apoA-I and BSA were iodinated in a similar fashion except that the sodium deoxycholate was omitted. The resultant ¹²⁵I-labeled proteins were counted on a Beckman Gamma 300 system and exhibited specific activities in the range 5–300 μCi/mg. Iodination of BSA did not change its surface activity as measured by the surface pressure it exerted at the air–water interface.

Throughout this work, protein concentrations were determined by the Lowry procedure [12] using albumin as the standard.

Lipids and Solvents

Chromatographically pure L-α-egg yolk phosphatidylcholine (grade A, Calbiochem, San Diego, Calif.) was used as supplied. Spectroscopic grade *n*-hexane (Applied Science Labs, State College, Pa.), absolute ethanol (Publicker Industries, Linfield, Pa.) and anhydrous isopropanol (A. H. Thomas Co., Philadelphia, Pa.) were used as supplied. The salts used for the various buffers were all reagent grade and dissolved in distilled water, which was further purified by passage through columns of activated carbon and ion exchange resin.

Methods

A Teflon Langmuir trough fitted with a horizontal float was used as described previously [13] to determine surface pressure (π)–molecular area (A) isothermal curves. The protein monolayers were spread at the air–water interface from 30% vol/vol isopropanol–phosphate buffer (pH 7, ionic strength = 0.1:0.08 M NaCl, 3.05 mM NaH_2PO_4, 5.65 mM Na_2HPO_4) solution (0.05–0.3 mg/ml protein) down a glass rod as described by Trurnit.[14] The general procedure for spreading has been described.[15, 16] The monolayers were compressed in a stepwise fashion with 1 minute allowed for relaxation after each barrier movement before the reading of π was noted; complete compression took ~15 min.

The changes in π during adsorption of the proteins at the air–water interface were measured using a roughened mica Wilhemy plate suspended from a Cahn recording microbalance.[17] The substrate (60 ml) was contained in a polypropylene dish so that the surface area was 60 cm^2; the appropriate volume of protein solution (~0.2 mg/ml) was injected and the substrate stirred with a small magnetic bar during the adsorption process, which took ~3 hr for completion. In order to measure the adsorption of protein to monolayers of egg phosphatidylcholine (PC) spread at the air–water interface, the lipid was initially spread from 9:1 vol/vol hexane/ethanol [13] to the desired π (the mica plate was removed during the spreading of lipid to prevent lipid adsorbing to the Wilhemy plate and changing the contact angle) before the protein was injected into the substrate through a narrow polypropylene tube fitted to the wall of the dish.

In order to determine the surface concentration of protein adsorbed at the air–water interface, the ^{125}I-labeled proteins were injected into the substrate as described above. Samples of the substrate were removed after 3 hr through a narrow tube mounted in the bottom of the polypropylene dish without disturbing the air–water interface. The decrease in substrate concentration was determined by counting 1 ml aliquots; the decrease was assumed to be entirely due to adsorption at the air–water interface as washing the surface of the polypropylene dish with a solution containing SDS did not release significant radioactivity.

Surface pressures exerted by the proteins were reproducible to ± 1 mN m^{-1} except in the presence of egg PC when the errors were doubled. The surface concentration of ^{125}I-labeled protein could be determined to ± 1 mg m^{-2}.

RESULTS

It has been demonstrated before [16, 18] that apoproteins can be spread as insoluble monolayers at the air–water interface, and FIGURE 1 shows the π-A

curves for rat apoA-I, rabbit apo E, and BSA. It is apparent that all three
proteins give similar curves with limiting areas at $\pi = 23$ mN m^{-1} in the range
0.55–0.7 m^2 mg^{-1}, corresponding to 10–13 Å^2/residue (assuming a mean
residue weight of 115 for all three proteins). Extrapolation to $\pi = 0$ gives
limiting areas of 0.8 m^2 mg^{-1} (15 Å^2/res) for rat apoA-I and 0.95 m^2 mg^{-1}

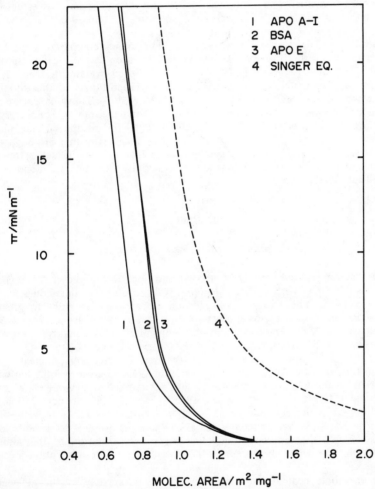

FIGURE 1. Plot of surface pressure (π) versus molecular area for monolayers of
rat apoA-I (curve 1), rabbit apoE (curve 3), and bovine serum albumin (curve 2)
spread on phosphate buffer (pH 7, I=0.1) at 22° C. Curve 4 is calculated from the
Singer Equation (see text) with $a_0 = 15$ Å^2/residue and $Z' = 4$.

(18 Å^2/res) for rabbit apoE and BSA. The curve for BSA is in excellent
agreement with a published curve for the same substrate,[15, 19] whereas that for
rat A-I is more condensed than an earlier curve for porcine apo-HDL obtained
by one of us by continuous compression of the film.[16] Probably the most
significant factor accounting for this discrepancy is the difference in rate of

compression because the rate of molecular relaxation in protein monolayers can be long with relaxation times in the range 1–8 hr.[4]

The two apoproteins have essentially the same effect on the surface tension of the phosphate buffer (FIGURE 2) and adsorb to maximum π values of about 23 mN m^{-1} at substrate protein concentrations (C_p) of 1×10^{-4} wt%.[16, 18] In contrast, BSA is significantly less surface active and exerts a maximum π of ~18 mN m^{-1} when $C_p > 5 \times 10^{-3}$ wt%.[5, 18] This difference in π arises despite the fact that the surface concentrations of all three proteins are similar when $C_p = 10^{-6}$–10^{-4} wt % (FIGURES 3–5).

The difference in surface activity of the apoproteins compared to BSA is also evident when the proteins are allowed to adsorb on to an insoluble liquid-expanded monolayer of egg PC [13, 20] spread at the air–water interface. It is well known that protein adsorption is inversely proportional to the initial π (π_i) at which the lipid monolayer is spread.[16, 18, 20, 21] Thus, as shown in FIGURE 6, when $C_p = 5 \times 10^{-5}$ wt%, BSA cannot penetrate a monolayer of egg PC at $\pi_i > 15$ mN m^{-1}, whereas the cutoff values for rat apoA-I and rabbit apoE are 28 and 35 mN m^{-1}, respectively. It is noteworthy that although the dependence of π on C_p at the clean air–water interface is the same for rat apoA-I and rabbit apoE, apoE has a greater affinity for the lipid-monolayer-covered surface than apoA-I.

DISCUSSION

Adsorption at the Air–Water Interface

The greater surface activity of apoA-I and apoE compared to BSA (FIGURE 2) is consistent with a higher degree of exposure of apolar residues in the former proteins. This exposure of hydrophobic groups also leads to greater self-association of apoproteins at low C_p values (for a review, see Reference 23) as compared to BSA. The formation of oligomers of apoA-I involves cooperative interactions between protein molecules and the steepness of the π-C_p curve for apoproteins suggests that the air–water interface effectively nucleates the removal of apoprotein molecules from solution. It is interesting that the concentration of apoA-I in solution when π attains its maximum value of 23 mN m^{-1} is about 10^{-3} mg/ml, which is similar to the monomer concentration of apoA-I found in the aqueous phase of HDL solutions.[24] The relatively wide concentration range over which π for BSA increases from 0 to 19 mN m^{-1} reflects the fact that adsorption involves surface denaturation of the soluble globular protein with greater unfolding occurring when adsorption occurs at low π.[4-6]

Water-soluble proteins such as BSA adsorb irreversibly at the air–water interface so that denatured, adsorbed molecules do not exchange freely with molecules in the aqueous phase.[5] In contrast, apoproteins have evolved to perform their biological function at fluid–fluid interfaces, and apoA-I, for example, can exchange between free and bound forms with HDL,[25] so it is not immediately obvious whether they will adsorb reversibly at the air–water interface. A convenient way to test this possibility is to check whether apoprotein adsorption fits the Gibbs adsorption equation; the reversible adsorption at the air–water interface of simple surfactants such as SDS is described by this thermodynamic equation.

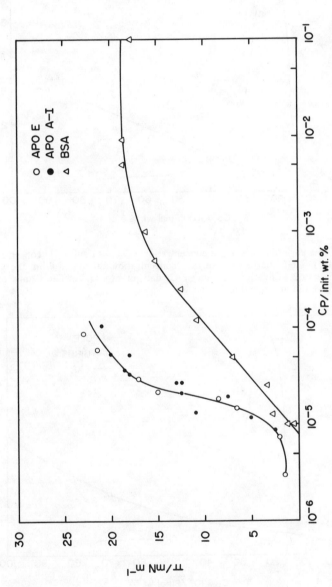

FIGURE 2. The variation of surface pressure (π) with initial substrate concentration (C_P) of rat apoA-I (●), rabbit apoE (○), and bovine serum albumin (△). The substrate was phosphate buffer (pH 7, $I = 0.1$) at 22°C.

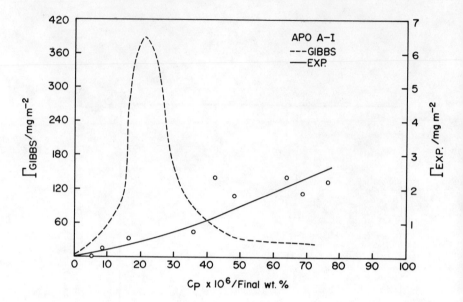

FIGURE 3. The variation of surface concentration (○) with substrate concentration of rat apoA-I. Dotted line denotes surface concentration calculated from the Gibbs Adsorption Equation (Equation 1) using π-C_p data in FIGURE 2. The details of the substrate are given in the legend to FIGURE 2.

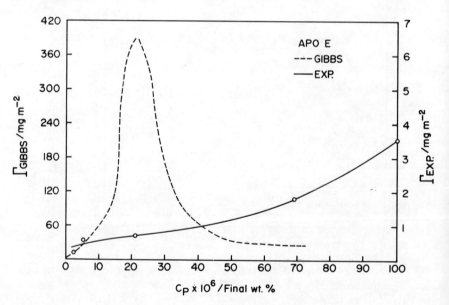

FIGURE 4. Comparison of the experimental surface concentration (Γ_{exp}) of apoE (○) with surface concentration Γ_{Gibbs} (−−−) calculated from the Gibbs Adsorption Equation. See legend of FIGURE 3 for further details.

In general, it is found that application of Gibbs adsorption equation to solutions containing synthetic polymers or biopolymers give unrealistically low values for the surface area per molecule.[2] For low protein concentrations the Gibbs equation reads

$$\Gamma = \frac{C_p}{RT} \frac{d\pi}{dC_p},$$ (1)

where C_p is the protein concentration and Γ is the surface excess of the protein. If equilibrium between surface and substrate is established, then the chemical potentials of protein molecules in the surface and substrate are equal, and, at

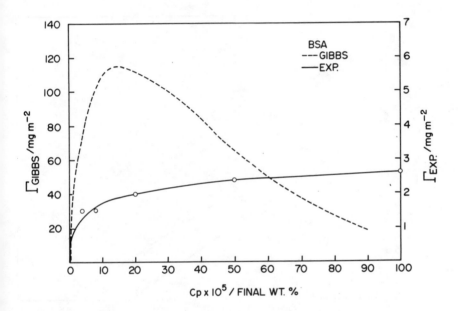

FIGURE 5. Comparison of the experimental surface concentration Γ_{exp} (O) of bovine serum albumin with surface concentration Γ_{Gibbs} (– – –) calculated from the Gibbs Adsorption Equation. See legend of FIGURE 3 for further details.

low C_p, it is reasonable to use protein concentration rather than activity. As discussed elsewhere,[26] the adsorption of water and salt can be neglected at low C_p so that application of Equation 1 to the π-C_p data in FIGURE 2 should yield the surface concentration of protein as it would be measured by a surface radioactivity experiment.

The values of Γ derived by application of Equation 1 to the π-C_p data for apoA-I, apoE, and BSA are shown in FIGURES 3–5, respectively. It is apparent that Γ_{Gibbs} is of the wrong form and up to two orders of magnitude too high compared to the experimental Γ. As has been discussed in detail for several other proteins,[5, 27] this discrepancy strongly suggests that the primary layer of apoprotein or albumin is adsorbed irreversibly. Thus, the protein molecules studied here appear not to exchange freely between the air–water interface and substrate although compression of the adsorbed film can lead to desorption of protein molecules.[17] This behavior contrasts with the lipoprotein surface, suggesting that the presence of phospholipid may play a special role in controlling apoprotein adsorption.

Adsorption at an Egg Phosphatidylcholine Monolayer

Studying the effects of an insoluble monolayer spread at the air–water interface on the adsorption of apoproteins and albumin provides a convenient

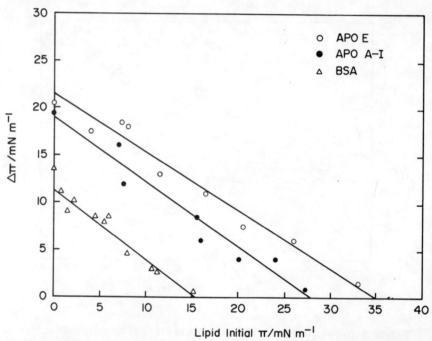

FIGURE 6. The change in surface pressure ($\Delta\pi$) when protein is injected beneath a monolayer of egg phosphatidylcholine spread to different initial pressures: ($\bullet$) rat apoA-I; ($\bigcirc$) rabbit apoE; ($\triangle$) bovine serum albumin. The initial protein concentration is 5×10^{-5} wt% and the substrate was as given in FIGURE 2.

model for the role of lipid and film pressure in determining the surface structure of lipoproteins. It is known that if a close packed lipid monolayer is present initially, then both π and Γ for a given C_p of protein are reduced significantly as compared to the clean air–water interface.[16, 21, 28] Indeed, at sufficiently high initial film pressures (π_i) the protein is prevented from reaching the interface so that the increase in π due to protein adsorption ($\Delta\pi$) is zero. Thus, the affinity of protein for the clean air–water interface ($\pi_i = 0$) is so strong that adsorption is irreversible, but when π_i is high enough, adsorption of protein can be eliminated. Clearly, reversible adsorption is possible at intermediate π values, and determining the π_i at which $\Delta\pi = 0$ for different proteins gives a comparison of their affinities for the lipid–water interface.

Changes in π with protein adsorption are due to penetration of amino acid residues from molecules in the first layer into the interface so that molecules in second or subsequent layers of any multilayer that may be present do not contribute to π. As a result, the points at which the linear plots of $\Delta\pi$ versus π_i (FIGURE 6) for apoA-I, apoE, and BSA extrapolate to $\Delta\pi = 0$ give a measure of the relative abilities of the three proteins to penetrate a liquid-expanded egg PC monolayer. It should be noted that the actual values of $\Delta\pi$ are a function of the C_p chosen, but the relative $\Delta\pi$ values are not a function of C_p. Combining the data in FIGURE 6 with the π-A curve for egg PC on this phosphate buffer [20] indicates that BSA is excluded from the egg PC monolayer when the lipid molecular area is less than 85 Å², while the equivalent figures for apoA-I and apoE are 70 and 65 Å², respectively.

The average molecular area for phospholipid in the surface of human serum lipoproteins has been estimated as about 65 Å²,[29] equivalent to $\pi \simeq 30$ mN m⁻¹ for dipalmitoyl PC spread at the n-heptane/water interface.[30] This suggests that apoA-I and apoE would only just be able to remain in the lipoprotein surface whereas BSA would be effectively excluded. This prediction is consistent with the observation that apoA-I on the surface of HDL is labile and can be removed by heating[31] or treatment with guanidine hydrochloride.[32] The above results also lead to the expectations that compression of a mixed monolayer containing PC and the three proteins formed at a low π would lead to sequential ejection of proteins from the interface with albumin leaving first and apoE last. Extrapolation of these data for the air–water interface to a lipoprotein surface suggests that when lipoprotein lipase acts on a triglyceride-rich lipoprotein and shrinks its core, any concomitant compression of the surface components would lead to ejection of apoA-I before apoE. Such a mechanism could control the apoprotein composition of a lipoprotein and be important in the interconversion of lipoproteins.

Interfacial Conformation

The conformations adopted by the apoproteins in mixed monolayers with egg PC are not known, but by analogy to their structure when recombined with phospholipid in bulk (for a review, see Reference 33), it is likely that significant amounts of amphipathic helix are present. The π-A curves for all three proteins under study here (FIGURE 1) are consistent with the monolayer comprising α-helices lying in the plane of the air–water interface. Spread monolayers of homopolypeptides which are α-helical assume areas of 13–19 Å²/residue;[34] the variation in area depends on the length of the amino acid sidechain with bigger groups causing greater separation of the α-helical rods lying in the surface. Since the close packed molecular areas lie in the range 10–18 Å²/residue for all three proteins, the interfacial conformation could be mainly α-helical, but it should be noted that the average molecular area for a peptide monolayer comprising a β sheet is about 16 Å²/residue.[35] However, since the average area per residue in HDL has been estimated as 15.6 Å²,[29] and in this situation the predominant secondary structure is α-helical, the most probable conformation at the air–water interface is the same. Since the mean residue weight is 115 for all three proteins, the average interhelix distance should be the same, so that the apoA-I monolayer is presumably more condensed because a greater proportion of the peptide chain forms loops or tails that protrude out of the plane of the interface; the reduction of 3 Å²/residue in the limiting area at $\pi = 0$ for apoA-I would arise if an extra 20% of the molecules ($\sim$50 residues) relative to apoE were in loops or tails and not in the plane of the interface. The redistribution of residues between these various locations in the monolayer occurs quite slowly, so that the π-A curve is highly dependent on the history of the monolayer and the rate of compression.[4-6]

The possibility that apoA-I, apoE, or BSA are completely denatured at the air–water interface and form a random coil structure with all residues in the surface can be eliminated by a comparison of experimental curves with the theoretical curve in FIGURE 1. Singer [35] derived an expression (Equation 2) for π for flexible macromolecules adsorbed flat to a surface. In the case of the proteins discussed here, π is given by:

$$\pi = \pi_0 \left[\frac{Z'}{2} \ln \left(1 - \frac{2\theta}{Z'} \right) - \ln \left(1 - \theta \right) \right], \tag{2}$$

where $\pi_0 = kT/a_0$, k is the Boltzmann constant, T is the absolute temperature, a_0 is the limiting, condensed area per statistical unit of the linear polymer, Z' is a number close to the coordination number of the lattice, and θ is the degree of surface coverage given by the ratio a_0/a where a is the observed area per statistical unit. Curve 4 in FIGURE 1 is calculated from Equation 2 using $Z' = 4$ and $a_0 = 15$ Å²/residue. Although adsorbed films of the highly disordered β-casein molecule give π-A curves that agree with curve 4 when $\pi < 8$ mN m⁻¹, it is clear that apoA-I, apoE, and BSA form spread films that are more condensed at all π values. This condensation is presumably due to the existence of helices; apoA-I and BSA are known to contain amphipathic helices, and the phospholipid-binding properties of apoE (D. Reijngoud, unpublished results) are consistent with this protein also containing an amphipathic helix.

CONCLUSIONS

Apolipoproteins A-I and E are more surface-active than BSA. All three proteins are irreversibly adsorbed at the air–water interface and can only leave the surface when the film is compressed. Raising the interfacial pressure (π) with a spread insoluble PC monolayer also inhibits protein adsorption. At a given substrate protein concentration, the initial lipid monolayer π at which protein penetration to the surface is prevented increases in the order BSA < apoA-I < apoE. These observations suggest that the lipid packing and pressure at the surface of a lipoprotein are critical in controlling the apoprotein composition by determining which apoproteins are squeezed out.

SUMMARY

Plots of surface pressure (π) versus molecular area for rat apolipoprotein A-I (apoA-I), rabbit apoE, and bovine serum albumin (BSA) spread at the air–water interface are similar. The curves are consistent with significant amounts of amphipathic helix lying in the plane of the air–water interface.

The dependence of π on the substrate concentration (C_p) of apoA-I and apoE is essentially the same with both proteins exhibiting maximum values of ~24 mN m^{-1} at $C_p > 10^{-4}$ wt%; these apoproteins are much more surface-active than albumin, which exerts a maximum π of 18 mN m^{-1} at $C_p > 10^{-3}$ wt%.

Application of the Gibbs Adsorption Equation to the π-C_p data for all three proteins predicts surface concentrations that are much greater than those measured directly by monitoring the adsorption of ^{125}I-labeled protein. This discrepancy suggests that apoA-I, apoE, and BSA molecules are adsorbed irreversibly at the air–water interface. The conformation of adsorbed protein molecules is sensitive to π and compression can lead to desorption. The proteins can penetrate monolayers of egg phosphatidylcholine (PC) spread at the air–water interface at low π but highly compressed lipid monolayers prevent adsorption of the proteins. When $C_p = 5 \times 10^{-5}$ wt%, BSA is excluded when the PC monolayer has $\pi > 15$ mN m^{-1}, whereas apoA-I and apoE are excluded at pressures of 28 and 35 mN m^{-1}, respectively. Since the isotherms suggest that the apoproteins behave qualitatively the same at the air–water interface and the lipoprotein surface, this difference in lipid interaction between apoA-I and apoE may be significant in the interconversion of lipoproteins.

ACKNOWLEDGMENTS

We are indebted to Mr. M. Forte, Mrs. A. Ritz, and Mr. B. LaMont for expert technical assistance.

REFERENCES

1. NEURATH, H. & H. B. BULL. 1938. Chem. Rev. **23**:391–434.
2. MILLER, I. R. & D. BACH. 1973. *In* Surface and Colloid Chemistry. E. Matijevic, Ed. Vol. 6: 185–260. Wiley Press, New York, N.Y.
3. PHILLIPS, M. C. 1977. Chem. Ind. (London): 170–176.
4. GRAHAM, D. E. & M. C. PHILLIPS. 1979. J. Colloid Interface Sci. **70**:403–414.
5. GRAHAM, D. E. & M. C. PHILLIPS. 1979. J. Colloid Interface Sci. **70**:415–426.
6. GRAHAM, D. E. & M. C. PHILLIPS. 1979. J. Colloid Interface Sci. **70**:427–439.
7. MARSH, J. B. & C. E. SPARKS. 1979. Metabolism. **28**:1040–1045.
8. LUX, S. E., K. M. JOHN & H. B. BREWER. 1972. J. Biol. Chem. **247**:7510–7518.
9. MARSH, J. B. 1976. J. Lipid Res. **17**:85–90.
10. MARCEL, Y. L., M. BERGSETH & A. C. NESTRUCK. 1979. Biochim. Biophys. Acta **573**:175–183.
11. BILHEIMER, D. W., S. EISENBERG & R. I. LEVY. 1972. Biochim. Biophys. Acta **260**:212–221.
12. DAUGHADAY, W. H., O. H. LOWRY, N. J. ROSEBROUGH & W. S. FIELDS. 1952. J. Lab. Clin. Med. **39**:663–665.
13. PHILLIPS, M. C. & D. CHAPMAN. 1968. Biochim. Biophys. Acta **163**:301–313.
14. TRURNIT, H. J. 1960. J. Colloid Sci. **15**:1–13.
15. EVANS, M. T. A., J. MITCHELL, P. R. MUSSELLWHITE & L. IRONS. 1970. *In* Surface Chemistry of Biological Systems. M. Blank, Ed. pp. 1–22. Plenum Press, New York, N.Y.
16. PHILLIPS, M. C., H. HAUSER, R. B. LESLIE & D. OLDANI. 1975. Biochim. Biophys. Acta **406**:402–414.

17. ADAMS D. J., M. T. A. EVANS, J. R. MITCHELL, M. C. PHILLIPS & P. M. REES. 1971. J. Polymer Sci. (Part C) **34**:167–179.
18. CAMEJO, G., G. COLACICCO & M. M. RAPPORT. 1968. J. Lipid Res. **9**:562–569.
19. MITCHELL, J., L. IRONS & G. J. PALMER. 1970. Biochim. Biophys. Acta **200**: 138–150.
20. PHILLIPS, M. C., M. T. A. EVANS & H. HAUSER. 1975. Adv. Chem. **17**:217–230.
21. COLACICCO, G. 1970. Lipids **5**:636–649.
22. QUINN, P. & R. M. C. DAWSON. 1970. Biochem. J. **119**:21–25.
23. OSBORNE, J. C., JR. & H. B. BREWER, JR. 1977. Adv. Protein Chem. **31**:253–337.
24. POWNALL, H. J., Q. PAO, M. ROHDE & A. M. GOTTO. 1978. Biochem. Biophys. Res. Commun. **85**:408–414.
25. SHEPHARD, J., A. M. GOTTO, JR., O. D. TAUNTON, M. J. CASLAKE & E. FARISH. 1977. Biochim. Biophys. Acta **489**:486–501.
26. DEFEIJTER, J. A., D. E. GRAHAM & M. C. PHILLIPS. 1975. Faraday Disc. Chem. Soc. **59**:254–256.
27. BENJAMINS, J., J. A. DEFEIJTER, M. T. A. EVANS, D. E. GRAHAM & M. C. PHILLIPS. 1975. Faraday Disc. Chem. Soc. **59**:218–229.
28. PHILLIPS, M. C., H. HAUSER & M. C. PHILLIPS. 1973. Proc. 6th Internat. Congress Surface Activity. Vol. 2: 381–391. Carl Hanser Verlag, Munich, W. Germany.
29. SHEN, B. W., A. M. SCANU & F. J. KEZDY. 1977. Proc. Natl. Acad. Sci. USA **74**:837–841.
30. TAYLOR, J. A. G., J. MINGINS, B. A. PETHICA, B. Y. J. TAN & C. M. JACKSON. 1973. Biochim. Biophys. Acta **323**:157–160.
31. TALL, A. R., R. J. DECKELBAUM, D. M. SMALL & G. G. SHIPLEY. 1977. Biochim. Biophys. Acta **487**:145–153.
32. NICHOLS, A. V., E. L. GONG, P. J. BLANCHE, T. M. FORTE & D. W. ANDERSON. 1976. Biochim. Biophys. Acta **446**:226–239.
33. MORRISETT, J. D., R. L. JACKSON & A. M. GOTTO, JR. 1977. Biochim. Biophys. Acta **472**:93–133.
34. MALCOLM, B. R. 1973. Prog. Surface Membrane Sci. **7**:183–229.
35. SINGER, S. J. 1948. J. Chem. Phys. **16**:872–876.

DISCUSSION OF THE PAPER

DR. R. L. JACKSON: Dr. Phillips, in your experiments, did you take any precautions when initially you added the apoproteins to the monolayer trough to make sure that they were in a monomeric form?

DR. M. C. PHILLIPS: Yes, we did take precautions by spreading protein from isopropanol–water mixtures. In adsorption experiments we were injecting a very small volume of relatively concentrated solution (~0.2 mg/ml) of the apoprotein, which became diluted to very low concentrations of less than 1 μg/ml. So, we think that we were finally in the monomeric state although it is difficult to be absolutely sure.

DR. JACKSON: Did you do the converse, namely, not take any precautions?

DR. PHILLIPS: We did not do that.

DR. JACKSON: The reason I asked the question is because a monolayer system, of course, is a very sensitive system to determine whether or not the state of aggregation of a protein has anything to do with the rate of interaction with lipids. In our experience when we do not treat apoA-I or apoE with guanidine HCL, we find that the surface pressure of the protein increases; the same is true when we pretreat the protein with 6 M guanidine HCl and then dilute it very highly in the Teflon trough, which indicates that at least this kind of monolayer study may not be the best to study lipid–protein interaction, since the phenomena that you observe may have nothing to do with the rate of interaction of the protein with the lipid.

DR. PHILLIPS: I agree with you. Extrapolating kinetics from this sort of system to what is going on in plasma would be extremely difficult. One thing I would say about the state of aggregation—you remember that I pointed out that the air–water surface saturates at about 1 μg of apoE and apoA per ml of substrate. This is just what Dr. Gotto and colleagues find with HDL, suggesting that it is the same monomer concentration of apoA-I which is in equilibrium with HDL. So, it is very interesting that when you saturate the surface with the apoprotein you are also saturating the substrate with monomeric protein and beyond that you may have aggregates.

DR. JACKSON: May I just add one more point here? We have also been studying the interaction of lipoprotein lipase with a model system using phospholipid vesicles as a substrate, and it is of interest that in that kind of system where the lipase does bind to phospholipid vesicle in the absence of apoC-II, if one starts putting cholesterol into those vesicles, the amount of lipase that is associated with those complexes is decreased. We do not know, of course, what the surface pressure in those model systems is. But, it may well reflect on your statement that as the VLDL particle gets smaller the surface pressure changes, and, as a result, lipoprotein lipase can then leave the interface of the particle.

DR. PHILLIPS: Certainly the effects of cholesterol that you describe are consistent with a condensation forcing protein molecules out of the surface. It is well established in a variety of experiments that cholesterol condenses or reduces the molecular area of the phospholipids.

DR. A. M. SCANU: But, if you are adding cholesterol to your vesicles then the geometry of the vesicle changes. Would this have an effect on the interactions.

DR. PHILLIPS: It may have an effect.

DR. F. T. LINDGREN: I want to ask you one question: Have you or anyone else put your kind of apparatus into a pressure chamber where you could generate the kind of pressures that Dr. Osborne and others have using the ultracentrifuge?

DR. PHILLIPS: The answer is no. It has not been done, and in principle it could be done but I would need a big grant to build a pressure chamber.

DR. B. SHEN: First, I have a comment on Dr. Jackson's question. In the case of apoA-I, the native protein obeys a diffusion-controlled process, whereas in the presence of guanidine hydrochloride the rate is much slower. So, maybe, the structure of the native protein has something to do with the surface absorption.

DR. PHILLIPS: Could I just make a comment on that too? I agree entirely that the state of aggregation of the protein will affect the rate of adsorption. Using a protein such as lysozyme where we know we have a monomeric state at given concentrations, we can calculate the rate of surface adsorption to see if it agrees with diffusion equations. This is the case. So, in that system adsorption is diffusion-controlled and we obviously could do the same sort of thing here with the apoproteins. If there is an initial disaggregation step that occurs before adsorption then the diffusion may not be rate-determining. I have not carried out experiments along these lines.

DR. SHEN: Actually, we did such an experiment. At very low concentration of apoA-I when the protein is mainly monomeric, we find that its adsorption is diffusion-controlled. My question is, in your work with apoA-I using fast compression, did you observe any aging effect?

DR. PHILLIPS: Yes, the kinetic effects in the protein monolayers are very marked. There are a variety of relaxation processes going on, and in the case of albumin, which we studied more, there are relaxation times of the order of an hour involved. So, you have to wait an extremely long time for equilibrium and continuous compression would not give you any equilibrium.

DR. SHEN: In our hands when we measured the force–area curve of apoA-I by fast compression and when we did it by aging the apoprotein at the surface for different time intervals, we found that the pressure–area curve moves upward as time increases to indicate unfolding of the protein at the interface. That comes back to the question of the irreversibility of apoA-I in your experiments. How long did it take to reach the end point of adsorption?

DR. PHILLIPS: In the adsorption experiments, 3 hours.

DR. SHEN: Maybe the protein that you are measuring is totally denatured. That is why it is not reversible. We find that the adsorbed protein monolayer can be desorbed by compression. But, if the protein sits at the interface at low pressure for too long, it becomes totally insoluble and has a kind of random structure, which does not obey the Gibbs equation.

DR. PHILLIPS: What I want to say is that I do not believe there is free exchange between apoprotein molecules adsorbed at the clean air–water interface and protein molecules in the substrate. I do believe that if you compress the protein monolayer then the apoprotein molecules will leave. But, I think you will get a free exchange between apoprotein molecules adsorbed to a lipid monolayer at high pressure and the solution because then they are in a different conformation, which we have yet to determine.

DR. SHEN: What is the pressure range you are measuring your absorption? Very low?

DR. PHILLIPS: No, up to the maximum pressure that exists. Putting the two pieces of information together suggests that you only get reversible adsorption when the final pressure is more than 25 dynes/cm and less than 35 dynes/cm. So, that is a rather narrow range. But, we need more information on this.

DR. D. STEINBERG: Well, this is just an observation I wanted to report since there is a lot of discussion about pressure and what it does to apoA-I self-association. We have been trying to make a derivative of apoA-I with a covalent modification using an activated sucrose molecule and we kept getting dimers. In the SDS gel we had a molecular weight twice what it should be. Jim told us about his pressure experiments and he suggested that if we could add the reactants under high pressure then we might get what we wanted which was a sucrose-tagged apoA-I monomer. The problem was that we did not have any gadget with which we could add the activated sucrose at 150 atmospheres and Jim suggested to do it in the centrifuge except then the reaction would be all over by the time we got up to speed. So, what we did instead was to freeze the apoA-I in solution, put the reactant on top, have the centrifuge head frozen, put it in the machine, and then when it got up to speed let it thaw. In doing so we got the apoA-I monomers. Whereas, if we did it at an atmospheric pressure we got apoA-I dimers.

DR. SCANU: The problem, of course, Dr. Steinberg, is that once you alter or modify apoA-I, its mode of self-association can significantly change and on this there is some evidence in literature. So, the prediction as to how the protein is modified may not be applicable to the native form. Freezing may have also something to do with your effect.

DR. STEINBERG: Well, doing the reaction in the same way at atmospheric pressure gave 80% plus apoA-I dimer. Now, maybe the freezing may have affected the reaction. We never tried to control freezing and this probably should be done.

GENERAL DISCUSSION

A. M. Scanu, *Moderator*

University of Chicago
Pritzker School of Medicine
Chicago, Illinois 60637

DR. D. M. SMALL: Dr. Phillips, you have made an interesting number of suggestions. The problem that I have is to really understand what surface pressure means in the *in vivo* system and this is a similar sort of problem with Richard Jackson's material and anybody who works with the Langmuir trough has. There are innumerable things that happen during the lipolysis reaction including the formation of products that have a very low surface free energy, i.e., fatty acids and monoglycerides or diglycerides. I wonder if we have any way of looking at the interfacial free energy of a more natural system?

DR. M. C. PHILLIPS: We can obviously try and mimic the complicated mixture you are describing at the air–water interface. But, I think that what you are really getting at is how do you measure the film pressure in a lipoprotein particle. The same sort of problem arises when you use insoluble monolayers as a membrane model. How do we make a comparison between the model and the real system. There is no clear way to answer your question and you are well aware of that. The best way, I think, to make the comparison is to consider molecular areas, and I like to think in terms of the area for phospholipid molecule. That is why I tried to stress that those pressures at which the various apoproteins are incorporated occur at certain lipid molecular areas.

I think it might be possible in terms of x-ray diffraction that when we get very accurate surface areas and very accurate chemical compositions we may be able to do a calculation and at least get an estimate of the molecular packing, the lipid packing, and from that infer what the film pressure is. I cannot at the moment think of a way where one can directly measure the film pressure.

DR. V. LUZZATI: About the protein in a monolayer, there is something which always bothered me in that it is supposed to lie at the interface. Now, in fact, if you look, say, at the membrane structure, proteins can span the membrane by virtue of specific associations which satisfy the chemical requirement.

DR. PHILLIPS: I agree entirely that the amphipathic helix can either lay in principle in the plane of the interface or can lay in some self-associated form perpendicular to the interface. My molecular areas are consistent with the protein being in the plane of the interface. That does not mean that in membranes it is always that way. Certainly not.

DR. A. M. SCANU: Dr. Phillips, what is the effect of the alkyl chains of the phospholipids on the protein packing?

DR. PHILLIPS: We have done the reconstitution in bulk using DMPC and the apoprotein; in the case of the monolayer we have used egg PC and the apoprotein. The reason we went away from using egg PC for the reconstitution in bulk is that we did not get discs. We got small spherical particles rather than the well-defined discs that everybody describes.

If your question is what is the role of fatty acid chain lengths or saturation on this interaction and the position at which the various proteins are incorporated, we do not know yet. That has to be done.

DR. SCANU: Which means that the usual general question remains, namely, when you try to simplify a system in order to derive accurate parameters, it is difficult to extrapolate the information to the real biological system. But, still those model studies are very worthwhile conducting.

DR. PHILLIPS: Well, I would not like to study monolayers in isolation. I think it is too far a removed system. The sort of questions that you are raising are too important. So, I always study the bulk system and the monolayer together.

DR. SMALL: Your calculation assigning 13–18 $Å^2$ per amino acid residue could mean that the helix is lying in the plane of the interface rather than having a random distribution. This would give you a larger area like 25 $Å^2$, indicating that perhaps you have actually a portion of the protein tightly packed along the perpendicular axis to the plane of the layer; the rest of it being in the aqueous phase.

DR. PHILLIPS: Certainly. I want to invoke an argument like that to explain the difference between the apoA-I and apoE force–area curves. I think that in the case of apoA-I there is more of the protein in loops and tails, as they are called.

DR. A. R. TALL: Do you also find, like Richard Jackson, that apoA-I does not remove any phospholipid from the interface?

DR. PHILLIPS: We have not done that particular experiment. What we should do is label the lipid and then inject the protein and watch the radioactivity.

DR. K. W. A. WIRTZ: I have a question for Dr. Jackson with respect to his experiment where the apoC catalyzes the transfer of the PC from a monolayer to a liposome. He shows that if he raises the surface pressure of his monolayer, the apoC will not remove the phosphatidylcholine molecule. On the other hand, when he adds the liposomes to the system he finds that the liposomes do function as a sink for the PC that is transferred from the interface. Now, the surface pressure of the liposomes I would expect to be on the order of about 30 dynes/cm² or perhaps even higher. How do you explain the effect that the liposomes have as acceptors for lipids, when, on the other hand, the apoC cannot interact effectively with the monolayer at about 30 dynes/cm²?

DR. R. L. JACKSON: The reason we started these experiments in the first place was to test the hypothesis whether or not the apoCs can serve as a phospholipid exchange protein. Of course, since Dr. Wirtz is the expert on phospholipid exchange proteins, that is why I went to his lab to test this; and we did find that the apoC proteins actually remove phospholipids from the interface. The phenomena that we showed, I think just go to prove what Dr. Small just said. You cannot use monolayer systems all the time and extrapolate the results to lipoproteins. But, is the surface pressure of the egg lecithin indeed 30 dynes/cm²? I thought it was a bit lower than that.

DR. B. SHEN: Dr. Jackson, in the kind of experiment where you just inject liposome underneath the monolayer or labeled phospholipid, is there any decrease in radioactivity?

DR. JACKSON: There is almost no decrease.

DR. SHEN: No decrease in the absence of apoC?

DR. JACKSON: That is right. Now, if you add the phospholipid exchange protein, a very fast exchange of phospholipids occurs. On the contrary, if you add liposomes first to the subphase and then apoC-II, this apoprotein binds to the liposomes very rapidly. Then you see no removal of phospholipids from the interface. So, the apoC-II or apoC-III does not come off, or if. it comes off it goes back on the liposomes much more quickly than the time that it takes for that apoprotein or apoprotein–phospholipid complex to go to the interface to exchange with radio-labeled phospholipids.

DR. SHEN: If you use a clean surface and inject the liposome into the solution, would the lipid adsorb to the surface?

DR. JACKSON: We have not done so many studies just at the air–water interface. Almost all of our studies have been with a phospholipid monolayer, or a cholesterol monolayer.

DR. SMALL: In studies that we carried out about 15 years ago, we observed a very slow adsorption of egg phospholipids to the surface at high concentrations like 4 g%. Thus the process is very slow, but it occurs.

DR. JACKSON: In our experiment, there was 1 mg of phospholipid per 15 milliliters.

DR. SMALL: This is what you put underneath?

DR. JACKSON: Yes. It is a very low concentration.

DR. SMALL: When you spread phospholipids on the surface with no phospholipid in the bulk system and you put the C peptides underneath, does the surface pressure decrease?

DR. JACKSON: Yes, there is a small decrease in surface pressure. We do not think that this is the reason why the phospholipid is leaving the interface, however, because we also see the same decrease in surface pressure when we add VLDL underneath the interface. In that case we do not see any removal of the phospholipids.

DR. SMALL: Can you remove it by increasing the concentrations of C peptides?

DR. JACKSON: You can. Eventually, if you go to a high enough concentration you can remove all the phospholipids from the interface, or, if you take that subphase and put it just into a new trough you can show that the radioactivity will go back to the interface as a function of time if the concentration is high enough. This process seems to be very specific for the apoCs, which I find to be very exciting because those are the ones that transfer during lipolysis. We do not see this phenomenon with apoA-I or apoE.

DR. SCANU: You are not claiming that you can explain *in vivo* phenomena from *in vitro* studies.

DR. JACKSON: We have not done anything with chylomicrons. All the work I have described today was with VLDL.

DR. SCANU: We know that apoA-I can dissociate from HDL and can be found in solution. The same appears to be true for apoE. Based on your studies, how do you explain this phenomenon?

DR. JACKSON: Dr. Scanu, may I just say one thing, and that is the amount of lipid that is associated with these apoproteins is very small. It may only be one or two molecules, and I am not sure that in the systems that people have used to date they could actually show that the apoA-I that comes off does not have any lipid associated with it.

DR. PHILLIPS: My question really relates to stoichiometry, in the system where the C peptides are removing phospholipid molecules from the air–water interface. Do you have any feel for what the stoichiometry is? I mean, do you envisage a disc or something like it forming and coming off, or do you envisage one C peptide molecule taking away one or two phospholipid molecules?

DR. JACKSON: I really do not have any information on that because I have not been able to separate the apoC-II that contains the phospholipid from the apoC-II that contains none. I do not have a method to separate those two because there is a relatively small amount of phospholipids there and, in fact, there is a relatively small amount of mass. My gut reaction is that the apoCs bind only one or two phospholipids. At least this is the kind of stoichiometry we get when we inject a limited amount of protein underneath the monolayer that contains only 6 nanomoles of phospholipid.

DR. A. JONAS (*University of Illinois, Urbana, Ill.*): We have to keep in mind what systems we are talking about. When apoCs from the bovine system are interacted with DMPC, we definitely observe a disclike particle with a stoichiometry of about 20 DMPC per equivalent apoC protein. At least in our system, we do not see a stoichiometry of one protein to one of lipid.

DR. JACKSON: I do not see a stoichiometry of one to one when I use DMPC and apoC-II in solution either.

DR. F. R. LANDSBERGER (*Rockefeller University, New York, N.Y.*): You showed a number of experiments whose basic design consisted of radio-labeled phospholipid spread at the air–water interface and a protein injected underneath. You then determined changes in surface pressure and surface radioactivity. This is a two-part question: When do you think you would see a perturbation of the surface pressure as a result of the interaction of the protein with the surface? Secondly, at the end of a reasonable period of time, would the net surface pressure be changed? I mean, how do you interpret that set of experiments?

DR. JACKSON: Using radio-labeled apoproteins we have shown that, indeed, all the apoproteins will interact with lipid. Now, when I say interact I mean that there is an increase in surface pressure when the apoprotein is there. Now, whether or not all the apoproteins that are there are interacting with the lipid, I cannot answer. There is no way to know whether or not that is true. But, even though apoA-I and apoE are at the interface they do not take phospholipid away from the interface. I feel that this phenomenon is specific for the apoCs.

DR. G. D. FASMAN: I would like to go back to my question to Dr. Osborne about his experiments, which were beautifully conducted but somewhat questionable in interpretation. You gave a perfect example where by adding phosphate your apoprotein assumed a higher secondary structure. The only sort of proteins that I know will act in that fashion are usually highly charged proteins, positively charged proteins, so that when you add phosphate you get some neutralization of charge and increase in structure. I would like to hear how you explain that.

DR. J. C. OSBORNE, JR.: First of all, phosphate, according to the Hofmeister series, is a structure-making salt. The interaction of inorganic ions with water is quite complex; Von Hipple has addressed this in the last few years.

Briefly, all inorganic salts, to some extent, favor hydrophobic interactions and I can provide references to that. I think that Dr. Tanford deals with this question in his book *The Hydrophobic Effect*. Dr. Edelhoch and I treated that in a manuscript in *Advances in Protein Chemistry*, Volume 30. Inorganic phosphate favors nonpolar interactions. To carry this a little further, the thermodynamics that we presented on the apoA-II system indicate that both the enthalpy and the entropy for the dimerization of apoA-II are very sensitive functions of temperature. And, this indicates that dimerization is associated with a large change in heat capacity and is thus hydrophobic in nature.

Brants, from 1966 through about 1967 while studying the thermal denaturation of globular proteins, addressed himself to the effect of the change in free energy with temperature for hydrophobic interactions. As I mentioned before, the studies by Dr. Tanford and our own studies on the temperature dependence of the enthalpy and entropy, indicate that there will be a maximum in stability at some temperature for hydrophobic interactions. For globular proteins this temperature is rather low, about, I think, 13° for ribonuclease. What this means is that when the temperature is decreased from about 10° that protein will unfold. For the dimerization of apoA-II all we have done is shift that temperature scale to about 30°. So, our free energy is highest at about 30°. This means that although the process is driven by hydrophobic interactions we get association with increasing temperature to about 30°, and then we get dissociation, which is really what one would predict for hydrophobic interactions.

DR. SCANU: We shall now go back to apoB and the problem of its molecular weight.

DR. BRADLEY: There are a number of things one has to consider in the molecular weight of this apoprotein. The best hydrodynamic data are from the laboratories of Dr. Reynolds and Dr. Tanford. In those studies there is no doubt that the minimum molecular weight of the species that one is looking at is 255,000, that is in guanidine hydrochloride. In a paper recently published by Dr. Reynolds' laboratory one notes that 20%–30% of the molecule has a higher molecular weight species, even in guanidine hydrochloride. So, what this says is that apoB aggregates also in the presence of guanidine hydrochloride. SDS, a detergent commonly used in the separation of the peptides, also promoted aggregation. A dimer formation appears to be preferred.

I am very glad that Dr. Reynolds is here because there are a few points about her SDS data that need discussion. I get the impression that the molecular weight is slightly biased in the sense that if one sees breakdown products in the starting materials using SDS gels, then that data is thrown out. The majority of material in the SDS gels has a molecular weight of 510,000, which is that of the whole apoprotein whatever the minimum molecular weight is. If you now transfer this material into guanidine you get a minimum molecular weight of 255,000 plus higher molecular weight species.

Now, if apoB really breaks down, then the existence of apoprotein hydrolysis must be considered. This means production of N terminals, and this has not been observed by all laboratories. I wonder whether it is this ability that makes Dr. Reynolds discard the data when smaller molecular weight species are seen. We too put apoB in the centrifuge and also get low molecular weights, down to 26,000 or perhaps a little smaller.

People have now developed new methods of delipidation, and I am speaking specifically of a paper by Camejo's laboratory in which apoB was supposedly mildly delipidated by binding it to a DEAE Sepharose column and then using a gradient of a nonionic detergent to strip the lipid. Under these conditions they see no production of N terminals in spite of the elution of low and high molecular weight species. Now if they took the low molecular weight delipidated material and treated it with guanidine hydrochloride, they again see the high molecular weight species.

My own data with the cyanogen bromide also suggest a low molecular weight. But this does not rule out the possibility of repeated sequences.

The other thing we need to address today is the possibility of cross-links that are covalent in nature. There have been at least two abstracts that I know of with one invoking cross-links between γ-Glu terminal and the ϵ-Lys and the other one perhaps involving lysine or norleucine.

DR. REYNOLDS: Dr. Bradley did a very good job of summarizing the problem on apoB, but he left out one very important thing and this is that the 250,000 minimum molecular weight of apoB in guanidine that was seen originally by Smith, Dawson, and Tanford and which was seen again by John Steele and myself is not just in the centrifuge. The hydrodynamic measurements say that if apoB is a subunit containing protein then the subunit association has to be end to end. The minimum hydrodynamic radius that one gets in guanidine for a species that in the centrifuge weighs 250,000 is close to 157Å, and that is exactly what you would predict for that length of a random coil. Moreover, as I understand from the people trying to sequence this protein, they find no labile bonds.

So, my question is, what kind of polypeptide chain is this? I do not care if you want to call them subunits but if they were hooked end to end by some covalent bond, then that is a single polypeptide chain.

Now, apoB is dimeric, that is 500,000 grams, so far in every detergent system that has been looked at, and it is not just our laboratory. My comment to the sequencers is that they are going to have a hell of a time separating all these peptides if they cannot even separate them in denaturing detergents. Everybody that I know who puts forth strenuous effort to store whole LDL by means of keeping out proteolytic enzymes, contamination from airborne spores, and so forth, keeping out oxygen and doing everything one can, sees nothing except for the single polypeptide chain. It is only after long periods of storage or hitting it with something like plasmin that one begins to see breakdown products.

DR. SCANU: I suppose the problem that we are having is that physical determinations have not led to unequivocal answers, and we are waiting for the chemist to help. You have to recognize that this protein is anomalous, and it may not be appropriate to approach it as a normal globular protein. Until such a time that the chemistry of apoB is resolved, I suppose that we should keep our minds open on its molecular weight.

DR. REYNOLDS: No, there is no way to keep the mind open on the fact that a random coil of 157 Å must weigh 250,000 and must be just that. But, it does not say anything about repetitive sequences, about the possibility of end-to-end linkages, which is up to the sequencers to resolve.

DR. R. M. WATT (*Duke University, Durham, N.C.*): I just wanted to add one thing. I have made 13 preps of apoB in the last year, thrown out about 2 of them, and made the following observation. A fresh preparation gives only one band on a gel. If I sterilize this preparation and put it in the refrigerator it will be good for at least four weeks. In regard to the use of SDS on cyanogen fragments, when I tried to repeat published data I got markedly different results when I delipidated the protein in SDS (this was also true for organic solvents). Cyanogen bromide fragmentation in the nonalkylated preparations gave somewhere between 18 and 20 bands in a one dimensional gel. On the other hand if I alkylated the protein, no matter how I delipidate it, and then use cyanogen bromide cleavage, I got a mess. I do not know if that helps you or hinders you but I thought I would tell you that anyway.

DR. SCANU: I suppose the question is whether it is reasonable for those involved in the sequence of apoB to keep going if the protein is indeed that large; but it is better to let this kind of philosophical question rest.

DR. LUZZATI: I am surprised that nobody said anything or almost anything on apoE and HDL_C because from my personal viewpoint about structure I think that in that direction we can find very useful information. What I know about the structure of HDL_C is very little; it seems to be very similar to LDL, and it would be extremely important at the present to know, for example, how many apoE molecules are in that particle. I am wondering to what extent the molecular weight of HDL_C is known, I mean, in an accurate way. If I use what is published by Dr. Mahley and his group, it comes out as something on the order of 15 protein molecules per particle. Now, with the model I have put forward I need 12 or a multiple of it since symmetry imposes very strict rules. Now, how close is 15 to 12? This is why the accuracy of the molecular weight of the whole HDL_C is so necessary.

DR. R. W. MAHLEY: We have been looking at the molecular weight of apoE–HDL_C with Dr. Nelson in Arkansas. The best data that we have now, I think, confirms what we published and this gives something like 15 or 16, not 12 molecules of apoE. But, I do not know how close 15 or 16 is to 12.

DR. SCANU: Is this particle homogeneous? Is it always the same from preparation to preparation or do you note differences?

DR. MAHLEY: We find that apoE–HDL_C is homogeneous by analytical ultracentrifugation.

DR. R. L. HEINRIKSON: Yes, I have to reveal myself as one of those people who has been trying to do the sequence of apoB. I can say that in general our findings parallel those of Dr. Bradley very closely. We have come down to same questions, namely, how do you solubilize these peptides, how do we separate them, and how do you sequence them? It is very hard to separate these things, as you have seen from the presentations today. We, however, proceed with them and hope that it is really a small molecular weight protein that we are dealing with, although we do not have any definitive proof.

Our results do fit with some of the data that Dr. Langdon presented at the

Federation Meeting a couple of years ago. That is, if apoB is exposed to performic acid oxidation and then is separated by gel electrophoresis, there is an accumulation of low molecular weight bands of about 12 to 20,000.

So, we proceed with the belief that apoB has a low molecular weight form that shows a tremendous capacity to aggregate, and we have additional data to this subject, which I will present later at the Poster Session.

DR. BRADLEY: I would like to address the point that just came up a minute ago about the similarity between apoE and apoB. First of all, I do not think they are very similar. One, the apoE protein is highly alpha helical (as high as 70%–75%) when bound to DMPC vesicles. That is quite different from the secondary structures seen in apoB as studied in the whole lipoprotein itself. There may be regions, let us say patches, in these two apoprotein that are similar, and this may be due to the arginine content and a highly positive surface charge. Thus the similarities are not related to secondary structure but perhaps more to the way this protein is laid on the surface.

DR. A. M. GOTTO, JR.: Dr. Luzzati and Dr. Small made some comments about the relationship between soluble apoproteins and membrane proteins that span the bilayer. I do not think that these proteins are similar. A typical membrane protein has one relatively long sequence or segments of hydrophobic amino acids. This is not true with the apolipoproteins.

I think that the question is unsettled as to how deeply the apoproteins may penetrate into the lipid phase, say, of HDL. The low-angle x-ray scattering data, for whatever they are worth, would only indicate a region between 12 to 15 Å. But, this is far from the protein spanning the membrane which represents quite a different type of amphipathic helical structure.

DR. SMALL: I agree with that, Dr. Gotto. However, I do not think we are making a strong analogy between an artificial surface such as a Langmuir trough and how the protein might be oriented at the lipoprotein surface. We are speculating on a number of possible conformations that could occur there. But we do not know what they are.

But, if you think of lipoproteins in general and then start with a discoidal lipoprotein, which is a small disc of phospholipid around which apoA-I or apoA-II is wrapped around, both of these apoproteins have very high helical contents. Their organization can be envisaged as an accordion-like structure with the hydrophobic parts of the α helices facing the hydrocarbon chains of the phospholipids along the edge of the disc.

Now, when that same protein is either in an aqueous solution or in the intact HDL molecules, then you see a tremendous difference in the overall conformation. The HDL are quasispherical particles in which the phospholipids are sticking out from a pseudomicellar structure. They are no longer aligned in a bilayer. Under those circumstances the protein has a very different free energy and that free energy is probably dictated by the geometry of the overall particle.

Now, if you carry this notion further to the surface of the chylomicrons, the surface is almost a plane when considered in molecular dimensions; i.e., it is almost like a Langmuir trough. Therefore, the orientation of the protein at that surface is going to be different from that in HDL, in a disc, or in solution. Their conformation is different depending upon the particle they are associated with even though they have the same primary structure.

DR. LUZZATI: In my opinion, I see very little useful information coming from model experiments on the components of systems as complex as lipoproteins. In the case of LDL, we have to crystallize it and know the chemistry of apoB. Only this information can prove or disprove the results proposed thus far, including our own.

DR. OSBORNE: I think we must emphasize that plasma lipoproteins are dynamic and not necessarily amenable to static descriptions.

I think that we should differentiate between plasma lipoproteins in the HDL density range from those that are in the LDL density range. LDL is a rigid particle, which can be treated rather drastically without changing its molecular properties. HDL is much different; HDL actually dissociates in solution. That is because its structure is governed by the laws of mass action and the rates of those reactions are such that in many instances we are dealing with a free equilibrium situation.

PREDICTION OF PROTEIN
CONFORMATION FROM THE PRIMARY STRUCTURE *

Gerald D. Fasman

Graduate Department of Biochemistry
Brandeis University
Waltham, Massachusetts 02254

The conformation of biologically active proteins and polypeptides is one of the main determinants of the high degree of specificity of their reactivity *in vivo*. In turn the native conformation of a protein is determined by its amino acid sequence.[1] X-ray diffraction techniques have successfully elucidated the three-dimensional structure (conformation) of over 60 proteins.[2, 3] However, this number is small compared to the number of protein sequences (>1000) that have been completed.[4] Many of these proteins, such as histones, membranes, and ribosomal proteins have not yet been crystallized so other techniques must be utilized to yield structural information. Because of this enormous backlog of proteins whose structure is unknown, and the conviction that the amino acid sequence determines conformation, many efforts have been made to predict protein secondary structure from sequence data. Many predictive methods are available and these have been reviewed in articles on protein folding and sequence analysis; two recent reviews summarize the various predictive algorithms and evaluate their efficacy.[5, 6] Since these reviews were written two other methods have been published.[7, 8]

No attempt will be made herein to discuss the relative merits of these predictive algorithms, but rather the Chou-Fasman method[9, 10] will be used as an example to demonstrate the general utility of this approach to assist in understanding the general phenomena of structure and function of polypeptides and proteins.

These predictive methods can locate α-helical, β-sheet, and β-turn regions in proteins with an 80% degree of accuracy. The predictive projections of protein conformation have been applied in the following ways:

1. Initial delineation of secondary structure in X-ray crystallographic studies.
2. Starting conformations for energy minimization procedures.
3. Detecting regions with potential for conformational changes.
4. Recognition of structural domains in homologous sequences.
5. Suggesting the rational design of synthetic analogs for experimental testing to see whether conservation or change in conformation will produce alteration or retention of biological activity, e.g., structure and biological function relationships.

A brief description of the Chou-Fasman method[9, 10] will be given and its utility demonstrated in terms of the above outlined potentials. A statistical

* This work was supported in part by grants from the United States Public Health Service (GM 17533) and the National Science Foundation (PCM-76–21856). This is Publication No. 1302 from the Graduate Department of Biochemistry, Brandeis University.

147

survey of 15 proteins, whose X-ray structure had been determined, was made and the helix and β-sheet conformation potentials of all 20 amino acids were established in their hierarchial order. Tables on the frequency of helical and β-sheet boundary residues in these 15 proteins were also published.[9] The helix and β-sheet conformational parameters P_α and P_β (where $P_\alpha = f_\alpha / \langle f_\alpha \rangle$ and $P_\beta = f_\beta / \langle f_\beta \rangle$; f_α and f_β are the frequency of residues in the helix and β regions; $\langle f_\alpha \rangle$ and $\langle f_\beta \rangle$ are the average frequency of residues in the helix and β regions) were utilized with a set of empirical rules to predict the α and β regions in proteins. The method's simplicity and relative degree of accuracy ($\simeq 75$) are the main reasons for its wide use (see approximately 90 examples in Appendix in Reference 5).

PREDICTION RULES

A more recent analysis of 29 proteins, containing 4741 amino acids, whose X-ray structure has been published has produced a slightly revised set of conformational parameters. These are shown in TABLE 1,[11] in their hierarchial order and classified as: H_α (strong helix former), h_α (helix former), I_α (weak helix former), i_α (helix indifferent), b_α (helix breaker), B_α (strong helix breakers), and H_β (strong β-former) and so forth as for the helix. Using the following empirical rules (abbreviated), one locates the secondary structures of proteins: (1) A cluster of four helical residues (h_α or H_α) out of six residues along the protein sequence will initiate a helix. The helical segment is extended in both directions until sets of tetrapeptide breakers $\langle P_\alpha \rangle < 1.00$ are reached (e.g., b_4, $b_3 i$, $b_2 i_2$, etc.). Certain amino acids have positional preferences; for example, proline, aspartic acid, and glutamic acid are found with a high frequency at the N-terminal helical end, and histidine, lysine, and arginine at the C-terminal helical end. Furthermore, proline cannot occur in the inner helix or at the C-terminal helical end. Any segment with the $\langle P_\alpha \rangle \geq 1.03$ as well as $\langle P_\alpha \rangle > \langle P_\beta \rangle$ is predicted as helical. (2) A sequence of three β-formers or a cluster of three β-formers out of four or five residues along the protein sequence will initiate a β sheet. The β sheet is propagated in both directions as long as the sheet contains less than $\frac{1}{3}$ β-breakers. It is terminated by the same set of tetrapeptide breakers as found for the helical sections (above). Any segment with $\langle P_\beta \rangle \geq 1.05$, as well as $\langle P_\beta \rangle > \langle P_\alpha \rangle$ is predicted as β sheet. (3) Any segment containing overlapping α and β residues is resolved through conformational boundary analysis. These three basic rules determine the prediction of protein secondary structures (helix, β sheet, and random coil).

β TURNS

There remains one additional important secondary structure, the β turn, which involves four consecutive residues in a protein where the polypeptide chain folds back on itself by nearly 180°. It is these chain reversals that give a protein its globularity. Venkatachalam[12] first characterized three types of turns in a tetrapeptide where there is a hydrogen bond between the CO group of residue i and the NH group of residue $i + 3$. Analysis of proteins revealed many β turns present in their secondary structures (for review, see Refer-

TABLE 1

Conformational Parameters for α-Helical, β-Sheet, and β-Turn Residues in 29 Proteins *

P_α		P_β		P_t	f_i	f_{i+1}	f_{i+2}	f_{i+3}
Glu 1.51		Val 1.70		Asn 1.56	Asn 0.161	Pro 0.301	Asn 0.191	Trp 0.167
Met 1.45	H_α	Ile 1.60	H_β	Gly 1.56	Cys 0.149	Ser 0.139	Gly 0.190	Gly 0.152
Ala 1.42		Tyr 1.47		Pro 1.52	Asp 0.147	Lys 0.115	Asp 0.179	Cys 0.128
Leu 1.21		Phe 1.38		Asp 1.46	His 0.140	Asp 0.110	Ser 0.125	Tyr 0.125
Lys 1.16		Trp 1.37	h_β	Ser 1.43	Ser 0.120	Thr 0.108	Cys 0.117	Ser 0.106
Phe 1.13	h_α	Leu 1.30		Cys 1.19	Pro 0.102	Arg 0.106	Tyr 0.114	Gln 0.098
Gln 1.11		Cys 1.19		Tyr 1.14	Gly 0.102	Gln 0.098	Arg 0.099	Lys 0.095
Trp 1.08		Thr 1.19		Lys 1.01	Thr 0.086	Gly 0.085	His 0.093	Asn 0.091
Ile 1.08		Gln 1.10		Gln 0.98	Tyr 0.082	Asn 0.083	Glu 0.077	Arg 0.085
Val 1.06		Met 1.05		Thr 0.96	Trp 0.077	Met 0.082	Lys 0.072	Asp 0.081
Asp 1.01		Arg 0.93		Trp 0.96	Gln 0.074	Ala 0.076	Thr 0.065	Thr 0.079
His 1.00	I_α	Asn 0.89	i_β	Arg 0.95	Arg 0.070	Tyr 0.065	Phe 0.065	Leu 0.070
Arg 0.98		His 0.87		His 0.95	Met 0.068	Glu 0.060	Trp 0.064	Pro 0.068
Thr 0.83		Ala 0.83		Glu 0.74	Val 0.062	Cys 0.053	Gln 0.037	Phe 0.065
Ser 0.77		Ser 0.75		Ala 0.66	Leu 0.061	Val 0.048	Leu 0.036	Glu 0.064
Cys 0.70	i_α	Gly 0.75	b_β	Met 0.60	Ala 0.060	His 0.047	Ala 0.035	Ala 0.058
Tyr 0.69		Lys 0.74		Phe 0.60	Phe 0.059	Phe 0.041	Pro 0.034	Ile 0.056
Asn 0.67	b_α	Pro 0.55		Leu 0.59	Glu 0.056	Ile 0.034	Val 0.028	Met 0.055
Pro 0.57		Asp 0.54	B_β	Val 0.50	Lys 0.055	Leu 0.025	Met 0.014	His 0.054
Gly 0.57	B_α	Glu 0.37		Ile 0.47	Ile 0.043	Trp 0.013	Ile 0.013	Val 0.053

* P_α, P_β, P_t are conformational parameters of helixes, β sheets, and β turns; f_i, f_{i+1}, f_{i+2}, f_{i+3} are bend frequencies in the four positions of the β turn; H_α, H_β, etc., are as defined previously.[10]. From Chou & Fasman.[5, 11]

ence 6). Utilizing the X-ray atomic coordinates from 29 proteins, Chou and Fasman [13] computed the $C_i^\alpha - C_{i+3}^\alpha$ distances of all 4651 tetrapeptides. Those whose distances were below 7 Å and not in a helical region were considered as β turns. A total of 457 β bends were located, and 32% of all the amino acid residues in the 29 proteins occurred in these bends. The α helix occupies 38% of the residues and 20% of the residues are found in the β sheet. These frequencies for all the amino acids, in the helix, β sheet, and β turns are obtained when their occurrence in each conformational state is divided by their total occurrences in the 29 proteins. The frequencies of residues in the 1st, 2nd, 3rd, and 4th positions of β turns for all the residues were obtained. These positional preferences of amino acids in β turns can be seen in TABLE 1, which are based on 408 turns.[5, 11]

Some residues are found to have a dramatic positional preference in the β turn: for example, proline in the 2nd (30%) but not in the 3rd position (3%); residues with the highest β-turn potential in all four positions (P_t values) are asparagine, glycine, proline, aspartic acid, and serine, with the most hydrophobic residues showing the lowest bend potential. On the other hand in regions adjacent to β turns many hydrophobic residues were found, in either α–α, α–β, or β–β interactions. The probability of β-turn occurrence at position i is calculated from

$$p_t = (f_i \times f_{i+1} \times f_{i+2} \times f_{i+3}),$$

and those tetrapeptides with $p_t > 0.75 \times 10^{-4}$, as well as $\langle P_t \rangle > 1.00$ and

$$\langle P_\alpha \rangle < \langle P_t \rangle > \langle P_\beta \rangle$$

are predicted as β turns.[14] The percentage of bend and nonbend residues predicted correctly for 29 proteins by this algorithm is $\%_{t+nt} = 70\%$, while 78% of the β turns were localized correctly within ±2 residues.[14] Applying the above conditions of prediction, the secondary structure, the α, β, random coil and β turns can be delineated. Since β turns are often located at the boundaries of both α and β regions, they may play an important role, initiating the tertiary folding of proteins.

APPLICATIONS OF THE PREDICTIVE METHOD

The predictive method may serve as a *guideline for the direction of folding* in low-resolution electron density maps of proteins, as in the case of tobacco mosaic virus (TMV) protein.[15] More recently, crystallographers have found the empirical rules of Chou and Fasman to be consistent with their X-ray results.[15, 16-19]

The conformation of proteins can be estimated by several physical-chemical techniques, e.g., circular dichroism, infrared spectroscopy, NMR, and so forth. The predictive method can supplement these experimental methods since it is able to locate where the secondary structural regions are in the amino acid sequence, as well as regions in proteins having both helical and β-forming potentials and therefore the potential for *conformational changes*. For example, the X-ray crystallographic studies of concanavalin A[20, 21] showed only 2% helix in the native structure. However, 55% helicity can be induced in concanavalin A with 70% chloroethanol.[22] The predictive scheme[10] correctly located all 12 β-sheet regions in concanavalin A with only one overpredicted

β region. In addition, it showed that a total of 47% of its residues in 13 regions also have α potential although many of these had still higher β potentials. Similarly, elastase has 7% helicity as shown from X-ray diffraction,[23] but circular dichroism studies showed that it assumed 35% helicity in sodium dodecyl sulfate.[24] The predictive method [10] showed that there are 79 residues in 15 regions with helical potential accounting for 33% helicity. Hence, the easily computed $\langle P_\alpha \rangle$ and $\langle P_\beta \rangle$ values for the α and β segments in proteins may assist in elucidating the regions potentially capable of undergoing conformational change. It is interesting to note that the B1–7 region of insulin was predicted as β sheet [10] with $\langle P_\beta \rangle = 1.15 > \langle P_\alpha \rangle = 1.07$ in agreement with the X-ray data. Since B1–7 also has α potential, it is not surprising that this region was found to be helical in 4-Zn insulin in 6% NaCl.[25] Thus, by computing $\langle P_\alpha \rangle$ and $\langle P_\beta \rangle$ values for the α and β segments in proteins, one may elucidate the regions potentially capable of undergoing conformational change.

The prediction of the conformation of *glucagon,* a hormone containing 29 amino acid residues, offers an excellent example of the potential of the method. Utilizing the conformational parameters for helix, β sheet, β turns, and random coil, Chou and Fasman [26] predicted two conformational states for glucagon. They showed that the conformational sensitivity of glucagon may be due to residues 19–27, which have both α-helical potential ($\langle P_\alpha \rangle = 1.19$) as well as β-sheet potential ($\langle P_\beta \rangle = 1.25$). Thus, in predicted form (a), residues 5–10 with $\langle P_\beta \rangle = 1.08 > \langle P_\alpha \rangle = 0.86$ adopt a β conformation, while residues 19–27 form a helical region (31% α, 21% β). In predicted form (b) both regions, residues 5–10 and residues 19–27 are β sheets (0% α, 52% β). Circular dichroism studies [27] of glucagon solutions (12.6 mg/ml) yield 33% α and 20% β, supportive of form (a). Infrared studies of glucagon gels and fibrils [28, 29] show a predominant β conformation, consistent with form (b). In addition, three reverse β turns were predicted at 2–5, 10–13, and 15–18, suggesting this small polypeptide has the potential to fold into a relatively compact structure. Thus, it appears that glucagon has different α and β conformations under different concentration conditions. Hence, residues 19–27 may be involved in an $\alpha \rightarrow \beta$ transition.

The *in vivo* concentration is probably too small to elicit the β conformation, but this conformational state may be induced upon binding of glucagon to its receptor site. As the conformational state of region 19–27 is sensitively balanced between α and β states, it is predicted that replacement of one or more residues of high β potential in this region with strong α formers would lock the conformation in the helical state. If this hypothesis for receptor binding is correct, namely, the necessity of the β structure, then this homolog of glucagon would be biologically inactive as a result of its inability to bind. It is also feasible to lock the β conformation by suitable substitutions. Thus, the predictive scheme offers a working hypothesis whereby the structure of the biologically active hormone may be arrived at. The $\alpha \rightarrow \beta$ transition of glucagon in solution has recently been followed by means of circular dichroism,[30] providing evidence for the potential conformational change predicted.

The conformational parameters P_α, P_β, and P_t (TABLE 1) are expedient for detecting regions in proteins with potential for *conformational changes due to mutations or changes in solvent conditions.* The *lac* repressor–*lac* operator interaction of *Escherichia coli* provides an excellent example of the specificity of protein binding to DNA.[31] The amino acid sequence of the *lac* repressor, a polypeptide subunit containing 347 amino acid residues has been determined.

Its secondary structure was predicted to contain 37% α helix and 35% β sheet while the trypsin-resistant core (residues 60 to 327) has 29% helix and 41% β sheet.[32] The extensive β sheets predicted in the 215–324 region may be responsible for tetramer stabilization found in both the *lac* repressor and the core. These β sheets are almost devoid of charge and would have an extremely hydrophobic nucleus. There are 23 predicted β turns in the *lac* repressor, made up of 50% charged and polar residues (serine and threonine) that would be found on the surface, conferring solubility.

Examination of five *lac* repressor mutants yields significant information regarding conformational requirements for repressor function. Mutant AP46 has an Ala[53] → Val[53] replacement and a loss of repressor activity, causing a predicted $\alpha \to \beta$ transition at residues 52–57. Several amber mutants at Gln[26] (Leu, Ser, Tyr) still cause repression and no conformational change is predicted. In mutant AP309 a Ser[16] → Pro[16] change is incurred with loss of biological activity and a predicted β turn at 14–17 is lost by this mutation. Thus, in these examples it is possible to correlate biological activity with definite secondary structures, and the loss of activity upon the induction of a conformational change brought about by a mutation.

Sickle-cell hemoglobin (Hb S) differs from normal adult hemoglobin (Hb A) in that there is a Glu[6] → Val[6] mutation in both β chains.[33] This mutation causes aggregation of Hb S inside the erythrocyte upon deoxygenation, resulting in the sickling phenomenon. The possible conformational consequence of this mutation has been predicted.[34] The region at the N-terminus of the β chains of Hb A, residues 1–6, has $\langle P_\alpha \rangle = 1.03 > \langle P_\beta \rangle = 0.99$ indicating α-helical potential and unfavorable β-sheet formation. However, the β-chain Glu[6] → Val[6] mutation involves not only the replacement of a charged polar residue by an uncharged hydrophobic residue, but more importantly it causes a drastic increase in the β-sheet potential. This region now has $\langle P_\beta \rangle = 1.21 > \langle P_\alpha \rangle = 0.96$. Hence, a single amino acid replacement could disrupt the first turn (residues 4–6) of the α helix and convert the 1–6 region into a β sheet. These β regions may be responsible for the aggregation phenomena found in Hb S.

The enthusiastic response to the predictive model of Chou and Fasman[9, 10] is evident by the numerous citations in the literature showing increasing usage of the method.[35] By means of this formulation, the coenzyme-binding domains of glutamate dehydrogenases were located with the aid of homologous sequence comparisons,[36] a model of the fd gene 5 DNA-binding protein was proposed as two long β sheets,[37] and a three-dimensional structure of proinsulin was constructed.[38] Durham and Butler[39] were gratified that the predicted secondary structure of tobacco mosaic virus fitted well with other data based on low resolution X-ray results as well as immunological and chemical evidence. Using the P_α, P_β, and P_c conformational parameters, Parry[40] showed that α-tropomyosin is almost 100% α-helical with possible nonhelical regions confined to the N- and/or C-terminals. He also noted that short portions of the amino acid sequence with low helical potential show a well-defined 40-residue period. The predictive method was also extensively applied to indicate the predominant α and β regions in many of the ribosomal proteins sequenced in Wittmann's laboratory (References 41, 42, and references therein). Experimental studies showed a correlation of the helical forming potential of synthetic ribonuclease-S (1–20) peptides with binding to the S-protein.[43] The helical residue Glu 9 of ribonuclease S-peptide was replaced by Leu and Gly. While the binding affinity of the Leu S-peptide to S-protein is only a factor of three less than that for RNase-S (1–20), that for the Gly peptide is about 20-fold less. The stronger binding of the Leu peptide than the Gly peptide corresponds to the higher helical potential of Leu ($P_\alpha = 1.34$) than Gly ($P_\alpha = 0.53$), so that the Leu peptide has the greater tendency to adopt the helical conformation, which is a prerequisite for complex formation.

Other applications of the Chou-Fasman method include the elucidation of β-sheet and helical regions in the biotin subunit of transcarboxylase,[44] the proposal of an elongated antiparallel β-pleated sheet in the hypothalamic (cyclic) tetradecapeptide, somatostatin,[45] the identification of α, β, and β-turn regions in the epidermal growth factor,[46] and the correlation of the predicted conformation of hemerythrin with circular dichroism and X-ray data.[47] More extensive analysis was applied to predicting the conformation of the α_1-acid glycoprotein,[48] where it was found that the carbohydrate moiety of nine glycoproteins are situated predominately in β-turn regions.[49] Upon analysis of 30 phosphorylated sites in 14 different proteins, it was found that 80% were found to exist in regions predicted as β turns, usually on Ser or Thr.[50] By a combination of four predictive methods,[51] a tertiary model of plastocyanin was constructed, More recently, the Chou-Fasman model was successfully applied to elucidating the structure of staphylococcal enterotoxin B, showing excellent agreement between the predicted conformation (11% α, 34% β, 55% coil) and circular dichroism studies (9% α, 38% β, 53% coil),[52] In addition, the method was used to examine the effect of mutational amino acid replacements on the secondary structure predicted for glutamate dehydrogenase,[53] as well as to propose the NAD-domain of aldolase based on a complete secondary structural prediction of the enzyme.[54] Furthermore, the *prior* conformational prediction of triose phosphate isomerase (D. C. Phillips, personal communication) and fl bacteriophage coat protein (Tanford, personal communication) correlated well with *later* experimental data from X-ray crystallographic [16] and physical chemical measurements.[55] Using the Chou-Fasman method, Low *et al.*[17] predicted three β regions (2–6, 12–16, and 33–37) and two of the β turns, 18–21 and 47–50, in erabutoxin b in agreement with their X-ray analysis (observed β: 4–9, 12–14, and 34–40). Hence, the relative accuracy and simplicity of the Chou-Fasman method have resulted in its extensive use in predicting the conformation of biological macromolecules.

The *β-turn conformation* can now be predicted with the same degree of accuracy as the α-helical and β-sheet regions in proteins.[14] As mentioned above the three-dimensional structure of proinsulin has been predicted.[38] Examining the C-peptide sequence of 10 mammalian species showed a remarkable conservation of predicted conformation with a β turn at residues 15–18 flanked by two helices. Utilizing data from 29 proteins,[5] it has been shown that a high β-turn potential exists in the 12–17 region for this series and more importantly none outside of it.[76] Although no biological role has been assigned to the C-peptide, the present prediction shows that the β-turn conservation in proinsulin is probably necessary for directing the proper folding of C-peptide helices, which possibly masks the receptor binding region of the hormone thus making the precursor, proinsulin, inactive.

The importance of the β turn is also seen in the predicted structure of seven homologous proteinase inhibitors. There are only five other invariant residues, as well as six half-cystine residues (of approximately 60 residues), however, the β turns are conserved with onset at residues 12, 25, 37, and 41, as shown by X-ray studies for the bovine pancreatic trypsin inhibitor.[76]

Conformational homologies were elucidated in growth hormones,[56] immunoglobulins,[57] and the neurotoxins. Fifty-seven snake venom toxins were predicted and common distribution of secondary structure was detected throughout these toxins. The results also highlight the contrasts between short and long neurotoxins and cytotoxins.[58-60] The conformational parameters have also been used to deduce the probable polypeptide conformation on prebiotic earth,[61] to test structural convergence during protein evolution[62] and to construct genealogical trees.[63] Recent phytogenetic studies include rubredoxins[64] and muscular parvalbumins.[65]

Finally, the predictive method may suggest the *rational design of synthetic analogs* for experimental testing to see whether conservation or changes in conformation will produce alteration or retention of hormonal or enzymatic activity (for example, ribonuclease S-peptide,[43] proinsulin C-peptide,[66] secretin,[67, 68] and the region 75–120 of human growth hormone.[56]

The structure of the pentapeptide enkephalins was predicted as a β bend[69] and this has recently been shown by X-ray crystallography to be true in the solid state.[70] The synthesis of a model β turn was based on the predictive rules and the circular dichroism spectra of this conformation was obtained from this model compound.[71] It has been suggested, based on the predictive scheme, that the polypeptide secondary structure may direct the specificity of prohormone conversion.[72]

Comparisons of the various predictive methods have been published for adenylate kinase[73] and T4 phage lysozyme.[74] The prediction of lysozyme was severely criticized;[74] however, in a more recent publication,[75] at a 2.4-Å resolution, it has been found that the predictive method[9, 10] yielded results of 70% accuracy.

Although unquestionably the function of a protein depends on its unique three-dimensional structure, one may still learn much from the prediction of the secondary structure of proteins. Although it might be considered judicious to wait for a perfect predictive algorithm to be developed, the wealth of knowledge accumulated during the last decade regarding protein conformational prediction should be continually tested, refined, and applied. Although great caution should be exercised in the application of predictive models, it would be ultraconservative not to utilize this knowledge of secondary structure to aid our further understanding of protein conformation and biological activity. The prediction of secondary structures should not be an end in itself, but a means for furthering our understanding of protein conformation through synthetic analogs, corroborative experimental studies, sequence and conformational homology comparisons, and tertiary structure model building. Such an approach will hopefully provide great insight into the principles of protein folding.

Acknowledgment

The author expresses his appreciation to Dr. Peter Chou, a former collaborator who contributed royally to the development of the method.

References

1. Anfinsen, C. B., E. Haber, M. Sela & F. H. White, Jr. 1961. Proc. Natl. Acad. Sci. USA **47:**1309–1314.

2. LILJAS, A. & M. G. ROSSMAN. 1974. Ann. Rev. Biochem. **43:**475–507.
3. MATTHEWS, B. 1976. Ann. Rev. Phys. Chem. **27:**493–523.
4. DAYHOFF, M. O. 1972. Atlas of Protein Sequence and Structure, Vol. 5 (and Suppl. 1, 2, and 3; 1973, 1976, 1978). Natl. Biomed. Res. Found. Silver Spring, Md.
5. CHOU, P. Y. & G. D. FASMAN. 1978. Adv. Enzymol. **47:**45–148.
6. CHOU, P. Y. & G. D. FASMAN. 1978. Ann. Rev. Biochem. **47:**251–276.
7. LEVITT, M. & J. GREER. 1977. J. Mol. Biol. **114:**181–293.
8. GARNIER, J., D. J. OSGUTHORPE & B. ROBSON. 1978. J. Mol. Biol. **120:**97–120.
9. CHOU, P. Y. & G. D. FASMAN. 1974. Biochemistry **13:**211–222.
10. CHOU, P. Y. & G. D. FASMAN. 1974. Biochemistry **13:**222–245.
11. CHOU, P. Y. & G. D. FASMAN. 1977. Peptides. Proc. 5th Am. Peptide Symp. M. Goodman & J. Meienhofer, Eds., pp. 284–287. John Wiley & Sons, New York, N.Y.
12. VENKATHACHALAM, C. M. 1968. Biopolymers **6:**1425–1436.
13. CHOU, P. Y. & G. D. FASMAN. 1977. J. Mol. Biol. **115:**135–175.
14. CHOU, P. Y. & G. D. FASMAN. 1979. Biophys. J. **26:**367–384.
15. DURHAM, A. C. H. & P. J. G. BUTLER. 1975. Eur. J. Biochem. **53:**397–404.
16. BANNER, D. W., A. C. BLOOMER, G. A. PETSKO, D. C. PHILLIPS, C. I. POGSON, I. A. WILSON, P. H. CORRAN, A. J. FURTH, J. D. MILMAN, R. E. OFFORD, J. D. PRIDDLE & S. G. WALEY. 1975. Nature **255:**609–614.
17. LOW, B. W., H. S. PRESTON, A. SATO, L. S. ROSEN, J. E. SEARL, A. D. RUDKO & J. S. RICHARDSON. 1976. Proc. Natl. Acad. Sci. USA **73:**2991–2994.
18. OLSEN, K. W., D. MORAS, M. G. ROSSMANN & J. I. HARRIS. 1975. J. Biol. Chem. **250:**9313–9321.
19. MAVRIDIS, I. M. & A. TULINSKY. 1976. Biochemistry **15:**4410–4417.
20. EDELMAN, G. M., B. A. CUNNINGHAM, G. N. REEKE, JR., J. W. BECKER, M. J. WAXDAL & J. L. WANG. 1972. Proc. Natl. Acad. Sci. USA **69:**2580–2584.
21. HARDMAN, K. D. & C. F. AINSWORTH. 1972. Biochemistry **11:**4910–4919.
22. McCUBBIN, W. D., K. OIKAWA & C. M. KAY. 1971. Biochem. Biophys. Res. Commun. **43:**666–674.
23. SHOTTON, D. M. & H. C. WATSON. 1970. Nature **225:**811–816.
24. VISSER, L. & E. R. BLOUT. 1971. Biochemistry **10:**743–752.
25. BENTLEY, G., E. DODSON, G. DODSON, D. HODGKIN & D. MERCOLA. 1976. Nature **261:**166–168.
26. CHOU, P. Y. & G. D. FASMAN. 1975. Biochemistry **14:**2536–2541.
27. SRERE, P. A. & G. C. BROOKS. 1969. Arch. Biochem. Biophys. **129:**708–710.
28. GRATZER, W. B., E. BAILEY & G. H. BEAVEN. 1967. Biochem. Biophys. Res. Commun. **28:**914–919.
29. EPAND, R. M. 1971. Can. J. Biochem. **49:**166–169.
30. MORAN, E. C., P. Y. CHOU & G. D. FASMAN. 1977. Biochem. Biophys. Res. Commun. **77:**1300–1306.
31. BOURGEOIS, S. & M. PFAHL. 1976. Adv. Protein Chem. **30:**1–99.
32. CHOU, P. Y., A. J. ADLER & G. D. FASMAN. 1975. J. Mol. Biol. **96:**29–45.
33. INGRAM, V. M. 1959. Biochim. Biophys. Acta **36:**402–411.
34. CHOU, P. Y. 1974. Biochem. Biophys. Res. Commun. **61:**87–94.
35. Current Contents. 1976. **19**(8):5.
36. WOOTTON, J. C. 1974. Nature **252:**542–546.
37. ANDERSON, R. A., Y. NAKASHIMA & J. E. COLEMAN. 1975. Biochemistry **14:**907–917.
38. SNELL, C. R. & D. G. SMYTH. 1975. J. Biol. Chem. **250:**6291–6295.
39. DURHAM, A. C. H. & P. J. G. BUTLER. 1975. Eur. J. Biochem. **53:**397–404.
40. PARRY, D. A. D. 1975. J. Mol. Biol. **98:**519–535.
41. STADLER, H. 1974. FEBS Lett. **48:**114–116.
42. YAGUCHI, M. & H. G. WITTMANN. 1978. FEBS Lett. **88:**227–230.
43. DUNN, B. M. & I. M. CHAIKEN. 1975. J. Mol. Biol. **95:**497–511.
44. WOOD, H. G. & G. K. ZWOLINSKI. 1976. Crit. Rev. Biochem. **4:**47–122.

45. HOLLADAY, L. A. & D. PUETT. 1976. Proc. Natl. Acad. Sci. USA **73**:1199–1202.
46. HOLLADAY, L. A., C. R. SAVAGE, JR., S. COHEN & D. PUETT. 1976. Biochemistry **15**:2624–2633.
47. KLOTZ, I. M., G. L. KLIPPENSTEIN & W. A. HENDRICKSON. 1976. Science **192**:335–344.
48. AUBERT, J. P. & M. H. LOUCHEUX-LEFEBVRE. 1976. Arch. Biochem. Biophys. **175**:400–409.
49. AUBERT, J. P., G. BISERTE & M. H. LOUCHEUX-LEFEBVRE. 1976. Arch. Biochem. Biophys. **175**:410–418.
50. SMALL, D., P. Y. CHOU & G. D. FASMAN. 1977. Biochem. Biophys. Res. Commun. **79**:341–346.
51. WALLACE, D. G. 1976. Biophys. Chem. **4**:123–130.
52. MUNOS, P. A., J. R. WARREN & M. E. NOELKEN. 1976. Biochemistry **15**:4666–4671.
53. BRETT, M., G. K. CHAMBERS, A. A. HOLDER, J. R. S. FINCHAM & J. C. WOOTTON. 1976. J. Mol. Biol. **106**:1–22.
54. STELLWAGEN, E. 1976. J. Mol. Biol. **106**:903–911.
55. NOZAKI, Y., B. K. CHAMBERLAIN, R. E. WEBSTER & C. TANFORD. 1976. Nature **259**:335–337.
56. PENA, C., J. M. STEWART, A. C. PALADINI, J. M. DELLACHA & J. A. SANTOME. 1975. In Peptides: Chemistry, Structure, and Biology. R. Walter & J. Meienhofer, Eds. pp. 523–528. Ann Arbor: Ann Arbor Science Publishers.
57. LOW, T. L. K., Y. S. V. LIU & F. W. PUTNAM. 1976. Science **191**:390–392.
58. ETEROVIC, V. A. & P. A. FERCHMIN. 1977. Int. J. Peptide Prot. Res. **10**:245–251.
59. HSEU, T.-H., Y.-C. LIU, C. WANG, H. CHANG, D.-M. HWANG & C.-C. YANG. 1977. Biochemistry **16**:2999–3006.
60. DUFTON, M. J. & R. C. HIDER. 1977. J. Mol. Biol. **115**:177–193.
61. BRACK, A. & L. E. ORGEL. 1975. Nature **256**:383–387.
62. SALEMME, F. R., M. D. MILLER & S. R. JORDAN. 1977. Proc. Natl. Acad. Sci. USA **74**:2820–2824.
63. GOODMAN, M. & G. W. MOORE. 1977. J. Mol. Evol. **10**:7–47.
64. VOGEL, H., M. BRUSHI & J. LEGALL. 1977. J. Mol. Evol. **9**:111–119.
65. GOODMAN, M. & J. F. PECHERE. 1977. J. Mol. Evol. **9**:131–158.
66. VOGT, H. P., A. WOLLMER, V. K. NAITHANI & H. ZAHN. 1976. Hoppe-Seyler's Z. Physio. Chem. **357**:107–115.
67. FINK, M. L. & M. J. BODANSZKY. 1976. J. Am. Chem. Soc. **98**:974–977.
68. BODANSZKY, M. & M. L. FINK. 1976. Bioorg. Chem. **5**:257–282.
69. BRADBURY, A. D., D. G. SMYTH & C. R. SNELL. 1976. Nature **260**:165–166.
70. SMITH, G. D. & J. F. GRIFFIN. 1978. Science **199**:1214–1216.
71. KAWAI, M. & G. D. FASMAN. 1978. J. Am. Chem. Soc. **100**:3630–3632.
72. Geisow, M. J. 1978. FEBS Lett. **87**:111–114.
73. SCHULZ, G. E., C. D. BARRY, J. FRIEDMAN, P. Y. CHOU, G. D. FASMAN, A. V. FINKELSTEIN, V. I. LIM, O. B. PTITSYN, E. A. KABAT, T. T. WU, M. LEVITT, B. ROBSON & K. NAGANO. 1974. Nature **250**:140–142.
74. MATTHEWS, B. W. 1975. Biochim. Biophys. Acta **405**:442–451.
75. REMINGTON, S. J., W. F. ANDERSON, J. OWEN, L. F. T. EYCK, C. T. GRAINGER & B. W. MATTHEWS. 1978. J. Mol. Biol. **118**:81–98.
76. CHOU, P. Y. & G. D. FASMAN. 1979. Biophysical J. **26**:385–400.

DISCUSSION OF THE PAPER

DR. E. T. KAISER: In the case of the toxins where you are dealing with very small molecules, in some instances at least, if you start putting in all your disulphides and all your predictions, you almost have what amounts to an x-ray structure. How is the analysis of these structures coming along?

DR. G. D. FASMAN: I think there is something like 30 or 40 of these molecules that have been sequenced, if not more. People have made predictions of their secondary structure. They are often very similar. There are the two groups: the long and the short neurotoxins. These groups all seem to fit together very nicely by having the same secondary structure.

DR. KAISER: Where would you say are the greatest failures of the prediction likely to be?

DR. FASMAN: Well, I think that the more highly structured your protein is, the more accurate will be the prediction. A larger percentage of randomness seems to give you a poorer result.

DR. J. A. REYNOLDS: Dr. Fasman, a criticism has often been raised against these predictions, and I do not happen to agree with it. Namely, can you apply them to intrinsic membrane proteins?

DR. FASMAN: At first I was very hesitant to apply our analyses to such proteins but then if you look at a globular protein and its interior, the polypeptides are really surrounded by very hydrophobic environment; if you look at a membrane from that point of view, they contain representative hydrophobic centers of a globular protein. With this concept, I think that one can apply our analysis to that situation.

DR. F. R. LANDSBERGER: I wonder if I can ask you to speculate a little bit on the signal sequence data that you talked about earlier. One of the components of the hypothesis is that there is probably a channel in the membrane through which the signal sequence is threaded. You indicated two examples, one of them is, if I recall correctly, an α helix and the other one is a β pleated sheet; so, what would the properties be of the protein along the channel?

DR. FASMAN: This is pure speculation, but what seems to be the unifying principle here is that the section of the polypeptide chain that is inserted into the membrane has to be very hydrophobic. When you look at the different dimensions between the helix and the β pleated sheet, it appears to me that perhaps all the channels are not of the same thickness. Depending upon the thickness, the channel assumes different structures, nevertheless the portion that penetrates the membrane is hydrophobic and has often been calculated as α helical.

DR. J. B. SWANEY (*Einstein College of Medicine, Bronx, N.Y.*): Two questions. First, do you find that there is a variability of the probabilities depending upon which proteins you use? Second, have you tried a much easier model like Sheraga's model to calculate some of the structures one has had trouble with, like gramicydin.

DR. FASMAN: We have taken complete sets of proteins. For instance, we had a number of cytochromes and hemoglobins. We then looked at all the parameters and they did not change a bit. So we have tried to remove a whole group to see if this would affect the parameters and it did not seem to. When we went from 15 proteins to 29, there was only one amino acid that seemed to change significantly. That was methionine. I think the reason for that is that there were so few methionines in the proteins that we sampled. It is difficult to answer your second question as to which method is best. Everybody's method has its faults. I think one just has to try various methods and satisfy himself as to which one gives the best answer. You have to keep in mind that this is an empirical method.

DR. R. L. HEINRIKSON: First of all I would like to congratulate you on this method. It has been very useful in predicting not only lipoprotein structures but also as you know a great many other structures. You are modest to say everybody's method is the best.

I thought it might be interesting to comment on some things that we have been doing in the lab in this context. Protein evolution clearly seems to conserve tertiary structure more than primary sequence structure. We are interested in this subject because we are comparing tertiary structures of domains that have little similarity in sequence yet are almost equivalent in terms of their three-dimensional structures. We wondered whether secondary structure can introduce bias in the sequences because as you point out, the probabilities apply best to α helix segments. So, if we take these residues and make up the so-called Fasman pools, we can make up β pools, and α pools, and β turn pools and then select randomly from these pools to see what kind of a bias one would find using a minimum base change per code as a criterion where 1.5 is approximately the random. The values fall into the range of 1.4 to 1.5 where the turn pool is the most effective. In fact, the more you refine your pools in terms of 1, 2, 3, and 4, the more the bias is effective and gets down to values as low as 1.3. That goes into the gray area of sequence comparison even for sequences that are probably derived from common ancestors. We are exploring this in detail to try to find out what really is the level of statistical significance.

DR. FASMAN: We are quite surprised to find that in sequences that had less than 20% conservation of residues, those turns practically turn up at the same positions, so that your overall three-dimensional structure can be maintained for a tremendous variety of different amino acid sequences.

DR. A. R. TALL: I just want to follow up on something that I guess Dr. Kaiser was getting at and I would like to ask you how useful your method has been, particularly for proteins that were subsequently crystallized.

Your method is based on a rather minute sample of the total number of proteins that there are in nature and one would have to wonder whether it sufficiently accounts for the extreme variability that probably exists.

DR. FASMAN: Well, I have not kept a really accurate score, but I have received a considerable amount of correspondence from people who have used the predicted scheme and then later the crystallographers have come along with the structure. There have been some notable examples where the prediction has been absolutely terrible, but I think that on the whole they have been between 75% and 80% correct.

I think that one of the reasons why this method maintains this percentage is that if we dissect a polypeptide chain into a number of segments, the segments do not maintain the same structure as they had in the native protein. This tells you that there is some conformational stability acquired through the interaction of the various segments. In consequence, often there is an increase of the helical contents of protein.

DR. W. A. BRADLEY: I guess you almost answered my question. The rules are based on relatively large globular proteins. Today, I think we will hear a number of discussions on model polypeptides that are relatively small. I was glad to see that the predictability applies to peptides as low as 29 residues. The question is would these rules apply to peptides of around 20 residues?

DR. FASMAN: Well, the smallest one that has been predicted is an enkephalin (five residues). That was predicted as a β turn and that is what was found by X-ray crystallography. I think, however, that one should not falsely gain too much confidence since when you predict a pentapeptide or something of that size all it tells you is that under a certain set of environmental conditions it can fold into that structure. That does not mean that that is the structure of that peptide in aqueous solutions. The environment of a small peptide chain is going to be terribly dependent upon the environment in which it finds itself. For instance, predictions about glucagon gives you just one of the several conformations that this peptide can take up and have a certain amount of stability.

DR. A. JONAS: Dr. Fasman, did you imply that in the case of the high concentrations of glucagon and hemoglobin the β pleated sheets that are not internally satisfied, become sticky points for protein interactions?

DR. FASMAN: Yes, that is what I was implying.

DR. JACKSON: In our initial discussion of the amphipathic helices it was clear that we could have very long helical segments. It seems from what you discussed today that the initiating point is very important and I wonder if you could comment on that aspect with regard to the active sites of proteins. Maybe it is not only the helical potential but also the first one, two, or three residues in that helix that can drive the reaction towards a helical segment.

DR. FASMAN: Well, what we did find by looking at any helical region in a protein it is that the highest probability of helix formation is always around the center of that region. This is why we decided to look at the nucleating center. I think that once the nucleation center is formed, other forces such as charge neutralization bring about stabilization of the secondary structure.

DR. JACKSON: I just wanted to say another thing. I do not believe that these predictions will say little as to where a nucleation site would be actually in a given solution. Would you comment on this?

DR. FASMAN: Well, you know that there are not much data on the kinetics of the folding of a protein at the time of synthesis. One says that it starts folding from the NH_2-terminus. I feel personally that you have to synthesize a certain length of a polypeptide chain and if that includes a nucleation center that chain will start folding up. In the case of lipoproteins, the conformation of the protein is going to change when it binds lipids. The only thing I can suggest in that case is to look at the various potentials, the various sections, so that you might see those areas that change their conformation as a function of environmental changes.

EFFECT OF APOLIPOPROTEIN A-II ON THE STRUCTURE OF HIGH-DENSITY LIPOPROTEINS: RELATIONSHIP TO THE ACTIVITY OF LECITHIN:CHOLESTEROL ACYL TRANSFERASE *IN VITRO* *

Angelo M. Scanu, Peter Lagocki,† and Jiwhey Chung

Departments of Medicine and Biochemistry
University of Chicago Pritzker School of Medicine
Chicago, Illinois 60637

INTRODUCTION

Although apolipoprotein A-I (apoA-I), a single 243 residue polypeptide (mol wt 28,171) is recognized to be the major apoprotein constituent of high-density lipoprotein (HDL), an additional major apoprotein, apoA-II, is found in the HDL of human subjects and nonhuman primates.[1-2] In human subjects [1] as well as in apes,[3] apoA-II is represented by two identical 77-residue chains (mol wt 8,500 each) linked together by a single disulfide bridge; in the non-human primates this chemical link is not present owing to the replacement of cysteine by serine in position 6 from the NH_2 terminus.[4] In the lower species, HDL has either no or insignificant amounts of apoA-II.[1, 3] In spite of these variations in apoprotein composition, the HDL particles of all of the animal species studied thus far have similar physico-chemical properties in terms of size and density. For instance, canine HDL, which has been rather extensively studied in this laboratory,[5] is relatively more homogeneous than its human counterpart with no evidence for the major HDL_2–HDL_3 subclasses described in the human subjects.

Another lipoprotein subspecies, HDL_1, which was first described by Mahley *et al.*[6] occurs only in very limited amounts in normolipidemic dogs. Since it does not represent a "true" HDL it will not be described here.

The notion that apoA-II only occurs in the HDL of higher animal species, raises the question of the general role of this polypeptide in HDL structure and function. In an attempt to shed some light on this problem we have been following several lines of approaches. In previous reports we have shown that when either apoA-I or apoA-II are exposed *in vitro* to the whole of the HDL lipids, the lipoprotein complexes that result are distinguishable in terms of size, density and degree of heterogeneity indicative of a difference in the intrinsic properties of these two apoproteins.[7] In the present studies we have examined the structural consequence of adding *in vitro* exogenous lipid-free, human apoA-II to HDL. As models we have chosen either canine HDL, a lipoprotein having about 97% of its protein moiety represented by apoA-I and no apoA-II,[5] or human HDL_3, known to contain apoA-I and apoA-II in addition to minor

* This work was supported by U.S. Public Health Service Grants HL-18577 and HL-15062.

† Predoctoral fellow under U.S. Public Health Service Training Grant 5T 32 HL 07237.

peptides.[1, 2] This account will summarize the properties of these HDL particles following their interaction with apoA-II and will also examine the capacity of these particles to serve as substrate for pure preparations of lecithin:cholesterol acyl transferase (LCAT) isolated from human plasma. Studies on artificial lecithin:cholesterol vesicles will also be presented. More detailed accounts of these studies are presented elsewhere.[8-10]

EXPERIMENTAL CONDITIONS

Canine HDL and lipid-free human apoA-II were incubated in various stoichiometric amounts at either 4° C or 23° C as a function of time.[11] The resulting products were resolved by density gradient ultracentrifugation and then characterized by physical and chemical means. In some experiments apoA-II was labeled with ^{125}I. Moreover, whenever indicated, a third component was added to the system, namely, mixed egg phosphatidylcholine(PC): cholesterol (molar ratio, 4:1) single bilayer vesicles in order to trap any lipid-free apoprotein present in the medium after the interaction between HDL and apoA-II had occurred. In the enzymatic studies, LCAT was isolated and purified from human plasma[9] and employed immediately after its isolation. In terms of substrate, mixed PC:cholesterol single bilayer vesicles containing various proportions of human apoA-I and apoA-II were prepared as previously described.[9] The addition of these apoproteins to the mixed vesicles had no appreciable effect on their geometry, at least until they had saturated the vesicle surface. Human HDL preparations of varying apoA-I:apoA-II ratios were also used as substrate; these particles were prepared by incubating at 23° C human HDL_3 with various amounts of lipid-free human apoA-II. As shown previously,[8, 11] under appropriate experimental conditions, apoA-II replaces progressively apoA-I at the HDL surface without loss of lipids to yield particles that contain increasing amounts of apoA-II. In some studies the HDL_2 and HDL_3 subclasses from normal subject and a patient with abetalipoproteinemia (ABL) were separated by rate zonal ultracentrifugation between densities of 1.0 and 1.4. For LCAT studies, these HDL particles or the mixed vesicles were equilibrated with [^{14}C]cholesterol. The enzymatic activity was followed for one hour at 37° C and was expressed in terms of cholesteryl ester production.[9]

RESULTS

Role of Apolipoprotein A-II in Modulating the Distribution of
A Apoproteins in HDL

Formation and Properties of Hybrids Resulting from the Interaction of Canine HDL and Human Apolipoprotein A-II.

In these studies variable amounts of human apoA-II were incubated with canine HDL in final apoA-II:HDL protein weight ratios ranging from 0.05 to 1.3 for one hour at 23° C in 0.15 M sodium bromide containing 0.05% EDTA, pH 8.0. Following incubation of the reactants, density gradient ultracentrifugation clearly resolved the HDL particles from the lipid-free apoproteins as indicated in a typical gradient shown in FIGURE 1. The results of the physico-

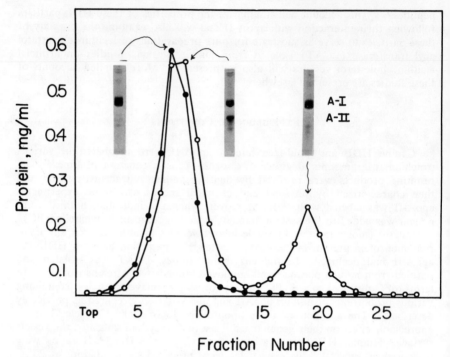

FIGURE 1. Density gradient ultracentrifugation of native canine HDL before
(●—●) and after (○—○) incubation with human apoA-II in the protein weight
ratio of apoA-II:HDL of 0.4. The incubation was carried out at 23° C in 0.15 M
NaBr containing 0.05% EDTA, pH 8.0 for one hour. The inset shows SDS polacryl-
amide gels of native canine HDL and fractions 9 and 19 from the gradient relative to
an HDL:apoA-II mixture.

chemical analyses of these products indicated that: (1) apoA-II displaced
apoA-I from HDL until all HDL particles contained essentially only apoA-II;
(2) per each molecule of apoA-I displaced there was an uptake by HDL of
two molecules of apoA-II, i.e., 28,000 per 34,000 daltons; (3) no lipid losses
occurred; in consequence, in spite of the slight increase in apoprotein mass, the
overall properties of the hybrid particles resembled those of the starting lipoprotein (TABLE 1).

The displacement reaction of apoA-I by apoA-II was found to be independent of temperature (4° C vs 23° C) and ionic strength ($\mu = 0.15$ to 3.0 M
NaBr) and to reach completion rapidly. A better definition of the time parameter was achieved by mixing first canine HDL and human apoA-II and then
adding, at various intervals, mixed PC:cholesterol (molar ratio 4:1) vesicles,
which in previous experiments we had shown to be able to take up both
apoA-I or apoA-II in predictable stoichiometric quantities.[9] In our current
system, the lipid vesicles, which could be readily separated from the other
components by density gradient ultracentrifugation, took up the apoA-I that
had been released from HDL as a consequence of the action of apoA-II. Of

interest, the latter exhibited a greater affinity for the HDL than for the vesicle surface.[11] By varying the time of addition of the mixed vesicles to the HDL-apoA-II system it was possible to determine that the uptake of apoA-II by HDL and thus the release of apoA-I occurred in less than one minute.

Products Formed From the Interaction Between Human HDL and Human Apolipoprotein A-II.

The addition of lipid-free human apoA-II to preparations of human HDL$_3$, resulted in the uptake of this apoprotein by the lipoprotein particle and a parallel release of apoA-I. Like the canine HDL-human apoA-II system, this process was attended by no loss of lipid and no substantial changes in the properties of the final particles. Thus, the addition of apoA-II afforded the production of human HDL particles that differed only in their apoA-I:apoA-II ratios.

Effect of Apolipoprotein A-II on the LCAT Reaction in Vitro

Mixed Lecithin:Cholesterol (4:1 Molar Ratio) Vesicles Used as a Substrate

Since a detailed account on these studies has appeared,[9] we will only summarize the data which are pertinent to this discussion. Vesicles when exposed to apoA-I, progressively take up this apoprotein to a maximum of 7–8 moles/vesicle. At this point these vesicles exhibit no changes in geometry and that portion of their surface that is unoccupied by the polar head group of phospholipids, can be calculated as being covered by 7–8 apoA-I molecules, if we consider the latter as total amphiphiles. The addition of lipid-free apoA-II to apoA-I laden vesicles leads to the displacement of apoA-I until the whole of the vesicle surface is replaced by apoA-II. Thus, by taking advantage of the

TABLE 1

COMPARATIVE CHEMICAL COMPOSITION AND PHYSICAL PARAMETERS OF
NATIVE CANINE HDL AND A REPRESENTATIVE HDL HYBRID CONTAINING
APPROXIMATELY 40% APOLIPOPROTEIN A-II BY WEIGHT

	HDL	
	Native	Hybrid
Composition (% by weight)		
Protein	40	40
Phospholipids	31	33
Cholesterol, unesterified	4	4
Cholesteryl esters	24	22
Triglycerides	1	1
Physical Parameters		
Electrophoretic mobility	α_1	α_1
Apparent molecular weight	214,000	219,000
Apparent partial specific volume	0.902	0.900
Buoyant density (g/ml)	1.12	1.12

greater affinity of apoA-II for the vesicle surface, it is possible to prepare, *in vitro,* vesicles that have comparable geometry and lipid composition but different apoA-I:apoA-II ratios. When these vesicles were tested as a substrate for LCAT, the LCAT activity was proportional to the number of apoA-I molecules in the vesicle. Vesicles containing only apoA-II did not affect LCAT activity; however, when apoA-II was added to the apoA-I-activated vesicles, the enzymatic reaction was inhibited via the displacement of apoA-I from the vesicle surface (FIGURE 2).

HDL with Varying Apolipoprotein A-I:A-II Ratios Used as a Substrate

The results of these studies were in keeping with those observed with the mixed lecithin:cholesterol vesicles, in that the LCAT activity was proportional to the content of apoA-I in HDL (FIGURE 3). Again apoA-II had no direct effect on the LCAT activity but caused inhibition of it by displacing apoA-I from the HDL surface.[10]

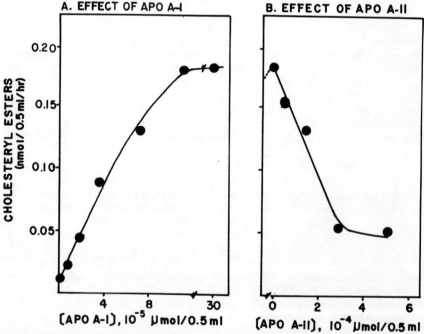

FIGURE 2. Effect of apoA-I and apoA-II on the activity of LCAT on mixed lecithin-cholesterol (molar ratio 4:1) single bilayer vesicles. (A) Effect of apoA-I. (B) Effect of apoA-II. In each case, substrate and apoA-I in concentration shown were incubated at 37° C for 30 minutes in the presence of 0.1 M sodium phosphate buffer, pH 7.1. The enzymatic reaction was initiated by adding 0.25 µg of lecithin:cholesterol acyltransferase (LCAT). In (B) apoA-II was added to apoA-I activated vesicles and the loss of enzymatic activity followed as a function of apoA-II added to the medium.

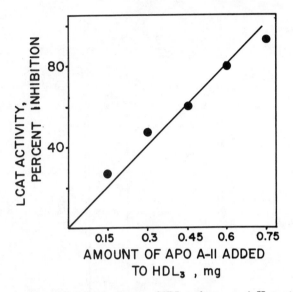

FIGURE 3. Action of LCAT in human HDL₃ whose apoA-II content had been modified by the addition of exogenous apoA-II. The enzymatic activity given in the ordinate was found to be proportional to the amount of apoA-II taken up by the human HDL₃ particle.

The Use of Naturally Occurring HDL with Differing Apolipoprotein A-I:A-II Ratios as a Substrate for LCAT

In the above studies the mixed vesicles or the HDL hybrids had the ratios of apoA-I:apoA-II modulated by the addition of exogenous lipid-free apoA-II. Since studies in this and other laboratories have shown that HDL particles differing in apoA-I:apoA-II ratios can be separated from the whole HDL class by density gradient ultracentrifugation [12] we have applied a previously described technique [13] to study the distribution of apoA-I and apoA-II within the whole of the lipoprotein profile. Two examples of typical ultracentrifugal runs applied to HDL from a normal human serum and a patient with abetalipoproteinemia (ABL) are presented in FIGURE 4 as continuous recordings of absorbance at 280 nm. In the normal serum two peaks corresponding to HDL₂ and HDL₃ are seen. In the ABL serum the HDL₂ peak is shifted towards a lower density and only a minor peak corresponding to HDL₃ is observed. Radioimmunoassay measurements indicated that within the peak area corresponding to HDL₂, the molar ratios of apoA-I:apoA-II in both normal and ABL serum were comparatively much higher than within the HDL₃ (TABLE 2). When representative samples from the HDL₂ and HDL₃ peaks were used as substrates for LCAT, the specimens with the highest apoA-I content and thus apoA-I:apoA-II ratios, were those that were the poorest substrate for LCAT as determined by the production of either cholesteryl esters or lysolecithin (TABLE 3). Therefore, the naturally occurring HDL particles, which, based on the *in vitro* displacement studies, we had anticipated to be most active as a substrate for LCAT, were

TABLE 2

MOLAR COMPOSITION OF HDL$_2$ AND HDL$_3$ SEPARATED BY DENSITY GRADIENT ULTRACENTRIFUGATION

Lipoprotein Subclass	Mol Wt 10^{-5}	ApoA-I	ApoA-II	Lecithin†	Cholesterol Unester.†	Cholesteryl Ester†	ApoA-I: ApoA-II Molar Ratio	Lecithin: ApoA-I Ratio	Lecithin: Unester. Cholesterol Molar Ratio
				(Moles/Mole Lipoprotein)					
HDL$_2$	4.1	4.9*	0.6	163.3	63.6	88.9	8.1	32	2.56
HDL$_3$	1.77	2.0	1.2	41.1	12.8	48.9	1.6	20	3.21

* Assuming that 90% of apoprotein is apoA-I (mol wt 28,000).
† Assuming that 78% of the total phospholipids is lecithin (mol wt 776). The molecular weights of cholesterol and cholesteryl esters are 387 and 650, respectively.

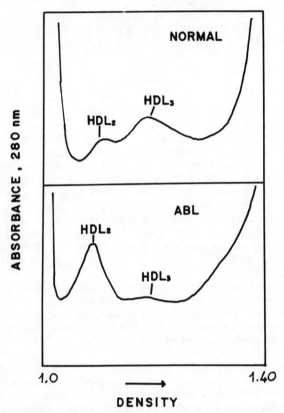

FIGURE 4. Density gradient ultracentrifugal profiles of HDL from a normal human serum (upper panel) and a serum from a patient with abetalipoproteinemia (lower panel).

TABLE 3

COMPARATIVE ACTIVITY OF LCAT ON HDL$_2$ AND HDL$_3$

Lipoprotein Class		LCAT Activity Cholesteryl Ester Produced %
Normal	HDL$_2$	3.2
	HDL$_3$	25.0
ABL	HDL$_2$	2.0
	HDL$_3$	17.4

instead those with the lowest activity. Obviously, these particles were struc-turally unsuited as LCAT substrate in spite of their relatively high content of apoA-I, the known LCAT activator.

DISCUSSION

The results of the studies outlined in this report indicate that the surface concentration of the two main A apolipoproteins can be regulated *in vitro* by the addition of exogenous lipid-free apoA-II to either HDL particles or artificial lipid vesicles. This process, which entails the preferential uptake of apoA-II and a concomitant displacement of apoA-I from these particles, appears to be dependent upon a higher affinity of apoA-II for the lipophilic-hydrophilic inter-face, this in turn an expression of a higher energy of stabilization of apoA-II at this interface. A remarkable feature of this process is that it is not attended by lipid losses. In addition it recognizes a precise stoichiometry, namely, the uptake-displacement reaction involves two molecules of apoA-II (total mass: 34,000 daltons) and one molecule of apoA-I (mass: ~28,000 daltons) and reaches completion so that at the end essentially all apoA-I molecules have been replaced by apoA-II.

From the measurement of the dissociation constants of apoA-I and apoA-II using single bilayer mixed PC:cholesterol vesicles we can estimate that the ΔG of association of two molecules of apoA-II with the interface is about twice that exhibited by a single molecule of apoA-I (ΔG assoc., apoA-I = -7.924 kcal/mole protein, apoA-II = -16.844 kcal/2 moles).

The fact that HDL or model vesicles can be induced to modify their surface concentration of the two main A apoproteins without significantly changing their physico-chemical properties invites comments on the relevance of this observation to the problem of HDL structure. Two main conclusions become apparent: in HDL there are neither strong interactions between apoA-I and apoA-II, nor between apoA-I and lipids. The data also suggest that both apoA-I and apoA-II occupy the same particle. All of these concepts are in keeping with our recent proposal [14, 15] in regard to a model of HDL structure which envisages this lipoprotein as being highly fluid, the major thermodynamic stabilization deriving from the hydrophobic boundary between the inner apolar portion of the surface monolayer surrounding the lipoprotein particle and the apolar surface of the core. According to this concept, the occupancy of apoA-I and apoA-II at the lipoprotein surface should be mainly dependent on the intrinsic structural properties of these apoproteins and particularly on their amphiphilic nature applied to both helical and nonhelical segments. The actual molecular basis for the ability of apoA-II to readily displace apoA-I and thus occupy the surface area previously occupied by the latter is unclear at this time. It is evident, however, that the process is the resultant of the differential be-havior of apoA-I and apoA-II in solution and at the hydrophilic-hydrophobic interface. For instance, it has been shown that, in solution, apoA-I is relatively more stable than apoA-II [1, 17] and that the opposite is true for the interface. Results at the air–water interface have shown that apoA-I, and in particular its monomer, is in equilibrium between the surface and the subphase and that this situation is likely to also apply between HDL and its aqueous environment.[18] In turn, apoA-II appears to prefer the interface, a fact which may explain why in biological fluids apoA-II is not found free in solution. From this knowledge we may infer that the exchange or transfer processes regulating the distribution of apoA-I or apoA-II among HDL particles recognize a different mechanism involving in the case of apoA-I a fluid step, and in the case of apoA-II a surface-to-surface collision reaction.

Our studies have also shown that the surface modulation of apoA-I and apoA-II has an important effect on the LCAT reaction, confirming the literature reports that apoA-I is the specific activator for LCAT.[1, 2] It is of interest that this dependence of LCAT activity on apoA-I was observed in mixed lecithin: cholesterol vesicles and HDL particles all having similar PC:cholesterol ratios ($\sim$4:1 molar ratio) and that there was no dependence on substrate size (diameters: vesicles $\sim$ 20 nm, HDL $\sim$ 10 nm). Therefore, in these lipid structures, their apoA-I:apoA-II ratio appeared to be a determining factor in LCAT activity. On the other hand this regulation does not seem to play a role in human HDL$_2$, which proved to be a poor substrate for LCAT. Literature data and previous work in this laboratory have shown that when either single bilayer vesicles or multilamellar liposomes are used as substrate, PC:cholesterol ratios and thus particle geometry influence markedly their response to LCAT action. For instance, vesicles with PC:cholesterol molar ratios below 3 do not serve as a good substrate for this enzyme (unpublished observations). If we now consider the molecular parameters of human HDL$_2$ as derived from the work of Anderson *et al.*[19] and our own laboratory (TABLE 2), based on an average mol wt of 4.2×10^5 for this lipoprotein one finds that the PC:cholesterol molar ratio is approximately 2.5. Thus, if the results of the vesicle studies could also apply to HDL, we may conclude that the PC:cholesterol organization of this lipoprotein is not suited for LCAT action in spite of this relatively high content in the specific LCAT activator, apoA-I. For instance, if one assumes that all PC and unesterified cholesterol are at the HDL$_2$ surface, the distance between each polar head group of PL and the hydroxyl function of cholesterol and/or their spatial orientation may not be suited for their interaction with LCAT and apoA-I. The ratio between apoA-I and PC molecules may also be an additional factor. This ratio was significantly higher in HDL$_2$ than in HDL$_3$ (TABLE 2). Moreover, the molar content of cholesteryl esters, one of the end products of the LCAT reaction was significantly higher in HDL$_2$ than HDL$_3$. Finally, the content and composition of minor peptides differ between HDL$_2$ and HDL$_3$ and there may be additional factors in determining the differential reactivity of these lipoproteins for LCAT.

CONCLUSIONS

Our present studies have shown that in HDL and artificial lipid vesicles wide variations of the contents of apoA-I and apoA-II can be induced by the addition of lipid-free apoA-II and that these variations have a profound effect on the LCAT activity. Although these *in vitro* data cannot be readily extrapolated to *in vivo* conditions, it is evident that factors such as particle surface potential, charge, chemical composition as well as the relative affinity of each apoprotein for the lipoprotein surface, can influence the physico-chemical and enzymatic processes that are involved in the interconversions among circulating lipoproteins. Studies directed at the definition of these factors both *in vitro* and *in vivo* are likely to provide a better understanding of the molecular basis of these interconversions and of lipoprotein metabolism in general.

ACKNOWLEDGMENTS

The authors wish to thank Mrs. Darla Abano for assistance in the performance of LCAT studies and Dr. B. W. Shen and Celina Edelstein for helpful discussions.

1. OSBORNE, J. C., JR. & H. B. BREWER. 1977. The plasma lipoproteins. Adv. Protein Chem. **31**:253–337.
2. SCANU, A. M., C. EDELSTEIN & P. KEIM. 1975. Serum lipoproteins. *In* The Plasma Proteins. F. W. Putnam, Ed. Vol. 1: 317–491. Academic Press, New York, N.Y.
3. SCANU, A. M. 1974. Apolipoprotein A-II: A protein of phylogenetic interest. PAABS Revista **4**:1–6.
4. EDELSTEIN, C., C. NOYES, R. HEINRIKSON, R. FELLOWS & A. M. SCANU. 1976. The covalent structure of apolipoprotein A-II from *Macaca Mulatta* serum high density lipoproteins. Biochemistry **15**:1262–1268.
5. EDELSTEIN, C., L. A. LEWIS, J. R. SHAINOFF & A. M. SCANU. 1976. Serum high density lipoproteins of normolipidemic dogs: A study of the *d* 1.063–1.21 g/ml particles. Biochemistry **15**:1934–1941.
6. MAHLEY, R. W. & K. H. WEISGRABER. 1974. Canine lipoproteins and atherosclerosis. I. Isolation and characterization of plasma lipoproteins from control dogs. Circ. res. **35**:713–721.
7. RITTER, M. & A. M. SCANU. 1979. Apolipoprotein A-II and structure of human high density lipoproteins: an approach by reassembly techniques. J. Biol. Chem. **254**:2517–2525.
8. LAGOCKI, P. & A. M. SCANU. 1978. *In vitro* hybrids of serum high density lipoproteins (HDL): displacement of apolipoprotein A-I (apo A-I) from canine HDL by human apolipoprotein A-II (apo A-II). Fed. Proc. **37**:1481.
9. CHUNG, J., D. A. ABANO, G. M. FLESS & A. M. SCANU. 1979. Isolation, properties, and mechanism of *in vitro* action of lecithin:cholesterol acyltransferase from human plasma. J. Biol. Chem. **254**:7456–7464.
10. CHUNG, J., P. LAGOCKI, D. ABANO & A. M. SCANU. 1979. Activity *in vitro* of lecithin-cholesterol acyltransferase (LCAT) in high density lipoproteins (HDL) of varying apo A-I:apo A-II ratios. Circulation. In press.
11. LAGOCKI, P. & A. M. SCANU. 1980. *In vitro* modification of the apoprotein composition of high density lipoprotein by lipid-free apoprotein A-II. Displacement of apoprotein A-I from the HDL surface by apoprotein apo A-II. J. Biol. Chem. In press.
12. CHUNG, M. C. & J. J. ALBERS. 1979. Distribution of cholesterol and apolipoprotein A-I and A-II in human high density lipoprotein sub-fractions separated by CsCl equilibrium gradient centrifugation: Evidence for HDL subpopulations with different A-I/A-II molar ratios. J. Lipid Res. **20**:200–207.
13. FOREMAN, J. R., J. B. KARLIN, C. EDELSTEIN, D. J. JUHN, A. H. RUBENSTEIN & A. M. SCANU. 1977. Fractionation of human serum lipoproteins in single-spin gradient ultracentrifugation: quantitation of apolipoprotein B and A-I and lipid components. J. Lipid Res. **18**:759–767.
14. SHEN, B. W., A. M. SCANU & F. J. KÉZDY. 1977. The structure of human serum lipoproteins inferred from compositional analysis. Proc. Natl. Acad. Sci. USA **74**:837–841.
15. SCANU, A. 1978. Ultrastructure of serum high density lipoproteins facts and models. Lipids **13**:920–925.
16. EDELSTEIN, C., F. J. KÉZDY, A. M. SCANU & B. W. SHEN. 1979. Apolipoproteins and the structural organization of plasma lipoproteins:human plasma high density lipoprotein-3. J. Lipid Res. **20**:143–153.

17. REYNOLDS, J. A. 1976. Conformational stability of the polypeptide components of human high density serum lipoprotein. J. Biol. Chem. **251**:6013–6015.
18. SHEN, B. & A. M. SCANU. Properties of human serum apolipoprotein A-I at the air-water interface. Biochemistry. Submitted.
19. ANDERSON, D. W., A. V. NICHOLS, T. M. FORTE & F. T. LINDGREN. 1977. Particle distribution of human serum high density lipoproteins. Biochem. Biophys. Acta **493**:55–68.
20. SHEN, B. W. Unpublished observations.

DISCUSSION OF THE PAPER

DR. EISENBERG: Those are fascinating studies. I would like to supplement your data with results of studies that we carried out in Houston.

We have consistently observed that under sudden situations where we generate a lot of C apoproteins from the lipolysis of VLDL, we end up with the displacement predominantly of A-I from HDL_3. What we really observed is that when apoA-I is really displaced from HDL_3, we found it in the bottom fraction. ApoA-II is largely retained in HDL_3. So this process is specific for apoA-I, where C apoproteins replace apoA-I accompanied by a structural transformation of the HDL particle. Inasmuch as this is a brittle system, we are observing a biological reaction, as an *in vitro* biological reaction.

My question is, you mentioned that you did look into displacement of apoA-I by apoC apoproteins. I want to know if you have any data on this? Also, does anything happen to apoA-II in this situation?

DR. A. M. SCANU: We have made a preliminary observation on it but we have not carried out detailed studies although we plan to do so.

DR. R. L. JACKSON: In your experiments where you add apoA-II to an apoA-I vesicle complex. Does the vesicle break down when you add apoA-II?

DR. SCANU: No, and we spent a lot of time in demonstrating this, including the use of radioactive labels such as [^{14}C]sucrose. Some of this work has recently been published in the *Journal of Biological Chemistry*.

DR. JACKSON: My other question is, in your experiments where you have cholesterol in your PC vesicles, does the apoprotein actually bind to that? The enzymatic activity is decreased as more cholesterol is added, but does the enzyme actually bind to those substrates?

DR. SCANU: We have not addressed ourselves directly to the question of LCAT binding to the vesicles. There is a recent paper, however, by T. Nishida of the University of Illinois. Apparently LCAT binds to the vesicles. The actual mechanisms of LCAT action are under intensive pursuit at our Institution.

DR. JACKSON: By the same token you can increase the cholesterol content of HDL, as described by Dr. Jonas, to show whether or not that inhibits the enzyme activity?

DR. SCANU: We have not done so in HDL, but we have carried out experiments with vesicles in which, as shown by others, the lecithin:cholesterol ratio appears to be crucial for enzymatic activity. In our system a lecithin:cholesterol 4:1 molar ratio appears to be optimal. But as you raise the cholesterol content in the vesicles, the enzymatic activity decreases. We like to believe that this is one of the reasons why HDL_2 is not an ideal substrate for LCAT.

DR. V. LUZZATI: When you have this hybrid population of canine HDL and human apoA-II, is this population homogeneous? I am presuming that the particles you are starting with are homogeneous; i.e., they contain the same number of apoA-I molecules.

DR. SCANU: The answer is yes at the end of the reaction when the three apoA-I that are estimated to be contained in canine HDL are replaced by six apoA-II molecules (MW ~17,500).

DR. LUZZATI: I understand that. But in between, you probably have a mixed particles population, do you have any data on this?

DR. SCANU: I cannot answer that question. In other words, when apoA-II is added below what we may call surface saturation of apoA-I, we do not know whether all HDL will have the same apoA-I:apoA-II ratio. In spite of this, we do have particle homogeneity in physical terms; that is, all exhibit homogeneous behavior in the analytical ultracentrifuge.

DR. LUZZATI: The reason why I am asking this question is because, from the structural viewpoint, objects like HDL are of great interest since you have a very small number of proteins. What can keep those particles together? We may think of a three-fold symmetry, in that particle. That is why I am a little uneasy when you look at these hybrid particles with different apoA-I:apoA-II ratios. If we could study these hybrids, they will be likely to show different types of symmetry.

DR. SCANU: What really struck us most is the precise stoichiometric replacement of apoA-I by apoA-II. This kind of precise substitution appears to say that the space occupied by one apoprotein was taken up by the other, involving about the same number of amino acids yet of two different proteins. In other words, the degree of occupancy of the HDL surface by the apoprotein has been respected. On the other hand, we do not know what one means by surface. The shell surrounding the HDL particle would have an inner and outer surface. How deep each apoprotein penetrates this layer we do not know. I do know, Dr. Luzzati, that you conceive HDL as having an undulated surface and I do not know whether this also applies to canine HDL. What impresses me about the system is the fact that it is more homogeneous than human HDL and is of interest to further structural pursuits.

DR. A. R. TALL: In your studies of LCAT activity versus cholesterol:phospholipid ratios in the vesicles, the activity goes up pretty sharply between molar ratios of about 0.2 and 0.3. This is also the approximate molarity of cholesterol which inhibits the breakdown of vesicles into apoA-I. I wonder if the change in LCAT between 0.2 and 0.3 is in fact a reflection of changes in the binding of A-I to vesicles.

DR. SCANU: According to the data by Wang, in those molar concentrations of cholesterol the vesicle geometry does not change significantly. We did not carry out a systematic study on the binding of apoA-I as a function of cholesterol concentration, but I suspect that the inhibitory effect of cholesterol on LCAT activity may recognize a more complex interpretation than simple vesicle binding by apoA-I.

DR. TALL: The other thing that I wanted to ask you about was in your density gradients of the human HDL and the abeta HDL you mentioned in passing I guess that you saw a greater variety of subclasses as those described by the Donner Laboratory dependent on how you prepared the sample. I just wondered if you could give more details on this.

DR. SCANU: This work is really in progress. As you probably noted, our gradients provided very broad HDL_2 and HDL_3 subfractions, which I think relates to heterogeneity. These observations are being pursued. The only point I wanted to make in this presentation is the subclass that we can broadly define as HDL_2 does not seem to represent a good substrate for LCAT.

DR. J. A. HUNTER (*University of California, Berkeley, Calif*): The exchange of apoA-II for apoA-I on the lipoprotein particles seems like a mass action. I was wondering if you looked at the displacement of apoA-II by apoA-I and the energetics of that reaction. My second comment is that I am somewhat surprised in the difference in phospholipid:cholesterol ratios between HDL_2 and HDL_3, given a lot of the literature data on the exchange of cholesterol between these lipoproteins.

DR. SCANU: I would like first to say that we cannot displace apoA-II by apoA-I. This is true for HDL_3 and mixed lecithin:cholesterol single bilayer vesicles. In regard to the displacement of apoA-I by apoA-II, I do not believe that we are dealing with a mass action phenomenon, but rather with relative affinities of apoA-I and apoA-II for the interface. This interpretation appears to be supported by studies at the air–water interface. In our calculations of free energy we made the assumption that we could extrapolate binding data from our own vesicle studies. Thus, our values must be considered as tentative only. In regard to our phospholipid:cholesterol ratios in HDL_2 and HDL_3 this is what we obtained in narrow cuts from those gradients since each of these subfractions appears to be heterogeneous. The final point I would like to make may not be strictly related to my presentation but does reflect on the importance of apoA-I:apoA-II ratios on the HDL surface. In work done with Dr. Mary Ritter, we have observed that when HDL is exposed to blood granulocytes *in vitro* in the absence of the bottom fraction, apoprotein hydrolysis occurs and this involves apoA-II most specifically. The same phenomenon has been shown by the Shores to occur when HDL is passed through a column where you have immobilized a proteolytic enzyme. It thus may be possible that the modulation of apoA-I:apoA-II ratios that we can induce *in vitro,* may have some biological implications as well.

BINDING STUDIES WITH APOLIPOPROTEINS

Jacqueline A. Reynolds

*Whitehead Medical Research Institute
and Department of Biochemistry
Duke University Medical Center
Durham, North Carolina 27710*

In June 1971 the New York Academy of Sciences sponsored a conference on biological membranes organized by Dr. David E. Green. Some of the participants present today also attended that meeting and may recall the following brief exchange.[1]

> D. E. GREEN: I had hoped you would come to grips with the question why one kind of protein interacts with phospholipid to form a membrane and another kind of protein interacts with phospholipid to form a highly dispersed lipoprotein. The bonding in both cases appears to be hydrophobic. Can you provide some basis for this distinction between membrane-forming proteins and lipoprotein(forming proteins?
>
> A. SCANU: I am not sure that I am in a position of providing a meaningful answer to your question. At present we do not have sufficient information on the nature of the proteins in membranes and circulating lipoproteins to allow for a careful comparison of their properties.

Eight years ago it was not possible to speculate on this subject. The enormous progress that has been made in the ensuing years is evidenced by the papers presented at this conference. Amino acid sequences have appeared for a number of membrane-bound proteins and apolipoproteins.[2] Solution properties of the individual components of the serum lipoproteins have been investigated in detail by a number of researchers.[2] The interactions among these components are beginning to be understood as is the dynamic nature of the serum lipoproteins *in vivo*.

This paper will summarize the results of studies designed to answer the question raised not only by Dr. Green, but by a number of us who were intrigued by the enormous solubilizing power of the serum apolipoproteins. We have used the rationale that a complex system is best understood by reducing it to a series of simpler systems. Ultimately, these reductions must be synthesized into the complete system to provide a thermodynamic and structural description.

I will address two of the reduced systems, summarizing briefly (1) the relevant properties of the apolipoproteins A-I, A-II, and B, in the absence of bound ligand and (2) the results of thermodynamic investigations of the interactions of these apoproteins with amphiphilic ligands containing normal alkyl chains. An underlying philosophy in these studies is that appropriate simple amphiphiles (such as detergents) can displace lipid without disruption of the native conformation since these compounds are capable of simulating the native hydrophobic environment.

SUMMARY OF THE RELEVANT PROPERTIES OF APOLIPOPROTEINS
A-I, A-II, AND B IN AQUEOUS SOLUTION IN THE ABSENCE OF
AMPHIPHILIC LIGANDS

The apoproteins from HDL, A-I and A-II, are water soluble in the absence
of bound amphiphiles. Investigations in a number of different laboratories
using different experimental approaches have demonstrated that these polypeptides possess a number of accessible conformational states that differ little
in free energy.[2, 3] These states are readily interconvertible and this conformational adaptability is undoubtedly important to the physiological function of
varying lipid composition as the HDL particles pass through the vascular system.

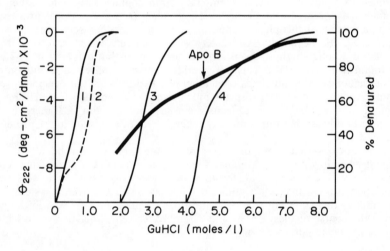

1. A II
2. A I
3. Polar Fragment of Cytochrome b5
4. Hydrophobic Fragment of Cytochrome b5

FIGURE 1. Guanidine hydrochloride denaturation of apolipoprotein A-I, A-II, B,
hydrophilic domain of cytochrome b5, and hydrophobic domain of cytochrome b5.

Apolipoprotein B from LDL displays quite different properties. It is soluble
only when amphiphilic ligands are bound or in high concentrations of guanidinum chloride (GuHCl).[2, 4] Preliminary studies on structural alterations as a
result of reduced ligand binding or denaturant concentration suggest that this
polypeptide forms a β-pleated sheet secondary structure when removed from
its native hydrophobic environment leading to irreversible aggregation.

FIGURE 1 demonstrates clearly one of the major differences between these
two classes of core proteins. The transition to random coil form is shown as a
function of GuHCl concentration for A-I, A-II, and B. Apolipoproteins A-I
and A-II undergo a highly cooperative transition at extremely low concentrations of denaturant. Apolipoprotein B does not show a cooperative transition,

but rather behaves as though it consists of independent regions of differing susceptibility such as would be expected if the primary sequence contained several groups of hydrophobic residues separated in space from the hydrophilic amino acids. For comparison, the denaturation curves of the water-soluble domain of cytochrome b5 and its hydrophobic anchor are included. Note the much higher GuHCl concentration required for conversion of this latter peptide to a random coil. In general, intrinsic membrane proteins that have been investigated exhibit broad denaturation curves in this solvent and resistance of the hydrophobic domains to conversion to a random coil.[5, 6]

Both A-I and A-II self-associate through hydrophobic interactions in the absence of bound amphiphile.[2] This observation is not in itself surprising since one would intuitively expect that hydrophobic regions on the protein normally occupied by lipids will remove themselves from contact with water either by intramolecular reorganization or intermolecular (self-association) processes. The relationship of this phenomenon to an *in vivo* state has been greatly over-emphasized. For example, A-I undergoes a relatively weak, reversible self-association to oligomeric states as large as an octamer, but octamers of A-I are not found in native HDL. This polypeptide is readily converted to monomers by interaction with amphiphiles containing one hydrophobic tail per polar head group. Apolipoprotein A-II displays much stronger association to a tetrameric form (mol wt: 34,800) in aqueous solutions, but as with A-I there is no evidence to suggest that this is directly related to an *in vivo* state in the presence of bound lipid.

It is obvious that these protein–protein interactions must be taken into account when investigating protein–amphiphile interactions. Experimental constraints may force the investigator to work under conditions where this self-association process makes a significant contribution to the overall system, but it is unlikely that sufficient free concentrations of either protein exist in the cell during the course of biosynthesis and assembly for self-association of this kind to be of *in vivo* importance.

SUMMARY OF THE INTERACTION PROPERTIES OF APOLIPOPROTEINS A-I, A-II, AND B WITH AMPHIPHILIC LIGANDS

A major research goal of the past few years has been to elucidate the difference in amphiphile binding properties among water-soluble proteins, apolipoproteins, and intrinsic membrane proteins. This problem has been approached by means of thermodynamic binding studies, which provide information as to (1) total number of binding sites, (2) energy of interaction, and (3) mode of interaction. One measures bound ligand as a function of increasing concentrations of unbound ligand and must demonstrate unequivocally the reversibility of the system because theoretical relations used apply only if the system is truly at equilibrium at all points on the binding isotherm. The total number of sites is seen as a plateau region at the highest unbound ligand concentrations. Energies of interaction can often be obtained from appropriate mathematical treatment of the data set. The mode of interaction is a particularly informative piece of information which can be obtained only when binding ratios have been measured over a wide range of unbound ligand concentrations.

Some proteins contain independent and identical binding sites, in which case the molar binding ratio is a hyperbolic function of free ligand concentration and this ratio increases from 10% to 90% saturation over a two-order-of-magnitude change in free ligand concentration. Only a very small number of water-soluble proteins have interaction sites of this type for amphiphilic ligands.[7]

It is also possible for ligands to bind cooperatively, i.e., the binding of one molecule facilitates the binding of the next. In this case, the binding ratio increases more steeply with increasing free ligand concentration since it is a higher order power function of the unbound ligand concentration. The formation of micelles and lipid bilayers are examples of a cooperative process. Similarly, membrane proteins containing hydrophobic domains bind amphiphiles in a cooperative manner at or near the critical micelle concentration of the ligand. This phenomenon resembles mixed micelle formation in that the membrane proteins do not significantly perturb the aggregation number of the pure amphiphilic ligand.[8]

Apolipoproteins A-I and A-II are quite different from both water-soluble proteins and intrinsic membrane proteins. Interaction with amphiphiles containing single hydrocarbon chains is described for these two proteins by the following sets of equations.[9-12] For A-I the equations are:

$$2(A\text{-}I) \rightleftharpoons (A\text{-}I)_2, \tag{1a}$$

$$\sum_{i=0}^{3} \{(A\text{-}I)L_i + L \rightleftharpoons {}^*(A\text{-}I)L_{i+1}\}, \tag{1b}$$

$${}^*(A\text{-}I)L_4 + mL \rightleftharpoons {}^*(A\text{-}I)L_{m+4}. \tag{1c}$$

1. All binding occurs below the CMC of the amphiphile.
2. AI contains four identical and independent sites in the monomeric form with maximum association constants of approximately 10^6 liter/mole (6 kcal/mol) for n-alkyl chains equal to or greater than 16 carbons. This process is described by Equation 1b above.
3. Binding to these sites promotes dissociation to the monomeric state and a conformational change.
4. Subsequent to this site occupancy, A-I binds amphiphilic ligands cooperatively with a maximal binding capacity of about 24,000 cm³ of hydrophobic volume.

For A-II the equations are:

$$2(A\text{-}II) \rightleftharpoons (A\text{-}II)_2, \tag{2a}$$

$$\sum_{i=0}^{n} \{(A\text{-}II)_2 L_i + L \rightleftharpoons {}^*(A\text{-}II)_2 L_{i+1}\}, \tag{2b}$$

$${}^*(A\text{-}II)_2 L_j + mL \rightleftharpoons 2{}^*(A\text{-}II)L_{m+j/2}. \tag{2c}$$

1. Binding occurs below the CMC of the amphiphile.
2. The tetrameric form of A-II (mol wt: 34,800) contains a set of independent and identical binding sites the occupancy of which leads to a conformational change. This is described by Equation 2b above.
3. Subsequent cooperative binding leads to dissociation of A-II to the dimeric form (mol wt 17,400).

4. A-II binds maximally approximately 15,000 cm³/mole of hydrophobic volume regardless of the polar head group of the amphiphilic ligand.

Since the independent sites on A-I must be occupied to induce the conformational change required for cooperative binding and since the free energy of this process cannot exceed about 6 kcal/mol, one would not expect A-I to interact with diacyl lipids which have free energies of self-association greater than 11 kcal/mol. Nichols,[13] Brewer,[14] and our own laboratory[15] have demonstrated that this is indeed the case. Cooperative binding of diacyl phospholipids to A-I occurs only when the independent sites have been filled by interaction with single tail amphiphiles which have higher monomer concentrations than their diacyl counterparts. The following equations describe the interaction between A-I and didecanoyl phosphatidylcholine.

$$2(\text{A-I}) \rightleftharpoons (\text{A-I})_2, \tag{3a}$$

$$\sum_{i=0}^{4} \{(\text{A-I})\,\text{B}_i + \text{B} \rightleftharpoons {}^*(\text{A-I})\,\text{B}_{i+1}\}, \tag{3b}$$

$$2^*(\text{A-I})\,\text{B}_j + m\text{L} \rightleftharpoons {}^*(\text{A-I})_2\text{B}_{2j}\text{L}_m. \tag{3c}$$

In these equations, B represents a single tail amphiphile binding to independent and identical sites and L represents the diacyl lipid. A particularly important observation resulting from this investigation is that A-I associates to a dimeric species in the presence of diacyl lipid, in marked contrast to its behavior in the presence of detergents, which promote the monomeric state. There is no effect on maximum hydrophobic volume bound when this ligand-induced association occurs, which confirms that this interaction is not between hydrophobic regions of the protein. This dimeric form is then unrelated to that observed in aqueous solution in the absence of ligands.

Unlike A-I, A-II interacts with didecanoyl phosphatidylcholine without prior binding by a single-tail amphiphile.

$$2(\text{A-II}) \rightleftharpoons (\text{A-II})_2, \tag{4a}$$

$$(\text{A-II})_2 + m\text{L} \rightleftharpoons {}^*(\text{A-II})_2\text{L}_m. \tag{4b}$$

However, A-II is not dissociated by the diacyl lipid as it is when the bound ligand is a single-tail amphiphile.

TABLES 1 and 2 summarize the saturation level binding data for A-I and A-II and demonstrate that within experimental error these two proteins interact with a fixed and specific hydrophobic volume of n-alkyl chains regardless of polar head group. Here we find the answer to Dr. Green's question. These core polypeptides from HDL are able to package a specific amount of n-alkyl hydrocarbon, while intrinsic membrane proteins indiscriminantly associate with preformed amphiphilic aggregates such as detergent micelles and lipid bilayers. In the case of these apolipoproteins, it is the protein that directs the final structure, while in cell membranes the final structure is dictated by the organization of lipid in aqueous solution.

The conformational changes which result from the binding to a set of identical and independent sites and lead to cooperative interaction can be

TABLE 1

MAXIMAL BINDING OF LIGANDS TO APOLIPOPROTEIN A-I

Ligand *	State of Association	Maximal Moles Ligand per Peptide Chain	Molar Volume of Bound Hydrophobic Moiety per Peptide Chain (cm^3/mol)
$C_{12}OSO_3^-$	monomer	138	$24,900 \pm 1000$
$C_{14}NMe_3^+$	monomer	117	$24,800 \pm 1000$
Lubrol WX	monomer	80 ± 10	$20,800 \pm 2600$
$C_{16}PC$	monomer	97 ± 10	$22,100 \pm 2000$
$diC_{10}PC$	dimer	95 ± 10	$25,000 \pm 2600$

* Abbreviations used are: $C_{12}OSO_3^-$, sodium dodecyl sulfate; $C_{14}NMe_3^+$, tetradecyl trimethyl ammonium ion; Lubrol WX, hexadecyl, and octadecyl ethers of polyoxyethylene glycol with an average of 16 oxyethylene groups per molecule; $C_{16}PC$, palmitoyl lysophosphatidyl choline; $diC_{10}PC$, didecanoyl phosphatidyl choline.

followed by circular dichroism measurements. Increases in ellipticity at 208 and 222 nm are observed as the result of ligand binding and the ratio of the ellipticity at 208 in the presence of amphiphile to that in its absence is presented in TABLE 3. A-I undergoes relatively small alterations in conformation by this criterion, but A-II is significantly changed. This latter increase does not appear to be related to the state of association of the protein since A-II is dimeric (mol wt: 17,400) in the presence of $C_{16}E_{20}$ but tetrameric when didecanoyl phosphatidylcholine is bound. The circular dichroic spectra for these two complexes are nearly identical.

Much less information is available with respect to the interaction of apoB with amphiphilic ligands. Indeed, as you have heard in this symposium there appears to be confusion even with respect to the polypeptide molecular weight. A discussion of this subject is not appropriate in the context of this paper and perhaps should be approached by a population geneticist. TABLE 4, for example,

TABLE 2

MAXIMAL BINDING OF LIGANDS TO APOLIPOPROTEIN A-II

Ligand *	State of Association	Maximal Moles Ligand per Peptide Chain	Molar Volume of Bound Hydrophobic Moiety per Peptide Chain (cm^3/mol)
$C_{12}E_8$	monomer	85 ± 10	$15,300 \pm 2,000$
$C_{12}OSO_3^-$	monomer	85 ± 7	$15,300 \pm 1,300$
$C_{14}NMe_3^+$	monomer	74 ± 7	$15,700 \pm 1,500$
$C_{16}E_{20}$	monomer	49 ± 7	$12,350 \pm 1,800$
$diC_{10}PC$	dimer	60 ± 10	$15,800 \pm 2,600$
Egg yolk PC †	n.d.	27 ± 3	$14,300 \pm 800$

* Abbreviations used: $C_{12}E_8$, n-dodecyl octaethyleneglycol monoether; $C_{12}OSO_3^-$, sodium dodecyl sulfate; $C_{14}NMe_3^+$, tetradecyl trimethylammonium ion; $C_{16}E_{20}$, n-hexadecyl eicosoethyleneglycol monoether; $diC_{10}PC$, didecanoyl phosphatidyl choline; egg yolk PC, egg yolk diacyl phosphatidylcholine.

† Assman & Brewer.[14]

TABLE 3

SPECTRAL PROPERTIES OF PROTEIN–AMPHIPHILE COMPLEXES

	$\Theta_{208}/\Theta_{208(\text{no ligand})}$	
Ligand *	A-I	A-II
none	1.0	1.0
$C_{12}OSO_3^-$	0.97	1.53
$C_{12}E_8$		1.47
$C_{14}NMe_3^+$	0.91	1.44
$C_{16}E_{20}$		1.68
$C_{16,18}E_{17}$	1.06	
$C_{16}PC$	1.16	1.65
$diC_{10}PC$	1.16	
Egg yolk PC		1.59 †

* Abbreviations as in TABLES 1 and 2.
† Assman & Brewer.[14]

presents the apparent molecular weights of apoB reported from various areas of the world and shows a pronounced geographical distribution. The form of apoB that I discuss herein comes from North Carolina and has a molecular weight of 255,000.

Bound lipid can be completely replaced on apoB by a number of different detergents which are used to mimic the native hydrophobic environment.[16, 17] In $C_{12}E_8$, sodium dodecylsulfate, and Triton X-100, the native dimeric state of 500,000 g/mole of complex is maintained, indicating direct protein–protein interaction. In the nonionic detergents the native circular dichroic spectrum is also retained (FIGURE 2). However, at saturating levels of sodium dodecyl-sulfate required for delipidation, a major conformational change is observed (FIGURE 3), which is completely reversible upon exchanging the anionic detergent for $C_{12}E_8$. The maximal binding of $C_{12}E_8$ and palmitoyl lysolecithin is

TABLE 4

REPORTED B POLYPEPTIDE "MOLECULAR WEIGHT"
BY GEOGRAPHICAL LOCATION.
A POPULATION DISTRIBUTION?

8,000	France
26,000	California (1)
27,000	Illinois
30,000	Texas
40,000	Virginia
64,000	California (2)
70,000	Oklahoma
80,000	Maryland
255,000	Florida
255,000	Japan
255,000	North Carolina

930 and 600 moles per 500,000 g protein, respectively—values far higher than the pure micelle aggregation numbers. One might interpret this data as independent micellar type binding to segregated hydrophobic domains, which were postulated earlier. ApoB is very asymmetric in the presence of bound detergents with a frictional ratio greater than 2.0.

There is not yet sufficient data relating to the interaction of apoB with

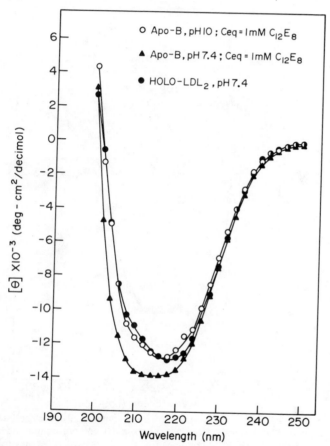

FIGURE 2. Circular dichroic spectra of LDL_2 and apoB:$C_{12}E_8$ complex at pH 7.4 and 10.0.

amphiphilic ligands to reach any conclusions regarding possible constancy of hydrophobic volume in the binding process such as was observed with A-I and A-II. Further, although the secondary structure of this polypeptide is retained in the presence of single-tail amphiphiles as is the association state, we cannot yet address the question of possible tertiary rearrangement as the result of diacyl lipid binding.

In the introduction to this paper I commented on the progress that has been made in the field of serum lipoproteins since 1971. This progress has been primarily an accumulation of a set of facts by different investigators using different methods of approach. There is more to be done at the level of reduced systems, which have been discussed briefly in this paper and by others attending this conference. Systematic binding studies with apoB and investigations of

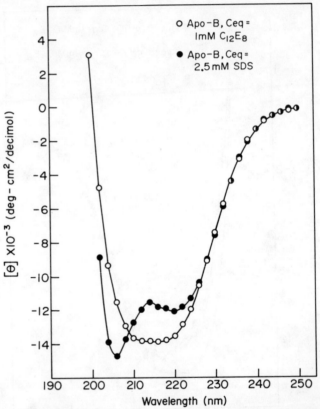

FIGURE 3. Reversibility of denaturation of apoB by sodium dodecylsulfate. Pooled fractions of apoB:SDS complex from a Sepharose 4B column equilibrated with 2.5 mM SDS in Tes buffer, pH 7.4 were concentrated and dialyzed either against 2.5 mM SDS or 1 mM $C_{12}E_8$.

ternary systems of protein–phospholipid–cholesteryl esters (or triglycerides) are obvious experimental approaches. However, the major task in the next few years will be the synthesis of all factual investigations into a complete understanding of each of the different types of human serum lipoproteins.

Henri Poincaré stated the problem clearly: "Science is built of facts the way a house is built of bricks; but an accumulation of facts is no more science than a pile of bricks is a house." [16]

REFERENCES

1. GREEN, D. E. 1972. Ann. N.Y. Acad. Sci. **195**:406.
2. OSBORN, J. C., JR. & H. B. BREWER, JR. 1977. Adv. Protein Chem. **31**:253–338.
3. REYNOLDS, J. A. 1976. J. Biol. Chem. **251**:6013–6015.
4. SMITH, R., J. R. DAWSON & C. TANFORD. 1972. J. Biol. Chem. **247**:3376–3379.
5. RIZZOLO, L. J. & C. TANFORD. 1978. Biochemistry **17**:4044–4048.
6. NOZAKI, Y., J. A. REYNOLDS & C. TANFORD. 1978. Biochemistry **17**:1239–1246.
7. STEINHARDT, J. & J. A. REYNOLDS. 1969. Multiple Equilibria in Proteins. Academic Press, New York, N.Y.
8. TANFORD, C. & J. A. REYNOLDS. 1976. Biochim. Biophys. Acta **457**:133–170.
9. REYNOLDS, J. A. & R. H. SIMON. 1974. J. Biol. Chem. **249**:3037–3940.
10. MAKINO, S., C. TANFORD & J. A. REYNOLDS. 1974. J. Biol. Chem. **249**:7379–7382.
11. STONE, W. L. & J. A. REYNOLDS. 1975. J. Biol. Chem. **250**:3584–3587.
12. HABERLAND, M. E. & J. A. REYNOLDS. 1975. J. Biol. Chem. **250**:6636–6639.
13. NICHOLS, A. V., T. FORTE, E. GONG, P. BLANCHE & R. B. VERDERY. 1974. Scand. J. Clin. Lab. Invest. **33**:147–156.
14. ASSMANN, G. & H. B. BREWER, JR. 1974. Proc. Natl. Acad. Sci. USA **71**:989–993.
15. REYNOLDS, J. A., C. TANFORD & W. L. STONE. 1977. Proc. Natl. Acad. Sci. USA **74**:3796–3799.
16. POINCARÉ, H. 1902. La Science et l'Hypothèse.

DISCUSSION OF THE PAPER

DR. J. C. OSBORNE, JR.: I am not sure that you intended to pass to the audience the concept that the problems encountered with the apoprotein in solution go away with dilution.

DR. J. A. REYNOLDS: That was my point when I said earlier that one has to keep in mind that self-association may badly perturb your data and complicate the mathematical calculations. I certainly did not intend to convey that impression. Not all problems are eliminated at high dilutions.

DR. OSBORNE: I would like to follow that up just one step further. Although we would be the first to admit that the concentration of lipid free apoproteins in plasma is very very low, we cannot underestimate their importance. Even one molecule of lipid-free apoA-I may prove of biological importance.

DR. REYNOLDS: I think I can agree with you from one standpoint. Three labs have measured the association constant of apoA-I, and while there are minor discrepancies, they are all in the same ballpark for $2A\text{-}I \rightleftharpoons (A\text{-}I)_2$ (dimerization). Henry Pownall has done a lot of work measuring how much apoA-I can dissociate into an aqueous solution from HDL. The concentrations are likely 10^{-10} M. At these concentrations you can calculate the effect of self-association and this is miniscule.

DR. OSBORNE: We do not know the mechanism of transfer of apoproteins among plasma lipoproteins during metabolism. We are dealing with a problem of rates.

DR. REYNOLDS: Do not confuse thermodynamics with mechanism. Thermodynamics only tells you about final states. If you want to talk about rates, then you talk about mechanisms and that is a separate story.

DR. OSBORNE: I just do not want people to be confused about the importance of lipid-free apoproteins in the *in vivo* state.

DR. REYNOLDS: Neither do I. That is why I made the statement. We agree.

DR. K. W. A. WIRTZ: You showed that SDS induces α helix formation in apoB. Is this induction dependent upon the pH of the medium?

DR. REYNOLDS: We have not investigated that parameter. I think what is happening is that SDS is inducing α helix formation on the water-soluble part of this protein, which is hanging out like little knobs; the rest of the structure is somehow associated with the lipid and is not being touched. That is my guess.

DR. J. T. SPARROW (*Baylor College of Medicine, Houston, Texas*): Dr. Reynolds, do you think that the amphiphiles are discretely binding, I assume that they are at different sites from the phospholipids in apoA-I and apoA-II?

DR. REYNOLDS: Are you talking about the cooperative ones?

DR. SPARROW: Yes.

DR. REYNOLDS: No, I do not. I think they are binding in the same place.

DR. SPARROW: Do you assume that in the case of the amphiphilic segments they are binding too?

DR. REYNOLDS: The model that I envisage without one piece of evidence other than the notion of a constant hydrophobic binding is that one is forming some sort of pocket within the amphipathic helix. You can see it if you build a model.

DR. SPARROW: Would you care to speculate on the differences between apoA-I and apoA-II?

DR. REYNOLDS: No. Because all we have are data on apoA-II and we are still working on it. You notice that I did not give you any interaction energies for apoA-II and this is because in the presence of detergents the dissociation to the 17,400 monomer is attended by conformational changes that set in before you have total saturation of the original sites. When you try to mathematically analyze these data you discover that you have too many unknown factors to consider.

DR. D. M. SMALL: I suppose I will play the advocate of controversy. I think that you said very clearly that in order to get apoA-I to bind cooperatively you have to fill up four sites within a single chain molecule.

DR. REYNOLDS: This is true in our laboratory and others.

DR. SMALL: Well, if you take reasonable care of apoA-I and add it to a very pure dimyristoyl lecithin preparation, it certainly clears, and forms definite structures. Is that binding?

DR. REYNOLDS: Yes, it is. We have not been able to reproduce that.

DR. SMALL: A lot of other laboratories have done those experiments. I think that what Dr. Scanu presented this morning suggests that apoA-I binds to an egg lecithin vesicle at a low concentration. Is that binding?

DR. REYNOLDS: That will also be binding. This is the point that I was bringing up yesterday, and which I brought up this morning. There are laboratories that had published discrepant data; and one does not understand why one laboratory sees one thing, and another sees another. Perhaps the best thing that we could all do in this field is to straighten things out, rather than forget that somebody else had done the other experiment.

COMMENT: The relevant question is under what conditions, temperature for example, did the binding in the DMPC system occur.

DR. REYNOLDS: That experiment was done a very long time ago, above and below the transition temperature. That is one of the reasons we did not like working with these systems and of course referring to Dr. Pownall's work, they showed a difference in the rate of association of apoA-I depending upon what temperature they worked at. We simply could not reproduce that. You cannot get any associations; unless one goes to such high lipid concentrations that one is in fact running the risk of having small amounts of contaminants affecting the results.

COMMENT: In regards to the purity of the material, the DMPC that Dr. Pownall has used, and I presume Dr. Small and his people have checked this out as well, excludes the possibility that there are any free fatty acids in it, although the commercially available DMPC does have a fair amount of free fatty acids in it.

DR. REYNOLDS: Before or after the reaction?

COMMENT: After the complex was isolated. The critical point here is to evaluate just exactly what the temperature is because Dr. Pownall has found that binding registers very high right after the transition temperature where one expects to have the largest number of defects.

DR. REYNOLDS: I would also point out that Dr. Scanu used ^{14}C phospholipids, or certainly Dr. Small has, and the association occurs at temperatures where Henry Pownall says it should not. This is part of the conflict that I am trying to point out to you; the people who are sitting in the audience who do not work in this field are going to believe every word we say when we get up here.

DR. SCANU: I just want to make a brief comment. Those of us who are working on apoA-I have recognized difficulties that are encountered not only in preparing apoA-I in a pure form but also in storing it. I know for instance that your data on its mode of self-association differ, and I do not know whether your approach is better or worse than ours. If we are going to really compare data, I think the smartest thing to do is to use one preparation and have various laboratories test it.

DR. D. ATKINSON (*Boston University, Boston, Mass.*): As one of the people who managed to study apoA-I both in England and Boston, there are one or two comments I would like to make. First, in the experiments that were carried out in England with Dr. Phillips, who is also here today, we were very careful to check both before and after the experiment that there were no single chain lipids in the complex resulting from the interaction with apoA-I. I have to add, however, that I have observed both cases of apoA-I interacting and not interacting with lipids.

DR. REYNOLDS: So we have seen a discrepancy in the same laboratory.

DR. ATKINSON: I put my apoprotein through a fairly standard preparative procedure. I take the apoprotein up in a solution pH 8.6 in Tris-HCl buffer and then dialyze that apoprotein very very slowly over a long period, against distilled water of pH 7. I then freeze-dry the apoprotein. What I end up with at the end of the dialysis is with a lot of insoluble irreversibly denatured apoprotein. I freeze and dry the supernatant, which is instantly put back into an aqueous environment. I have never had any trouble binding lipid with such preparations.

DR. REYNOLDS: The only comment I would make on that is that it is very strange because in the hands of everybody who has worked with apoA-I and apoA-II, almost anything you do to these proteins is completely reversible. I have never seen apoA-I or apoA-II precipitate. When I am talking about binding measurements, I am talking about demonstrated reversibility, not just throwing some lipid in and shaking it up with a protein and saying that a complex has been formed. In the paper you refer to on your work in England, which was published originally with Hauser as the senior author, I truly do not know how to interpret your binding data. You had a high excess of lipid in those experiments. If indeed a reversible process was going on as one would have expected, then why did you not obtain a homogeneous species? This is a problem that one sees with apoA-I, but not apoA-II.

DR. G. D. FASMAN: I was wondering about your curves where you showed a breakdown of secondary structure as a function of concentration. If you have a complex, does that shift the curve considerably?

DR. REYNOLDS: Yes, it does, at least with apoA-I. With apoA-II, we can never see 17,400-dalton forms in the absence of ligands. We only see the polymeric form. There you notice a little hump in the curve, and I assume that it is due to the dissociation. In the case of apoA-I, the curve is highly cooperative, but it is not a two-state process.

DR. FASMAN: Do you think that it would be more comparable to the protein binding to vesicle?

DR. REYNOLDS: That I really do not know. I do not think those proteins are contacting each other in the vesicle.

PHOSPHOLIPID BINDING STUDIES WITH SYNTHETIC APOLIPOPROTEIN FRAGMENTS *

James T. Sparrow † and Antonio M. Gotto, Jr.

Department of Medicine
Baylor College of Medicine
and The Methodist Hospital
Texas Medical Center
Houston, Texas 77030

INTRODUCTION

The plasma lipoproteins are macromolecular complexes of lipids and proteins and are the major carriers of triglycerides, cholesterol, cholesteryl esters, and phospholipids in the blood stream (TABLE 1) (see Reference 1 for a recent review). Several of the apoproteins, in addition to associating with lipids, have been shown to interact with enzymes and cell surface receptors to control lipid metabolism. The role of apolipoprotein B (apoB) and low-density lipoproteins (LDL) in cholesterol synthesis has been extensively studied by Brown and Goldstein and others.[2] The role of apoC-II in the activation of lipoprotein lipase for hydrolysis of chylomicron and very-low-density lipoprotein (VLDL) triglycerides is also well established.[3, 4] Apolipoproteins A-I and C-I are known to activate lecithin:cholesterol acyltransferase, the enzyme believed to be primarily responsible for the synthesis of cholesteryl esters.[5, 6]

The serum apolipoproteins have been shown by many investigators to interact with phospholipids, cholesterol, cholesteryl esters, and triglycerides to reform stable protein–lipid complexes.[7] In the process of binding lipids, the apoproteins show increases in their circular dichroic (CD) spectra at 208 and 222 nm, characteristic of the formation of an α helix. The intrinsic tryptophan fluorescence spectrum shifts from ~350 nm to ~335 nm; this shift has been interpreted as the tryptophan being placed in a more hydrophobic environment. These spectroscopic changes have been used as criteria of lipid binding.[7] In addition, phospholipid binding has been evaluated by differential scanning calorimetry, microcalorimetry, by measuring the decrease in lipid turbidity, and by the ability to isolate stable lipid–protein complexes by density gradient ultracentrifugation or agarose column chromatography.[7]

In 1971, as the sequences of the apolipoproteins became available, we began a program of peptide synthesis, the goal of which was to determine the structural features necessary for lipid binding. In addition, as the sequences became known of the three apoproteins that interact with the enzymes responsible for the metabolism of lipids, we undertook the additional task of defining the minimum sequence requirements for enzymic activation.

* This work was supported by the Atherosclerosis, Lipids, and Lipoproteins Section of the National Heart and Blood Vessel Research and Demonstration Center, Baylor College of Medicine, a grant-supported research project of the National Heart, Lung, and Blood Institute, National Institutes of Health, Grant HL–17269; and by the American Heart Association.

† Established Investigator of the American Heart Association.

TABLE 1

TABLE 1

COMPOSITION OF HUMAN PLASMA LIPOPROTEIN

	Chylomicrons	VLDL	LDL	HDL
Density range	<0.95	0.95–1.006	1.006–1.063	1.063–1.210
Major lipids	Exogenous triglycerides	Endogenous triglycerides	Cholesterol Cholesteryl esters	Phospholipids Cholesteryl esters
% Protein	2	10	25	50
Major apoproteins	ApoA-I * ApoB ApoC	ApoB ApoC-I * ApoC-II † ApoC-III ApoE	ApoB	ApoA-I * ApoA-II
Minor proteins	ApoA-II ApoE ‡ PRP §	ApoA-I * ApoA-II ApoD ¶	ApoC	ApoC-I * ApoC-II † ApoC-III ApoD ¶ ApoE ‡

* Activator of lecithin:cholesterol acyltransferase.
† Cofactor for lipoprotein lipase.
‡ Also termed arginine-rich protein (ARP).
§ Proline-rich protein.
¶ Also termed thin-line protein and apoA-III.

From the information obtained from the lipid binding of synthetic peptides and fragments of the native proteins, Segrest et al.[8] proposed the amphipathic helical hypothesis to explain the interaction of these proteins with phospholipids. Using Chou-Fasman analysis [9] and model building of the sequence of the apoprotein, Segrest et al. postulated that the mechanism of apolipoprotein–phospholipid interaction involved the formation of an amphipathic helix, i.e., a helical segment forms such that the acidic, basic, and hydrophilic amino acids occupy an 180° face of the helical cylinder and the hydrophobic residues are located along the remaining 180° face (FIGURE 1). It was observed that there was a high frequency of acidic and basic amino acid pairs formed with the acidic residues at the center of the polar face and the basics at the edge. In addition on the apolar face, there was a preponderance of highly hydrophobic amino acids often with pairings of aromatic residues. These authors postulated that there could be an ionic interaction between the pairings of acidic and basic residues and the zwitterionic polar head group of phospholipids. In addition, they proposed that the large hydrophobic surface of the apolar face could interact strongly with the fatty acyl chains of the phospholipids. With the above-described structure, the protein could organize lipids such that the hydrophobic regions were protected from the aqueous environment of the plasma by a surface of phospholipid polar head groups and the hydrophilic face of the apoprotein. Experimental evidence from several laboratories [1, 7] supports the role of hydrophobic interactions in lipoprotein structure but as yet fails to support the ionic interactions proposed by Segrest et al. Our studies of the interaction of synthetic peptide fragments of apolipoproteins with phospholipid strongly support the role of hydrophobicity in binding proposed in the amphipathic helical model. These peptides have also been used to define the regions of the apoproteins responsible for enzyme activation. We report here a summary of what we have learned about this family of important plasma proteins using synthetic peptide fragments.

APOLIPOPROTEIN C-III

The amino acid sequence of apolipoprotein C-III (apoC-III) from human serum very-low-density lipoprotein (VLDL) was first reported by Brewer et al.[10] The protein contains 79 amino acids with a carbohydrate chain attached to Thr_{74} (FIGURE 2) and exists in several forms differing in sialic acid content. Since there was no apparent hydrophobic region that might be associated with the known lipid-binding properties of this protein, we started the synthesis at the carboxyl terminal and removed resin samples periodically in order to establish where the lipid-binding regions occur. We began the synthesis on the classical Merrifield polystyrene resin [11] and quickly realized the difficulties involved in synthesizing hydrophobic helical proteins. Therefore, a modified resin was developed using a spacer arm and a more acid stable linkage, which

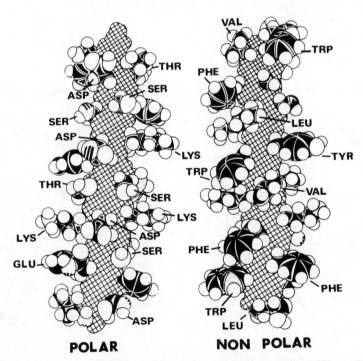

FIGURE 1. The amphipathic helical region of apolipoprotein C-III predicted by Segrest et al.[8] The polar face contains the aspartic acids at the center paired with lysine residues at the edge separating the polar and nonpolar faces. The nonpolar face contains all the hydrophobic amino acid.

improved the yield and purity of the final products.[12] The synthetic peptides used in our studies have been purified by gel permeation and ion exchange chromatography. The purity of the synthetic fragments has been determined by amino acid analysis, tryptic mapping, polyacrylamide gel electrophoresis, isoelectric focusing, and more recently, by high performance liquid chromatography (HPLC).

Peptides representing sequence positions 61–79, 55–79, 48–79, and 41–79 (FIGURE 2) were synthesized.[13] The purified peptides were evaluated for their ability to bind phospholipid by measuring the circular dichroic spectrum and the intrinsic tryptophan fluorescence spectrum. In the presence of phosphatidylcholine, we observed increases in the ellipticity at 222 nm in the circular dichroic spectrum and a blue shift of ~10 nm in the fluorescence spectrum (TABLE 2) with peptides 48–79 and 41–79. In contrast, the two shorter peptides displayed no change in their CD or fluorescence spectra in the presence of phospholipid.

H₂N-SER-GLU-ALA-GLU-ASP-ALA-SER-LEU-LEU-SER-PHE-MET-GLN-GLY-TYR-MET-LYS-HIS-ALA-THR-
                       10   20

LYS-THR-ALA-LYS-ASP-ALA-LEU-SER-SER-VAL-GLN-SER-GLN-GLN-VAL-ALA-ALA-GLN-GLN-ARG-
                       30   40

(GLY)-TRP-VAL-THR-ASP-GLY-PHE-(SER)-SER-LEU-LYS-ASP-TYR-TRP-(SER)-THR-VAL-LYS-ASP-LYS-
                       50   60

(PHE)-SER-GLU-PHE-TRP-ASP-LEU-ASP-PRO-GLU-VAL-ARG-PRO-THR-SER-ALA-VAL-ALA-ALA-COOH
                       70   CHO

FIGURE 2. Amino acid sequence of apolipoprotein C-III reported by Brewer et al.[10] The hydrophobic amphipathic helical region predicted by Segrest et al.[8] occurs between residues 40 and 67. The circled residues are the amino termini of the four synthetic peptides of apoC-III used to establish the lipid binding region.

The peptide–lipid mixtures were subjected to ultracentrifugation and the two larger peptides were found associated with the lipid vesicles whereas the shorter peptides were in the bottom of the centrifuge tubes. Therefore, we concluded that the 48–79 and the 41–79 peptides contained the necessary requirements for binding phospholipids. Subsequently, Segrest et al.[8] proposed an amphipathic helical segment between residues 40 and 67 of apoC-III (FIGURE 1 & 2).

To explain the lipid binding by the various synthetic fragments, we attempted to calculate the average hydrophobicity of the peptides. Using the hydrophobicity scale for the amino acids developed by Bull and Breese,[14] we estimated the mean residue hydrophobicity (MRH) of these peptides as well as the native protein (TABLE 2) as follows:

$$ MRH = \frac{\Sigma \Delta f_{AA}}{\text{no. of AA}}, $$

where $\Sigma \Delta f_{AA}$ is the summation of the free energies of transfer for each amino acid in cal/mole. The MRH for residues 1–40 was very low, −609 cal/residue

TABLE 2

PROPERTIES OF APOLIPOPROTEIN C-III

Residues	Mean Residue Hydrophobicity (cal/residue)	$[\Theta]_{222}$ (deg cm²/dmole) *		λ_{max} (nm)	
		Peptide Alone	Peptide+DMPC †	Peptide Alone	Peptide+DMPC †
1–79	−752	−5639	−17062	350	337
1–40	−603	−2690	−2690	—	—
41–79	−904	−1510	−10940	352	341
Synthetic Peptides					
61–79	−907	−1500	−1500	350	348
55–79	−824	−2900	−2900	350	349
48–79	−895	−2500	−6100	350	344
41–79	−904	−2400	−10400	350	338

* Molar ellipticity = $[\Theta]_{222}$ = MRW·Θ_{222}/l·c·100.
† Dimyristoylphosphatidylcholine.

but it was apparent that the MRH for the 41–67 amphipathic segment was large, −1039 cal/residue and that for the 41–79 and 48–79 fragments somewhat less. The 55–79 fragment had a lower MRH of −824 cal/residue but the shortest fragment 67–79, which did not bind, had a hydrophobicity of −907 cal/residue. Therefore, although these latter two peptides are hydrophobic and have helical potential, from our lipid binding experiments we must conclude that these shorter fragments had insufficient length of helix to form stable complexes.

We have subsequently shown that thrombin cleavage at Arg_{40}–Gly_{41} produces two fragments of apoC-III which are easily purified by DEAE-Sephadex chromatography.[15] We have studied the ability of these fragments to bind phospholipid and have found that the native 41–79 peptide was similar in its properties to the synthetic material; i.e., there was an increase in ellipticity at 222 nm and a shift in the fluorescence maximum of 11 nm. We were also able to isolate a complex by density gradient ultracentrifugation. However, the amino terminal 1–40 residues does not bind to phospholipid as evidenced by the absence of CD spectral changes and by the inability to isolate a peptide–lipid complex. Although residues 1–40 contain an amphipathic helical segment, we conclude from the failure to isolate a complex that the total hydrophobicity of this peptide is insufficient to permit stable complex formation.

APOLIPOPROTEIN C-I

Apolipoprotein C-I (apoC-I) is also isolated from human serum VLDL and has been sequenced by ourselves [16] and Shulman et al.[17] and contains 57 amino acids (FIGURE 3). Our laboratory [18, 19] has shown that the protein is able to bind phospholipid and to activate lecithin:cholesterol acyltransferase (LCAT), the enzyme thought responsible for the synthesis of plasma cholesteryl ester. Harding et al.[20] and our laboratory [21] have reported the synthesis of apoC-I and have shown that the synthetic protein activates LCAT to the same extent as the native protein. In addition, we have established that the total sequence is not needed for enzymic activation. We have demonstrated that residues 17–57 activate the enzyme to the same extent as apoC-I, whereas residues 24–57 and 32–57 had only 50% of the activity; the 39–57 peptide was inactive.[22, 23]

H₂N-THR-PRO-ASP-VAL-SER-SER-ALA-LEU-ASP-LYS-LEU-LYS-GLU-PHE-GLY-ASN-⟨THR⟩-LEU-GLU-ASP-
                                            10   20

LYS-ALA-ARG-⟨GLU⟩-LEU-ILE-SER-ARG-ILE-LYS-GLN-⟨SER⟩-GLU-LEU-SER-ALA-LYS-MET-⟨ARG⟩-GLU-
                                           30   40

TRP-PHE-SER-GLU-THR-PHE-GLN-LYS-VAL-LYS-GLU-LYS-LEU-LYS-ILE-ASP-SER-COOH
                                         50

FIGURE 3. Amino acid sequence of apolipoprotein C-I as determined by Jackson et al.[16] and Shulman et al.[17] The amphipathic helices are predicted to occur in 7–14, 18–29, and 33–53. The amino termini of the synthetic peptides used to confirm the lipid binding and determine the LCAT activating regions are circled.

H₂N-THR-GLN-GLN-PRO-GLN-GLN-ASP-GLU-MET-PRO-SER-PRO-THR-PHE-LEU-THR-GLU-VAL-LYS-GLU-
          5   10   15   20

TRP-LEU-SER-SER-TYR-GLN-SER-ALA-LYS-THR-ALA-ALA-GLN-ASN-LEU-TYR-GLU-LYS-THR-TYR-
       25   30   35   40

LEU-PRO-(ALA)-VAL-ASP-GLU-LYS-LEU-ARG-(ASP)-LEU-TYR-SER-LYS-(SER)-THR-ALA-ALA-MET-(SER)-
      45   50   55   60

THR-TYR-THR-GLY-ILE-(PHE)-THR-ASP-GLN-VAL-LEU-SER-VAL-LEU-LYS-GLY-GLU-GLU-COOH
      65   70   75

FIGURE 4. Amino acid sequence of apolipoprotein C-II according to Jackson et al.[24] Chou-Fasman analysis and model building of the protein sequence indicates amphipathic helices to occur between 13–22, 28–38, and 43–51. The circled residues are the amino termini of the synthetic peptides used to investigate the lipoprotein lipase activation and phospholipid binding.

Segrest et al.[8] predicted phospholipid binding regions in residues 7–14, 18–29, and 33–53 of apoC-I. We have studied the lipid binding properties of the synthetic fragments 39–57, 32–57, 24–57, 17–57, and 1–57.[22] When the peptides were mixed with phospholipid, we found that the 32–57, 24–57, and 17–57 peptides showed a blue shift of ~12 nm in their tryptophan fluorescence spectra (TABLE 3). In addition, there was a large increase in the ellipticity at 222 nm in the CD spectra; peptide 39–57 showed none of these changes (TABLE 3). Density gradient ultracentrifugation of the peptide–lipid mixtures permitted isolation of a stable peptide–lipid complex with peptides 32–57, 24–57, 17–57, and 1–57; a complex was not isolated from peptide 39–57.

In TABLE 3, we have given the MRH of each peptide and find them all to be moderately hydrophobic. Peptide 39–57, although hydrophobic, does not contain the complete amphipathic region proposed by Segrest et al. between residues 33 and 53 while the 32–57 and larger peptides contain this region; the 17–57 peptide also contains a second amphipathic region between 18 and 29. These results suggest that there is a critical length of amphipathic helix necessary for stable peptide-lipid complex formation.

APOLIPOPROTEIN C-II

Apolipoprotein C-II is one of the most interesting of the VLDL apoproteins since several laboratories [3, 4] have reported that it is a potent cofactor of the enzyme lipoprotein lipase (LPL), which is responsible for triglyceride hydrolysis in chylomicrons and VLDL. The sequence of apoC-II has been determined in our laboratories [24] and it contains 78 residues (FIGURE 4). We have shown, using the synthetic peptides 66–78, 60–78, 55–78, 50–78, and 43–78, that residues 55–78 contain the necessary structure for the full activation of lipoprotein lipase.[25]

Chou-Fasman analysis of apoC-II and model building indicate a high probability for amphipathic helices between residues 13–22, 28–38, and 43–51. In

TABLE 3

PROPERTIES OF APOLIPOPROTEIN C-I

Residues	Mean Residue Hydrophobicity (cal/residue)	$[\Theta]_{222}$ (deg cm²/dmole)		λ_{max} (nm)		Activation of Lecithin: Cholesterol Acyltransferase
		Peptide Alone	Peptide+DMPC	Peptide Alone	Peptide+DMPC	
1-57	-825	-11000 *	-16500	348	339	100%
		-19000 †	-25500	345	339	—
1-38	-797	-10700	-22400	—	—	0
39-57	-879	-2900	-3500	351	349	0
Synthetic Peptides						
39-57	-879	-1914	-1914	351	351	0
32-57	-863	-3829	-11104	351	339	50
24-57	-890	-4427	-10034	351	340	60
17-57	-839	-7452	-14664	351	339	100
1-57	-825	-8000	-12000	344	339	100

* Reference 20.
† Reference 17.

addition, there is a high probability for β turns at residues 9–12, 23–26, 52–55 and a weak β-turn at 60–63 followed by a region of β sheet to residue 74. We hypothesize that the interaction of this β-sheet region and the 60–63 β-turn with lipoprotein lipase are responsible for activation. We have shown that peptides 55–78 and 50–78 do not bind phospholipid.[26] However, the addition of the amphipathic helical segment 43–49 generates a peptide that does bind as evidenced by increases in the circular dichroic spectrum (FIGURE 5 and TABLE 4) at 222 nm and the isolation of a complex by density gradient ultracentrifugation (FIGURE 6). We have demonstrated that the hydrophobic peptides 66–78, 60–78, 55–78, 50–78 do not associate with phospholipid.[26] We attribute this lack of binding to the high β-sheet potential in this region of the protein. With the addition of the 43–51 region with a high hydrophobicity and helix probability, we generate one of the amphipathic lipid binding regions of apoC-II. Clearly we have demonstrated, for the first time, the separation of functions in one of the serum apolipoproteins, i.e., residues 55–78 are responsible for enzymic activation while residues 43–51 are involved in lipid binding.

APOLIPOPROTEIN A-I

Apolipoprotein A-I is the major protein constituent of human high-density lipoproteins (HDL) and is known to bind phospholipid and phospholipid–cholesterol as well as activate LCAT.[19] Two sequences of apoA-I have been published and differ somewhat in the sequence of the amino terminal cyanogen bromide fragment.[27, 28] Several authors [29, 30] have proposed that there are 11 or 22 residue repeating units in apoA-I, which have a close sequence homology and are thought to represent the lipid binding regions. Recently, we have synthesized parts of the carboxyl terminal cyanogen bromide fragment (FIGURE 7) that is known to activate LCAT and to bind phospholipid.[19] We have shown by CD (TABLE 5) and by density gradient ultracentrifugation that residues 220–245, 213–245, and 204–245 and 197–245 bind phospholipid (FIGURE 8) but do not activate LCAT; residues 227–245 do not bind.[31] From these results we conclude that an amphipathic helical segment of sufficient length and hydrophobicity for lipid binding is located in residues 224–242 of apoA-I.

By comparing the predicted structure of apoC-I with that of apoA-I we have identified two regions of apoA-I which might activate LCAT; these regions are residues 16–53 and 145–185. Since there are differences in the published sequences of the 16–53 region, we initially chose to synthesize fragments of the 145–185 region and study their activation of LCAT. We have recently found that peptides 157–185, 152–185, 148–185, and 145–185 activate LCAT 8%, 6%, 19%, and 24%, respectively, of that found for apoA-I; peptides 164–185 and 197–245 were inactive.[32] In addition, we find that peptides 164–185, 157–185, and 152–185 formed complexes with phospholipid and phospholipid–cholesterol mixtures; the larger peptides 148–185 and 145–185 formed somewhat more stable complexes (FIGURE 9). Kroon et al.[33] have also reported the phospholipid binding by part of this latter fragment of apoA-I. Although this region 145–185 of apoA-I contains an amphipathic helix, the hydrophobicity is low, therefore the peptides bind weakly to phosphatidylcholine. These studies with apoA-I fragments demonstrate that residues 148–185 are involved in the activation of LCAT and lipid binding where residues 197–245 are involved only in lipid binding.

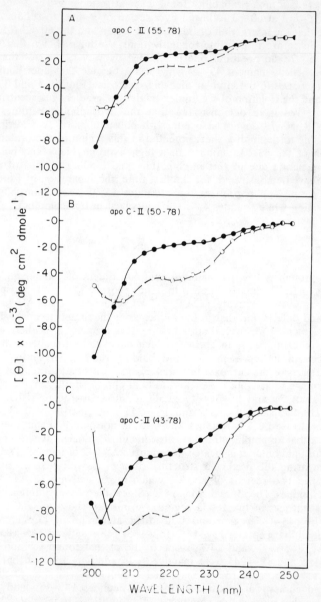

FIGURE 5. Circular dichroic spectra of synthetic peptides of apolipoprotein C-II. The CD spectra were recorded on a Cary 61 Spectropolarimeter in a 0.5 mm cell at 24° C. The peptide concentration was ~0.5 mg/ml. (A) Peptide 55–78: alone (●—●); with dimyristoylphosphatidylcholine (DMPC) (○—○). (B) Peptide 50–78: alone (●—●); with DMPC (○—○). (C) Peptide 43–78: alone (●—●); with DMPC (○—○).

TABLE 4

PROPERTIES OF APOLIPOPROTEIN C-II

Residues	Mean Residue Hydrophobicity (cal/residue)	$[\theta]_{222}$ (deg cm²/dmole)		Activation of Lipoprotein Lipase
		Peptide Alone	Peptide + DMPC	
1–78	−844	−5935	−20024	100%
60–78	−945	—	—	30%
1–59	−807	—	—	0
Synthetic Peptides				
66–78	−945	—	—	0
60–78	−937	—	—	25%
55–78	−874	−1630	−2865	100%
50–78	−818	−2096	−5545	100%
43–78	−884	−4270	−10540	100%

APOLIPOPROTEIN A-II

The other major apoprotein of HDL, apolipoprotein A-II (apoA-II) contains 77 residues connected by a disulfide bond at cysteine 6 (FIGURE 10).[34] Segrest et al. predicted residues 18–30 and 39–47 to bind lipid. We[35] and others[33] find that peptide 17–31 does not bind and we believe the length of the peptide to be insufficient to form a stable complex. However, the addition of five amino acids gives a peptide that, upon interaction with DMPC, shows an increase in the ellipticity at 222 nm (TABLE 6); peptide 7–31 behaves in a similar manner. Density gradient ultracentrifugation permits isolation of a stable complex with these two longer peptides while the shorter peptide (17–31) does not bind phospholipid. We also find that peptides 50–77, 47–77, and 40–77 show increases in their ellipticity[36] but that peptides 52–77, 54–77, and 56–77 do not.[37] A peptide–lipid complex with the three longer peptides was isolated by density gradient ultracentrifugation while there were no complexes formed with the shorter peptides. Thus we have identified a lipid binding region of apoA-II, contained in residues 50–77, that was not predicted by Segrest et al.[8] Space filling models of this segment of apoA-II indicate an amphipathic helix can form between residues 51 and 62.

TABLE 5

PROPERTIES OF SYNTHETIC FRAGMENTS OF APOLIPOPROTEIN A-I

Synthetic Peptide	Mean Residue Hydrophobicity (cal/residue)	$[\theta]_{222}$ (deg cm²/dmole)	
		Peptide Alone	Peptide+DMPC
227–245	−1016	−4300	−4700
220–245	−1136	−6800	−11100
213–245	−1060	−10300	−15200
204–245	−975	−13500	−17200
197–245	−922	−5300	−15800

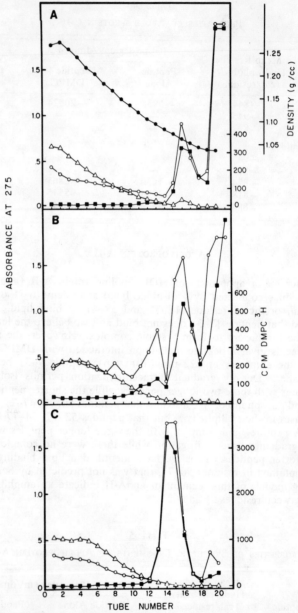

FIGURE 6. Density gradient ultracentrifugation of synthetic peptide DMPC mixtures. The gradients were formed with cesium chloride in a Beckman SW 50.1 rotor and were centrifuged at 45,000 rpm for 72 hrs at 24° C. The gradients were fractionated and analyzed for peptide by measuring the A_{275} and for phospholipid by liquid scintillation counting of the [^{3}H]DMPC. (A) Peptide 55–78: alone ($\triangle$—$\triangle$); with DMPC (O—O), [^{3}H]DMPC (■—■). (B) Peptide 50–78: alone ($\triangle$—$\triangle$); with DMPC (O—O), [^{3}H]DMPC (■—■). (C) Peptide 43–78: alone ($\triangle$—$\triangle$); with DMPC (O—O); [^{3}H]DMPC (■—■).

Lys-Val-Glu-Pro-Leu-Arg-Ala-Glu-Leu-Gln-Glu-Gly-Ala-Arg-Gln-Lys-Leu-His-Glu-Leu-

130   140

Gln-Glu-Lys-Leu-Ser-Pro-Leu-Gly-Glu-Glu-Met-Arg-Asp-Arg-Ala-Arg-Ala-His-Val-Asp-

150   160

Ala-Leu-Arg-Thr-His-Leu-Ala-Pro-Tyr-Ser-Asp-Glu-Leu-Arg-Gln-Arg-Leu-Ala-Ala-Arg-

170   180

Leu-Glu-Ala-Leu-Lys-Glu-Asn-Gly-Ala-Gly-Arg-Leu-Ala-Glu-Tyr-His-Ala-Lys-Ala-Thr-

190   200

Glu-His-Leu-Ser-Thr-Leu-Ser-Glu-Lys-Ala-Lys-Pro-Ala-Leu-Glu-Asp-Leu-Arg-Gln-Gly-

210   220

Leu-Leu-Pro-Val-Leu-Glu-Ser-Phe-Lys-Val-Ser-Phe-Leu-Ser-Ala-Leu-Glu-Glu-Tyr-Thr-

230   240

Lys-Leu-Asn-Thr-Gln-COOH

245

FIGURE 7. Amino acid sequence of residues 121–245 of apolipoprotein A-I reported by Baker *et al.*[27]

TABLE 6

PROPERTIES OF APOLIPOPROTEIN A-II

Residues	Mean Residue Hydrophobicity (cal/residue)	$[\Theta]_{222}$ (deg cm²/dmole)	
		Peptide Alone	Peptide+DMPC
1–77	−863	−16277	−21784
1–26	−826	−1000	−1000
27–77	−861	−4000	−12000
56–77	−951	−3900	−4100
Synthetic Peptides			
56–77	−951	−3500	−4000
54–77	−901	−8200 *	−8200 *
52–77	−1013	−8500 *	−11000 *
50–77	−993	−5500	−13500
47–77	−982	−7200	−15200
40–77	−968	−6300	−15700
17–31	−831	−1630	−1630
12–31	−856	−1170	−5150
7–31	−935	−1170	−8240

* The CD spectrum showed a trough at 215 nm with a $\Theta = -12600$ and no trough at 208 nm indicating a large β-structural component.

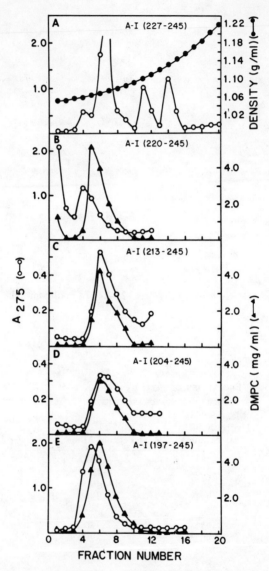

FIGURE 8. Density gradients of synthetic apoA-I peptides. The gradient conditions were the same as those in FIGURE 6. The peptide (O—O) was estimated by the absorbance at 275 nm and by amino acid analysis and phospholipid (▲—▲) by the method of Bartlett. (A) Peptide 227–245. (B) Peptide 220–245. (C) Peptide 213–245. (D) Peptide 204–245. (E) Peptide 197–245.

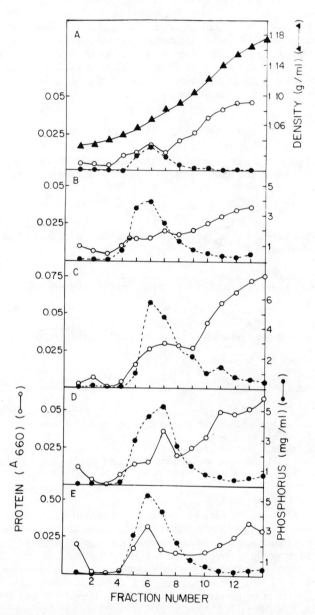

FIGURE 9. Density gradient of synthetic apoA-I peptides. (A) 164–185. (B) 157–185. (C) 152–185. (D) 148–185. (E) 145–185. The peptide (O—O) was estimated by the Lowry procedure and by amino acid analysis; the phospholipid (●—●) by the Bartlett procedure.

More recently we have investigated the role of the lysines and adjacent hydrophobic residues in lipid binding using the 50–77 peptide.[38] Replacement of $Lys_{54}Lys_{55}$ with Ser does not affect the binding (FIGURE 11C), whereas replacement of $Leu_{52}Ile_{53}$ with Ala destroys phospholipid binding (FIGURE 11B) as evidenced by the inability to isolate a complex of peptide and lipid. These results suggest that the hydrophobicity of the residues adjacent to the paired charged residues is more important for binding than ionic interaction with the polar head group of the phospholipid.

MODEL PEPTIDES

Several years ago we realized that if the amphipathic hypothesis were correct that peptide models for lipid–protein interaction could be designed.[22, 39] Using

$$S$$
PCA-Ala-Lys-Glu-Pro-Cys-Val-Glu-Ser-Leu-Val-Ser-Gln-Tyr-Phe-Gln-Thr-Val-Thr-Asp-
                                        10   20

Tyr-Gly-Lys-Asp-Leu-Met-Glu-Lys-Val-Lys-Ser-Pro-Glu-Leu-Gln-Ala-Gln-Ala-Lys-Ser-
                                        30   40

Tyr-Phe-Glu-Lys-Ser-Lys-Glu-Gln-Leu-Thr-Pro-Leu-Ile-Lys-Lys-Ala-Gly-Thr-Glu-Leu-
                                        50   60

Val-Asn-Phe-Leu-Ser-Tyr-Phe-Val-Glu-Leu-Gly-Thr-Gln-Pro-Ala-Thr-Gln-COOH
                                        70

FIGURE 10. Amino acid sequence of apolipoprotein A-II determined by Lux *et al.*[34] The predicted amphipathic helices occur between residues 17–30, 39–47, and 51–62. The circled residues are the amino termini of the synthetic peptides. The square around residues 31 indicates the carboxyl terminus of the first series of synthetic peptides, i.e., 17–31, 12–31, and 7–31.

the constraints of the amphipathic model, i.e., a potential helix with a sequence such that the acidic and basic residues were properly aligned on the polar face and that the hydrophobic residues formed a nonpolar face, we arrived at a sequence that would permit us to test several aspects of the amphipathic hypothesis. The sequences of several of these peptides are given in FIGURE 12 and Reference 39. We found that Peptide I, although hydrophobic, was not of sufficient length to form very stable complexes, Peptide II and III were too hydrophilic, while Peptide IV had sufficient length and hydrophobicity to form very stable complexes with phospholipids. Indeed, the helicity of this peptide, upon binding phospholipid increased from 28% to 70% while the tryptophan fluorescence maximum shifted from 350 nm to 331 nm (TABLE 7). Complexes of phospholipid and phospholipid–cholesterol have been isolated by density gradient ultracentrifugation [39, 40] and by agarose column chromatography.[40] The

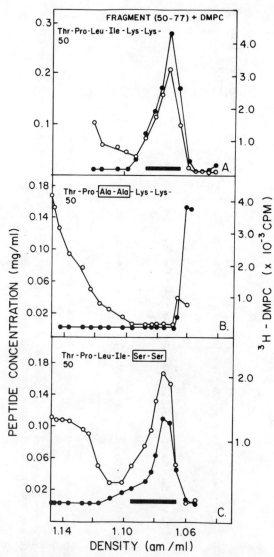

FIGURE 11. Density gradients of synthetic fragments of apolipoprotein A-II containing substitutions in the sequence between 52 and 55. (A) Peptide 50–77 with the natural sequence. (B) Peptide 50–77 with a substitution of Ala for $Leu_{52}Ile_{53}$. (C) Peptide 50–77 with a substitution of Ser for $Lys_{54}Lys_{55}$. The peptide (○—○) concentration was determined by amino acid analysis and the phospholipid (●—●) by counting the [³H]DMPC.

Hydrophobicity Index	
Val – Ser – Ser – Leu – Lys – Glu – Tyr – Trp – Ser – Ser – Leu – Lys – Glu – Ser – Phe – Ser I	– 1092
Val – Ser – Ser – Leu – Lys – Glu – Ala – Ala – Ser – Ser – Leu – Lys – Glu – Ser – Phe – Ser II	– 852
Val – Ser – Ser – Leu – Lys – Glu – Ala – Trp – Ser – Ser – Leu – Lys – Glu – Ser – Phe – Ser III	– 965
Val – Ser – Ser – Leu – Leu – Ser – Ser – Leu – Lys – Glu – Tyr – Trp – Ser – Ser – Leu – Lys – Glu – Ser – Phe – Ser IV	–1120

FIGURE 12. Amino acid sequences of four peptides designed to model phospholipid binding. The peptides have a high Chou-Fasman helix potential and form amphipathic helices when a space filling model of the sequence is built.

TABLE 7

PROPERTIES OF MODEL PEPTIDES

Peptide	Mean Residue Hydrophobicity (cal/residue)	$[\theta]_{222}$ (deg cm^2/dmole)		λ_{max} (nm)	
		Peptide Alone	Peptide+DMPC	Peptide Alone	Peptide+DMPC
I	−1092	−3210	−7782	351	342
II	−852	−2355	−2107	—	—
III	−965	−3625	−5870	351	346
IV	−1120	−5931	−24218	351	332

α helicity of the peptide in these complexes as calculated from the CD spectrum was ~90%.

Using peptide IV as a model, we have made substitutions of different amino acids in the sequence. We find that disruption of binding occurs with substitution of Glu for both Lys_9 and Lys_{16},[41] whereas the substitution of a single Glu for Lys_6 or Lys_{16} does not effect binding. Substitution of two alanines into the hydrophobic face at either positions 4,5,8,11, and/or 15 disrupts binding. Therefore, we conclude that hydrophobicity, helix potential and peptide length are more important in phospholipid binding than ionic interactions with the polar head groups.

SUMMARY AND CONCLUSIONS

With synthetic and native fragments, we have demonstrated that the lipid binding region of apoC-III resides in residues 48–79. Although the helix potential of the amino terminal segment is high, region 1–40 lacks sufficient hydrophobicity and therefore it does not meet the requirements for binding. The amphipathic helical region 40–67 does meet the requirements and is responsible for apoC-III binding to phospholipid.

We have identified residues 17–57 as the minimum sequence of apoC-I required for LCAT activation; at present, we have not identified specific residues responsible for activation. In addition, we have shown that the amphipathic helical region 32–53 is required for phospholipid binding.

From our investigations of synthetic fragments of apoC-II, we suggest that the β turn at residues 60–63 and the β sheet from 64–74 are involved in activation of lipoprotein lipase. The amphipathic helix between 43 and 51 constitutes one of the lipid binding regions of apoC-II. Therefore, we have demonstrated for the first time a clear separation of functions in an apolipoprotein.

We have identified a lipid binding region of apoA-I between residues 220 and 245. From comparison of the sequence of apoC-I and apoA-I we have identified a region (145–185) in the carboxyl terminal cyanogen bromide peptide responsible for LCAT activation. This region, which contains an amphipathic helix, also forms complexes with phospholipid and phospholipid–cholesterol dispersions.

We have shown that residues 12–31 and 50–77 of apoA-II contain two of the lipid binding regions of the protein. We believe these regions to be the amphipathic helices in residues 17–30 and 51–62. In addition, we have demonstrated that $Lys_{54}Lys_{55}$ are not needed for binding but the hydrophobic center formed by $Leu_{52}Ile_{53}$ is critical for binding.

Using the amphipathic helical hypothesis as a guide, we have designed and synthesized a large series of peptides to further establish criteria for phospholipid binding. From our studies of these model peptides as well as synthetic fragments of the native proteins, we suggest that the criteria for binding are (1) the potential to form a helical segment based on Chou-Fasman predictions, (2) a critical length of ~20 amino acids to stabilize the helix, and (3) a minimum hydrophobicity of the nonpolar face of the amphipathic helix of ~ −850 cal/residue.

ACKNOWLEDGMENTS

The authors wish to thank Ms. Sarah Myers for typing the manuscript and Ms. Kaye Shewmaker for drawing the figures.

REFERENCES

1. SMITH, L. C., H. J. POWNALL & A. M. GOTTO, JR. 1978. Ann. Rev. Biochem. **47:** 751–77.
2. GOLDSTEIN, M. & M. S. BROWN. 1977. Ann. Rev. Biochem. **46:**897–930.
3. LaROSA, J. C., R. I. LEVY, P. HERBERT, S. E. LUX & D. S. FREDRICKSON. 1970. Biochem. Biophys. Res. Commun. **41:**45–62.
4. HAVEL, R. J., V. G. SHORE, B. SHORE & D. M. BIER. 1970. Circ. Res. **27:**597– 600.
5. FIELDING, C. J., V. G. SHORE & P. E. FIELDING. 1972. Biochem. Biophys. Res. Commun. **46:**1493–98.
6. SOUTAR, A. K., C. W. GARNER, H. N. BAKER, J. T. SPARROW, R. L. JACKSON, A. M. GOTTO, JR. & L. C. SMITH. 1975. Biochemistry **14:**3057–64.
7. MORRISETT, J. D., R. L. JACKSON & A. M. GOTTO, JR. 1975. Ann. Rev. Biochem. **44:**183–207.
8. SEGREST, J. P., R. L. JACKSON, J. D. MORRISETT & A. M. GOTTO, JR. 1974. FEBS Lett. **38:**247–253.
9. CHOU, P. Y. & G. D. FASMAN. 1978. Ann. Rev. Biochem. **47:**251–76.
10. BREWER, H. B., JR., R. SHULMAN, P. HERBERT, R. RONAN & K. WEHRLY. 1974. J. Biol. Chem. **249:**4975–84.
11. MERRIFIELD, R. B. 1969. Adv. Enzymol. **32:**221.
12. SPARROW, J. T. 1976. J. Org. Chem. **41:**1350–53.
13. SPARROW, J. T., A. M. GOTTO, JR. & J. D. MORRISETT. 1973. Proc. Natl. Acad. Sci. USA **70:**2124.
14. BULL, H. B. & K. BREESE. 1974. Arch. Biochem. Biophys. **161:**665–70.
15. SPARROW, J. T., H. J. POWNALL, F.-J. HSU & A. M. GOTTO, JR. 1977. Biochemistry **16:**5427–31.
16. JACKSON, R. L., J. T. SPARROW, H. N. BAKER, J. D. MORRISETT, O. D. TAUNTON & A. M. GOTTO. 1974. J. Biol. Chem. **249:**5308.
17. SHULMAN, R., P. HERBERT, K. WEHRLY & D. S. FREDRICKSON. 1974. J. Biol. Chem. **250:**182–190.
18. JACKSON, R. L., J. D. MORRISETT, J. T. SPARROW, J. P. SEGREST, H. J. POWNALL, L. C. SMITH, H. F. HOFF & A. M. GOTTO, JR. 1974. J. Biol. Chem. **249:**5314.
19. SOUTAR, A. K., C. W. GARNER, H. N. BAKER, J. T. SPARROW, R. L. JACKSON, A. M. GOTTO, JR. & L. C. SMITH. 1975. Biochemistry **14:**3057.
20. HARDING, D. R. K., J. E. BATTERSBY, D. R. HUSBANDS & W. S. HANCOCK. 1976. J. Am. Chem. Soc. **98:**2664–65.
21. SIGLER, G. F., A. K. SOUTAR, L. C. SMITH, A. M. GOTTO, JR. & J. T. SPARROW. 1976. Proc. Natl. Acad. Sci. USA **73:**1422–26.
22. SPARROW, J. T., H. J. POWNALL, G. F. SIGLER, L. C. SMITH, A. K. SOUTAR & A. M. GOTTO, JR. 1977. Peptides. Proc. 5th Am. Peptide Symp. M. Goodman & J. Meienhofer, Eds. pp. 149–52. John Wiley, New York, N.Y.
23. SOUTAR, A. K., G. F. SIGLER, L. C. SMITH, A. M. GOTTO & J. T. SPARROW. 1978. Scand. J. Clin. Lab. Inves. **38**(Suppl. 150):53–58.
24. JACKSON, R. L., H. N. BAKER, E. B. GILLIAM & A. M. GOTTO, JR. 1977. Proc. Natl. Acad. Sci. USA **74:**1942–45.
25. KINNUNEN, P. K. J., R. L. JACKSON, L. C. SMITH, A. M. GOTTO, JR. & J. T. SPARROW. 1977. Proc. Natl. Acad. Sci. USA **74:**4848–51.

26. SPARROW, J. T. & A. M. GOTTO, JR. 1978. Circulation **58**, Part 2, Abst. 294.
27. BAKER, H. N., T. DELAHUNTY, A. M. GOTTO, JR. & R. L. JACKSON. 1974. Proc. Natl. Acad. Sci. USA **71:**3131–34.
28. BREWER, H. B., T. FAIRWELL, A. LaRUE, R. RONAN, A. HOUSER & T. J. BRONZERT. 1978. Biochem. Biophys. Res. Commun. **80:**623–30.
29. BARKER, W. C. & M. O. DAYHOFF. 1977. Comp. Biochem. Physiol. **57B:**309–15.
30. FITCH, W. M. 1977. Genetics **86:**634–44.
31. SPARROW, J. T., A. H. WARMAN & A. M. GOTTO, JR. 1979. Proc. 6th Am. Peptide Symp. In press.
32. SOUTAR, A. K., H. J. POWNALL, J. J. ALBERS, A. M. GOTTO, JR. & J. T. SPARROW. 1979. Proc. 5th Int. Symp. Atherosclerosis, Houston, Texas. Abstract No. 110.
33. KROON, D. J., J. T. KUPFERBERG, E. T. KAISER & F. J. KEZDY. 1978. J. Am. Chem. Soc. **100:**5975–77.
34. LUX, S. E., K. M. JOHN, R. RONAN & H. B. BREWER. 1972. J. Biol. Chem. **247:**7519–27.
35. CHEN, T. C., J. T. SPARROW, A. M. GOTTO, JR. & J. D. MORRISETT. 1979. Biochemistry **18:**1617–22.
36. MAO, S. J. T., J. T. SPARROW, E. B. GILLIAM, A. M. GOTTO, JR. & R. L. JACKSON. 1977. Biochemistry **16:**4150–56.
37. MAO, S. J. T., J. T. SPARROW, A. M. GOTTO, JR. & R. L. JACKSON. 1978. Fed. Proc. **37**, Abstract 1164.
38. MAO, S. J. T., R. L. JACKSON, A. M. GOTTO, JR. & J. T. SPARROW. Manuscript in preparation.
39. SPARROW, J. T., J. D. MORRISETT, H. J. POWNALL, R. L. JACKSON & A. M. GOTTO, JR. 1975. Peptides: Chemistry, Structure, and Biology. Proc. 4th Am. Peptide Symp. R. Walter & J. Meienhofer, Eds. pp. 597–602. Ann Arbor Science, Ann Arbor, Mich.
40. POWNALL, H. J., A. HU, A. M. GOTTO, JR., J. J. ALBERS & J. T. SPARROW. 1980. Proc. Natl. Acad. Sci. USA. In press.
41. BHATNAGAR, P. K., A. M. GOTTO, JR. & J. T. SPARROW. Manuscript in preparation.

DISCUSSION OF THE PAPER

COMMENT: I was wondering if you have characterized the structure of these phospholipid–peptide complexes.

DR. J. T. SPARROW: They tend to be discoidal complexes.

QUESTION: I wonder if you looked at the protein alone as a function of temperature, and perhaps concentration. I also wonder whether the dissociation from the lipid at around 40° may be a function of the protein conformational change. Does it lose its ellipticity at that point?

DR. SPARROW: There are very small changes in ellipticity as a function of temperature. So it really seems to be more an expression of the dissociation of the lipid from the protein instead of a change in helical structure, if you can believe that the peptide had very little structure to begin with.

DR. A. R. TALL: In your summary you did not make any conclusions about what is being proposed as ionic interactions between the phospholipid polar groups and the hydrophilic surface of the amphipathic helix; I gather from your experiments that the replacement of the charged groups did not make a great difference in binding. Does one conclude that the originally proposed ionic interactions are no longer important?

DR. SPARROW: I believe that this is the case. This internal neutralization of charges among polypeptides may be important in stabilizing the structure. I also feel that the hydrophobic center near the ion pairs is probably more critical to binding than the actual ion pairs. If you put alanine in that position beneath those ion pairs you destroy the binding.

DR. C. EDELSTEIN: In a study of lipid–protein interactions, we are always worried about the state of both the lipid and the protein before we start. I was just wondering if you had looked at these peptide fragments alone in solution. What are their associative properties, and their solubility in the buffers used?

DR. SPARROW: Before lipid binding we treat the peptides with guanidine HCl and then we remove it. The larger peptide does indeed aggregate very much like apoproteins do in solution; we have not studied in detail the mechanism of the association at this point. We have looked at the fluorescence and CD spectra as a function of guanidine HCl concentration and disaggregation does occur at fairly low concentrations.

DR. R. L. JACKSON: I would like to follow up on Dr. Sparrow's comment to Alan Tall. In our original description of the amphipathic helix we felt that we had to have as a requirement two ion pairs. Based on the subsequent results, some of which were discussed today, it seems as if the ion pairs are not so important if you have a hydrophobic index which is high enough to start forming a helix. There are two contributions in other words, one is the ion pairs and the other is the degree of hydrophobicity. I think your elegant peptide syntheses will answer those questions. Now I have a question: In your small peptides, what was the stoichiometry between the phospholipid and peptides?

DR. SPARROW: It depends on how you do the experiment; we changed the stoichiometry from 2 to 1 up to 20 to 1. If you have very low salt concentrations, you can actually isolate the complex by column chromatography having 2 or 3 phospholipids per peptide. If you increase the salt concentration, the complexes that you get are more like 10 or 12 to 1.

DR. SCANU: I recall a time when we discussed these issues with Dr. Segrest, particularly in regard to ion pairs. If ion pairs do not play a role, then the question arises is there a difference between an amphipathic helix in a lipoprotein and the helical segments of other proteins, for instance, cytochrome C. The question really boils down to the issue as to whether the amphipathic helices in apolipoproteins are specific in terms of determining the binding to lipids. I personally would be pleased to know that there is in fact something different between the so-called amphipathic helices in apolipoproteins and those in other proteins.

DR. SPARROW: I think that the helical potential is quite critical as well. It has got to be the hydrophobicity of certain regions in the protein and not hydrophobicity of the total protein. I feel that these amphipathic segments are involved in the stabilization of a lipoprotein complex, and I would also like to think that they are involved in controlling the apoprotein exchange say between VLDL and HDL, and in regard to your particular studies, in displacing apoA-I by apoA-II in HDL.

DR. V. LUZZATI: I think that it would be very interesting to test this wide spectrum of peptides against some physiological phenomenon of any kind. I sense that by staying only with physiochemical reactions we would be just going around in circles to some extent.

DR. SPARROW: We have begun some experiments along these lines. We are trying to look at the association of some of these model peptides with the lipoproteins. Indeed they will associate with lipoproteins, particularly HDL. We have looked at the activation of LCAT, and at the ability of these model peptides to form complexes with DMPC-cholesterol and then used these as a substrate for LCAT. These model peptides are very good detergents, and there is a lot of work that we need to do with them.

DR. GOTTO: I am not sure that I understood DR. Luzzati's question. The work that Dr. Sparrow presented did help to delineate a region in apoC-II that is involved in lipoprotein lipase activation. Other than assessing the enzymatic activation within segments of one apoprotein, and phospholipid binding, I am not sure at this point what else we can do physiologically; apoC-I, a protein which also contains a large amount of amphipathic helices, has been completely synthesized by Dr. Sparrow and his colleagues. This protein also activates LCAT, and a careful delineation is being made between those regions within the protein which are involved in phospholipid binding and in the activation of the enzymes. The fact that synthetic material activates the enzyme, and also contains amphipathic helixes, is about as close as we can come to a physiological test. We have also done some other studies with the synthetic peptides, testing various modifications and their ability to promote cholesterol removal from cells. As for Dr. Scanu's question, we never postulated that the amphipathic helical model was the only way that interactions take place between apoproteins and phospholipids or lipids in lipoproteins. What we did suggest as an hypothesis is that it was a frequent structure in apolipoproteins, and I believe that the evidence accumulated to date from a variety of different procedures and laboratories, as well as studies from evolutionary studies, indicates that this type of basic structure is being preserved. Now, just what the charged ion pairs are doing at this point, we still cannot say. One possibility that has not been mentioned is that it has something to do with the evolution of the interaction of the apoproteins with phospholipids. From evidence obtained from several laboratories using a variety of techniques, those ion pairs do not seem to play a significant role in maintaining the structure of the intact or native lipoprotein. There are differences between the amphipathic structures in apolipoproteins and other proteins. There are many other α helical proteins that do not bind lipid and detailed reasons for this have been given in previous accounts by Segrest and Jackson.

DR. JACKSON: I would also like to reply to Dr. Luzzati's question. After we had built a space-filling model for these various segments, it was clear that we could write down a sequence of amino acids that potentially could generate an amphipathic helix. Dr. Segrest, in collaboration with his colleagues when he was still at the NIH, did a computer search to find out whether or not there were other proteins that indeed had that kind of structure. One of the proteins that we came up with was amyloid A. So, Jerry and I, and Henry Pownall did lipid binding studies on amyloid A, which has never been shown before to be associated with lipid in a system containing DMPC. We found that it exhibited the same type of lipid binding as the apoproteins. That in itself made us all very excited; but what made us even more excited was the report a couple of years later from a group in Seattle that HDL has amyloid A associated with it. So that is another physiological system, which demonstrates that these kinds of structures do exist.

DR. J. B. SWANEY: The current theme this morning has been the discussion of both thermodynamics, which is an equilibrium property, and kinetics, which is a mechanistic property. I am interested in the mechanism by which these peptides bind; for example, do you have any feeling as to whether the initiating event, that is, the interaction of the protein to the lipid bilayer, might occur in the middle of the chain as opposed to the ends? For example, have you carried out any experiments modifying the ends perhaps by charge neutralization to try to define whether they might have a role in the mechanism of the binding of these peptides to lipid?

DR. SPARROW: We have not done those specific experiments. What we have done with model peptides were very careful titration experiments to see how the addition of lipids changed the fluorescence spectrum. Changes were noted when the first two to three moles of phospholipids were added per mole of peptide. So it would appear that ionic interactions initiate the binding. After this initial binding a much larger structure forms. We do not have really good evidence to say that if we were to neutralize the charges that binding will still take place.

Thus, the ion pairs may be very important in controlling the rates of transfer. We also know that helix propagation is important for binding. Helix propagation is illustrated by the studies with apoC-III.

DR. B. SHEN: It seems that everybody agrees here that an amphiphilic helix is one of the necessary factors for lipid binding. The question is, what is sufficient for an α helix to bind lipid? Should we think in terms of just one or a few segments of α helix or of the whole protein in general. For instance, in the case of apoA-I one sees a series of short α-helical segments which appear to give to the apoprotein a great degree of flexibility. Would this be a factor in ligand binding?

DR. SPARROW: I agree and disagree in some respects. In some instance, segments of α helix bind lipids and in some instances not.

DR. FASMAN: Do you have any evidence that the ion pairs are on the outside surface or buried? The reason I ask this is that in many protein structures when you get ion pairs the purpose of the pair is to neutralize the charge, because you do not like to bury your charge in a hydrophobic region. That is not energetically favorable.

DR. SPARROW: A lot of work has been done with the apoproteins as well as with some of the synthetic peptides. It does appear that they orient themselves with the polar face towards the aqueous environment. Fluorescence energy transfer measurements with small peptides seem to indicate that the hydrophobic region is buried and the ion pairs are facing the aqueous environment. Several investigators have demonstrated that these residues are accessible.

GENERAL DISCUSSION

E. T. Kaiser, *Moderator*

University of Chicago
Chicago, Illinois 60637

DR. A. M. GOTTO, JR.: I have a question for Dr. Sparrow. The known increase in helicity of many of the apolipoproteins when they complex with phospholipid may be explained on the basis of hydrophobicity. You are, however, down-playing ionic interaction. Do you believe that the polar portion of the amphipathic helix plays a role in increasing the affinity for the interaction?

DR. J. T. SPARROW: I think that the affinity or the potential is already there. The driving force is the initial association of small amounts of amphiphiles with the protein. In such a case it becomes helical. Henry Pownall, I believe, has demonstrated that the thermodynamic changes that he sees can be attributed to helix formation. Certainly a large amount of the energy released in the microcalorimeter can be attributed to helix formation.

DR. GOTTO: Dr. Pownall has carried out a very careful series of calorimetric experiments measuring enthalpy or ΔH versus not the total amount of helicity in the protein but the delta in helicity, that is, the change in helicity that occurs in a protein as a consequence of its binding to phospholipid. Whether or not the ion pairs contribute to this delta helicity, I do not think it has been established. However, to make a long story short, in the plot of ΔH versus delta helicity when applied to apoC-II, apoA-II, apoA-I, or apoC-I, the intercept is almost but not quite zero. This indicates that virtually all of the energetic components of the association of the apoprotein with phospholipid can be accounted for by the coil to helix transition.

DR. R. L. JACKSON: With respect to Dr. Fasman's question concerning the ionic interactions, we do not feel that they are close to each other; in fact, the spacing is quite significant. They are ion pairs in the sense of each other, but whether or not they are close enough to lead to charge neutralization I do not know.

ACTIVATION OF LIPOPROTEIN LIPASE BY
SYNTHETIC FRAGMENTS
OF APOLIPOPROTEIN C-II *

Louis C. Smith,† John C. Voyta,‡ Alberico L. Catapano,
Paavo K. J. Kinnunen, Antonio M. Gotto, Jr., and
James T. Sparrow §

Departments of Medicine and Biochemistry
Baylor College of Medicine
Texas Medical Center
Houston, Texas 77030

Department of Medicine
The Methodist Hospital
Houston, Texas 77030

Fatty acids released from dietary fat during digestion, except for short chain fatty acids, enter the circulation in the form of chylomicrons. Circulating triglycerides also originate from the liver as very-low-density lipoproteins (VLDL), which carry triglycerides to nonhepatic tissues for utilization or storage. One of the most important metabolic interconversions of lipoproteins occurs in the vascular compartment of the body and involves lipoprotein lipase, which catalyzes the hydrolysis of triglyceride. This enzymatic process at capillary endothelium is the key event in the removal of circulating triglyceride from the plasma. In humans, there appears to be little, if any, uptake of intact triglyceride-rich lipoproteins.[1-4]

Lipoprotein lipase has an additional essential role in the formation of the cholesteryl-ester-rich low-density lipoproteins (LDL), the lipoproteins most closely associated with atherosclerosis.[5] The metabolic precursors of LDL are secreted from the intestine or from the liver in response to cellular synthesis of triglyceride. In man under normal circumstances, greater than 95% of the circulating LDL originates from the triglyceride-rich lipoproteins by the action of lipoprotein lipase.[6] Another metabolically important role has been identified by recent studies that demonstrate the conversion *in vitro* of high-density lipoprotein-3 (HDL$_3$) to HDL$_2$ in the presence of VLDL and lipoprotein lipase.[7] These latter results provide a reasonable explanation for the frequently observed reciprocal relationship of plasma VLDL and HDL levels. Thus, lipo-

* This work was supported by the Robert A. Welch Foundation (Grant Q-343), the National Heart and Blood Vessel Research and Demonstration Center at Baylor College of Medicine (a grant-supported research project of the National Heart, Lung, and Blood Institute, Grant HL-17269), the U.S. Public Health Service (Grant HL-15648), the American Heart Association, Texas Affiliate, and a grant from the Finnish Cultural Foundation to P.K.J.K.
† Address for correspondence: Department of Medicine, The Methodist Hospital, A-601, Room A-654-A, Alkek Tower, 6565 Fannin, Houston, Texas 77030.
‡ Robert A. Welch Predoctoral Fellow.
§ Established Investigator of the American Heart Association.

213

protein lipase has unique roles in lipid metabolism: the uptake of fatty acid into tissue, and the formation of LDL, and the production of HDL_2.

The activation of lipoprotein lipase by apolipoprotein C-II (apoC-II), a protein component of the surface film of chylomicrons, VLDL, and HDL, has been known for some years [8, 9] although the precise mechanism by which this activation occurs has not yet been established. Since lipoprotein lipase does hydrolyze triglyceride in the absence of apoC-II,[10–12] a true coenzyme function for the apoprotein can be excluded.

As a working hypothesis, we assume there is a specific protein-protein interaction of apoC-II with lipoprotein lipase at the lipoprotein surface. Initial support for this postulate has been obtained with monomolecular surface films of apoC-II.[13] At 10 ng/ml and in the absence of lipid, apoC-II forms a stable surface film with a conformation that is biologically active, as shown by the ability of the isolated apoprotein surface film to activate lipoprotein lipase. When apoC-II and lipoprotein lipase are allowed to interact in the absence of lipid, a stable apoprotein:enzyme complex forms at the interface. This surface film complex can be isolated by physical transfer from one subphase to another. This association of lipoprotein lipase and apoC-II has been shown to be extremely strong. The calculated equilibrium dissociation constant for the enzyme:apoC-II complex is 10^{-8} M from one laboratory [14] and 3×10^{-13} M from another.[15] The rate of hydrolysis increases as a function of apoC-II concentration and is maximal at a molar ratio of enzyme to apoC-II of 1:1.[14, 15] Formation of this surface film complex is prevented by sodium chloride,[13] specifically by the chloride anion.[16] The inability to activate in the presence of salts apparently results from the failure to form this enzyme:apoprotein complex.

The minimum sequence of apoC-II required for activation of lipoprotein lipase and identification of functionally important regions of apoC-II have been established in studies [17, 18] with both native and synthetic fragments of apoC-II. Cyanogen bromide (CNBr) fragments of apoC-II corresponding to residues 1–9 and 10–59 do not activate lipoprotein lipase. However, the carboxyl terminal CNBr fragment corresponding to residues 60–78 increases hydrolysis 4-fold, compared to an average of 9-fold activation for the same concentration of apoC-II. The combination of CNBr fragments is no more effective than the COOH-terminal peptide alone. The synthetic peptide containing residues 60–78, prepared by solid-phase techniques, enhances the lipolysis 3-fold, compared to 4-fold by the CNBr fragments 60–78. Addition of five residues produces a synthetic fragment apoC-II(55–78) that gives activation equal to that produced by intact apoC-II. By contrast, removal of the carboxyl terminal residues, Gly-Glu-Glu, from CNBr fragment 60–78 decreases the ability to activate lipoprotein lipase by greater than 95%. Therefore, activation of lipoprotein lipase by apoC-II requires a minimal sequence contained with residues 55–78.

The involvement of the lysine residue at position 75 (Lys_{75}) of apoC-II in activation of lipoprotein lipase has been studied by Musliner et al., who find that acylation of the ϵ-amino group reduces activation about 90%.[19, 20] Half-maximal activation by the maleylated COOH-terminal peptide requires a concentration of about 1.0 μM, a concentration comparable to that required for the succinylated COOH-terminal peptide and about 10-fold greater than that of native apoC-II. Maximal stimulation with both the maleyl and citraconyl COOH-terminal peptides can be achieved at much higher concentration, 10 μM. Activation is about the same as that observed with native apoC-II and roughly twice that obtained with the corresponding succinylated peptide.

A discrete α-helical lipid binding region in apoC-II has been identified in studies of lipoprotein lipase action on VLDL from an individual with a genetically determined absence of apoC-II.[12] Normal rates of ester cleavage could be achieved *in vitro* with native apoC-II and by three shorter synthetic peptides, apoC-II(55–78), apoC-II(50–78), and apoC-II(43–78). At 0.5 μM concentration, each peptide produced a 7-fold activation. ApoC-II(43–78), but not apoC-II(55–78), bound VLDL as shown by separation of unbound ^{125}I peptides and the lipoproteins. Thus, residues 43–50 of apoC-II are part of a lipid binding region. Since the synthetic peptides differ significantly from each other and from apoC-II in their abilities to bind to the apoC-II-deficient VLDL, high-affinity binding of the apoprotein to the lipoprotein surface is not required for hydrolysis of triglyceride by lipoprotein lipase. The formation of easily dissociated complexes of the two shorter apoC-II fragments (lipoprotein lipase and apoC-II-deficient VLDL) seems to be a reasonable possibility, although they are not detected by this experimental technique. The lipid binding region of the peptide makes no apparent contribution to the enhancement of lipoprotein lipase activity. The identity of the lipid binding region has also been established by isolation and characterization of a complex of apoC-II(43–78) and dimyristoylphosphatidylcholine.[21] Under the same experimental conditions, shorter fragments do not form isolatable complexes.

Synthesis of a series of related peptides that differ by a single amino acid or in the number of amino acid residues has been used as an experimental approach to the study of the structure–function relationships in apoC-II. The studies contained in this report are related to the following areas: (a) the functional importance of Tyr at position 62 in apoC-II and (b) the role of the amino acid residues between Tyr_{62} and the carboxyl terminal Glu_{78}. To determine a requirement for the phenolic hydroxyl group of Tyr_{62}, modified peptides, apoC-II(50–78 Phe_{62}), apoC-II(50–78 Trp_{62}), and apoC-II(50–78 Gly_{62}) with phenylalanine, tryptophan, and glycine, respectively, substituted for tyrosine at position 62 were synthesized. The role of the amino acids in the sequence region between Asp_{68} and Glu_{78} was explored with peptides with the sequence of the native peptide apoC-II(35–68), apoC-II(43–68), apoC-II (50–68), apoC-II(55–68), and apoC-II(60–68).

EXPERIMENTAL PROCEDURES

The peptides were prepared by solid-phase peptide synthesis as described previously [17] and after preparative isoelectric focusing had purities greater than 99% and the appropriate amino acid composition. The apparatus and procedures for monolayer assays using tri([1-^{14}C]octanoyl)glycerol [13, 22] and purified bovine milk lipoprotein lipase [23] have been published. In some experiments, assays systems with tri([1-^{14}C]oleoylglycerol dispersed in phosphatidylcholine were employed.[20] Other experimental details are given in the FIGURES.

RESULTS AND DISCUSSION

The substitution of Phe, Trp, or Gly in apoC-II(55–78) for Tyr reduces the activation of lipoprotein-lipase-mediated triglyceride hydrolysis about 60%–70%. The lower activity of apoC-II(55–78 Phe_{62}) may have reflected the functional importance of the phenolic hydroxyl group in the activation of lipo-

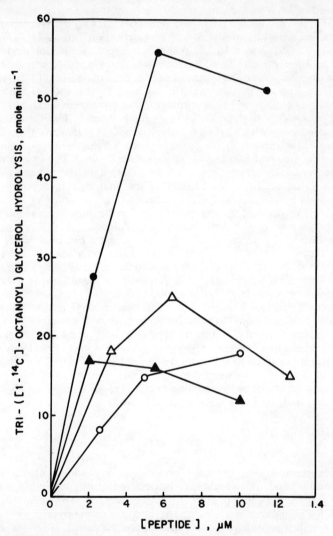

FIGURE 1. Effect of amino acid substitution at position 62 of apoC-II (55–78) on activation of lipoprotein lipase. Lipoprotein lipase, 110 ng, was injected into the stirred subphase to which indicated amounts of activator had been added 10 min previously. The values for decrease in surface radioactivity were obtained from the initial rates, i.e., less than 15% of the substrate had been hydrolyzed. Other experimental details are described in the text.

protein lipase, serving most likely as a hydrogen-bond donor or acceptor. Alternatively, insertion of Phe in lieu of Tyr may have precluded formation of a β turn involving residues 60–63 in apoC-II(55–78), thereby minimizing the ability to activate lipoprotein lipase. To exclude the latter possibility, apoC-II(55–78 Gly_{62}) was also synthesized and tested. This substitution was chosen because of the extremely high conformational potential of Gly in this position to stabilize a β turn.[24, 25] ApoC-II(55–78 Gly_{62}) was able to activate by only ⅓ as much as the native sequence and was comparable to that of apoC-II (55–78 Phe_{62}) and apoC-II(55–78 Trp_{62}). The extent to which Phe and Trp might destabilize a putative β turn is not known; however, the presence of an aromatic nucleus at position 62 is not sufficient for activation of lipoprotein lipase. The similar but lower level of activation by all three substituted peptides indicates that a part of activation can be accomplished by residues adjacent to Tyr_{62} in apoC-II(55–78), and also suggests that multiple residues of the activator peptide interact with the enzyme.

Since the apoC-II(60–75) derived from CNBr apoC-II(60–78) by tryptic removal of the terminal tripeptide was not active, apoC-II(50–75) was synthesized and tested. This fragment was fully active.[26] Furthermore, the activation by apoC-II and the synthetic peptide apoC-II(43–78), apoC-II(50–78), and apoC-II(50–75) was abolished by 1 M NaCl in the reaction mixture. These results exclude competition of the salt anion with the carboxyl terminal Glu residues as a simple explanation for the inhibition of lipoprotein lipase by high salt concentrations.

The empirical rules developed by Chou and Fasman [24, 25] for prediction of the secondary structure of proteins from their amino acid sequence have been used to identify possible structural domains in the carboxyl terminal region of apoC-II. The following secondary structure for apoC-II(35–78) serves as a working hypothesis and provides the rationale for synthesis of the individual synthetic fragments.

$$
\begin{array}{cccc}
 & \alpha\ \text{helix} & \text{nucleates} & \\
 & \text{terminator} & \alpha\ \text{helix} & \\
\alpha\ \text{helix} & & & \alpha\ \text{helix}
\end{array}
$$

Leu-Thr-Glu-Lys-Thr-Tyr-Leu-Pro-Ala-Val-Asp-Glu-Lys-Leu-Arg-Asp-Leu

35   43   50

α helix terminator β breaker β sheet nucleation

Tyr-Ser-Lys-Ser-Thr-Ala-Ala-Met-Ser-Thr-Tyr-Thr-Gly-Ile-Phe-Thr-Asp-

55   60   66   68

β turn β turn

β sheet β breaker

Gln-Val-Leu-Ser-Val-Leu-Lys-Gly-Glu-Glu

75   78

Differences in the activity of apoC-II(60–78) and apoC-II(60–75), the inhibition by high salt and the inactivity of apoC-II(66–78) suggest that a minimum critical length of the activator sequence between residues 60–78 is required for activation. This possibility is supported by the pattern of activation obtained with a series of synthetic peptides with Asp_{68} as the carboxyl terminus, apoC-II(60–68), apoC-II(55–68), apoC-II(50–68), apoC-II(43–68), and apoC-II(35–68) (FIGURE 2).

At low concentrations of peptides, where there was a linear increase in triglyceride hydrolysis with increasing amounts of activator, apoC-II(60–68) and apoC-II(55–68) gave virtually no enhancement of lipoprotein lipase

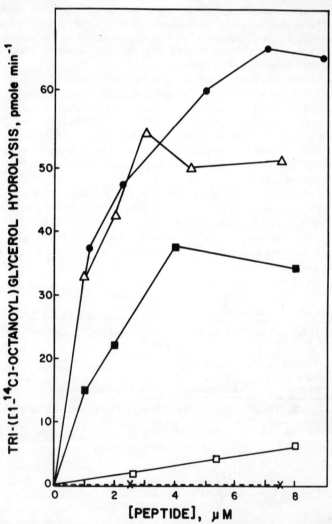

FIGURE 2. Dependence of activation of lipoprotein lipase on inclusion of lipid binding region in apoC-II fragments. The experimental procedures were those described in FIGURE 1.

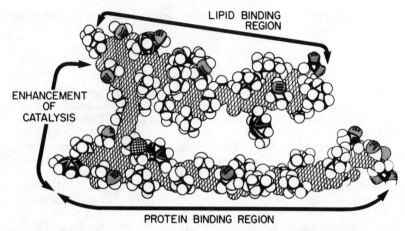

FIGURE 3. Proposed structure–function relationships in apoC-II (35–78).

activity. By contrast, apoC-II(55–78) gave complete activation, identical to that produced by the entire apoC-II. Extension of the peptide chain, as in apoC-II(50–68), apoC-II(43–68), and apoC-II(35–68), increases the ability to activate. The stimulation by these peptides at concentrations up to 4 μM was 50%, 100%, and 100%, respectively, of that of the native peptide. The presence of residues 50–55 in apoC-II(50–78) has no detectable effect on lipoprotein lipase catalysis, since apoC-II(55–78) gives complete activation. Whether the increased activity of apoC-II(50–68), as compared to apoC-II (55–68), results from stabilization of β turn comprised of Ser_{60} Thr_{61} Tyr_{62} Thr_{63} or from direct interaction of Asp_{50} Leu_{51} Tyr_{52} Ser_{53} Lys_{54} with the enzyme remains to be established in future studies of peptide:enzyme equilibrium.

The inclusion of a lipid binding region in the activator peptide gives complete activation, even when the sequence region 69–78 is absent. Thus, in terms of the ability of the peptide to enhance lipoprotein lipase catalysis, full activation can be achieved if two different sequence regions are present. As depicted in FIGURE 3, we postulate that the putative β sheet of residues 63–74 of apoC-II forms hydrogen bonds with a corresponding β sheet of the enzyme. Because the peptide backbone is most likely oriented parallel to the plane of the interface, hydrophobic interactions between the carboxyl terminal region of the apoprotein and the enzyme would seem to be sterically prohibited. Through electrostatic and hydrogen bond interactions, this peptide has sufficiently high affinity for the enzyme to juxtapose the sequence region including Tyr_{62} and lipoprotein lipase, thereby enhancing catalysis. Alternately, if the carboxyl terminal of the putative β sheet of apoC-II is too short for high affinity interaction with the enzyme, the presence of a lipid binding region consisting of residues 43–52 could increase the concentration of the activator at the surface of the macromolecular substrate, where the lipoprotein lipase could interact laterally with the activator. We conclude that enhancement of lipoprotein lipase catalysis depends on specific structural features in apoC-II that concentrate the apoprotein at the interface with the enzyme and the substrate. Both protein–protein and lipid–protein interactions appear to contribute to this process.

SUMMARY

Peptides with different amino acids substituted for the Tyr residue at position 62 were prepared by solid-phase synthesis to identify functionally important amino acids in apoC-II, the activator of lipoprotein lipase. These peptides were apoC-II(55–78 Phe_{62}), apoC-II(55–78 Trp_{62}), and apoC-II(55–78 Gly_{62}). In an assay system of tri-([1-^{14}C]octanoyl)glycerol monolayers and homogeneous bovine lipoprotein lipase, the peptides containing either Phe, Trp, or Gly at position 62 had only $\frac{1}{3}$ the activity of equal molar amounts of either apoC-II(55–78) or native apoC-II. Thus, the phenolic hydroxyl group of Tyr_{62} is necessary for complete activation. ApoC-II(60–75) was inactive while apoC-II(50–75) was fully active. This finding suggested that residues 50–59 in some way compensated for the absent carboxyl terminal residues. This view is supported by the results with apoC-II(60–68), apoC-II(55–68), apoC-II (50–68), apoC-II(43–68), apoC-II(35–68), which gave 0%, 10%, 25%, 100%, and 100% activation, respectively. We postulate that enhancement of catalysis can be achieved in two ways. A putative β sheet of residues 63–74 may form hydrogen bonds with a corresponding β sheet of the enzyme. Alternatively, if this region of the peptide is too short for high-affinity interaction with lipoprotein lipase, inclusion of a lipid binding region gives complete activation, as observed with apoC-II(43–68) and apoC-II(35–68). We conclude that activation depends on structural features in apoC-II that concentrate the apoprotein at the interface with the enzyme and the substrate. Both protein–protein and lipid–protein interactions contribute to this process.

ACKNOWLEDGMENTS

We are indebted to Drs. William A. Bradley and William M. Mantulin for valuable discussions and to Mrs. Karen Pogue for preparation of the manuscript.

REFERENCES

1. ROBINSON, D. S. 1970. The function of the plasma triglycerides in fatty acid transport. Comprehensive Biochem. **18:**51–116.
2. JACKSON, R. L., J. D. MORRISETT & A. M. GOTTO, JR. 1976. Lipoprotein structure metabolism. Phys. Rev. **56:**259–316.
3. SCOW, R. O. 1977. Metabolism of chylomicrons in perfused adipose and mammary tissue of the rat. Fed Proc. **36:**182–185.
4. FIELDING, C. J. & R. J. HAVEL. 1977. Lipoprotein lipase. Arch. Pathol. Lab. Med. **101:**225–229.
5. FREDRICKSON, D. S., J. L. GOLDSTEIN & M. S. BROWN. 1978. *In* Metabolic Basis of Inherited Disease. J. B. Stanburg, J. B. Wyngaarden & D. S. Fredrickson, Eds. 4th Ed. pp. 604–655. McGraw-Hill Book Company, New York, N.Y.
6. SIGURDSSON, G., A. NICOLL & B. LEWIS. 1975. Conversion of very low density lipoprotein to low density lipoprotein. J. Clin. Invest. **56:**1481–1490.
7. PATSCH, J. R., A. M. GOTTO, JR., S. EISENBERG & T. OLIVECRONA. 1978. Formation of high density lipoprotein-like particles during lipolysis of very low density lipoproteins *in vitro*. Proc. Natl. Acad. Sci. USA **75:**4519–4523.

8. LAROSA, J. C., R. I. LEVY, P. N. HERBERT, S. E. LUX & D. S. FREDRICKSON. 1970. A specific apoprotein activator for lipoprotein lipase. Biochem. Biophys. Res. Commun. **41:**57–62.

9. HAVEL, R. J., C. J. FIELDING, T. OLIVECRONA, V. G. SHORE, P. E. FIELDING & T. EGELRUD. 1973. Cofactor activity of protein components of human very low density lipoproteins in the hydrolysis of triglycerides by lipoprotein lipase from different sources. Biochemistry **12:**1828–1833.

10. EGELRUD, T. & T. OLIVECRONA. 1973. Purified bovine milk (lipoprotein) lipase: Activity against lipid substrates in the absence of exogenous serum factors. Biochim. Biophys. Acta **306:**115–127.

11. KINNUNEN, P. K. J., J. K. HUTTUNEN & C. EHNHOLM. 1976. Properties of purified bovine milk lipoprotein lipase. Biochim. Biophys. Acta **450:**342–351.

12. CATAPANO, A. L., P. K. J. KINNUNEN, W. C. BRECKENRIDGE, A. M. GOTTO, JR., R. L. JACKSON, J. A. LITTLE, L. C. SMITH & J. T. SPARROW. 1979. Lipolysis of ApoC-II deficient very low density lipoproteins: Enhancement of lipoprotein lipase action by synthetic fragments of ApoC-II. Biochem. Biophys. Res. Commun. **89:**951–957.

13. MILLER, A. L. & L. C. SMITH. 1973. Activation of lipoprotein lipase by apolipoprotein glutamic acid. J. Biol. Chem. **248:**3359–3362.

14. CHUNG, J. & A. M. SCANU. 1973. Isolation, molecular properties, and kinetic characterization of lipoprotein lipase from rat heart. J. Biol. Chem. **252:**4202–4209.

15. FIELDING, C. J. & P. E. FIELDING. 1977. The activation of lipoprotein lipase by lipase co-protein (apoC-2). *In* Cholesterol Metabolism and Lipolytic Enzymes. J. Polonovski, Ed. pp. 165–172. Masson Publishing Co., New York, N.Y.

16. FIELDING, C. J. & P. E. FIELDING. 1976. Mechanism of salt-mediated inhibition of lipoprotein lipase. J. Lipid Res. **17:**248–256.

17. KINNUNEN, P. K. J., R. L. JACKSON, L. C. SMITH, A. M. GOTTO, JR., & J. T. SPARROW. 1977. Activation of lipoprotein lipase by native and synthetic fragments of human plasma. Proc. Natl. Acad. Sci. USA **74:**4848–4851.

18. SMITH, L. C., P. K. J. KINNUNEN, R. L. JACKSON, A. M. GOTTO, JR. & J. T. SPARROW. 1978. *In* International Conference on Atherosclerosis, L. A. Carlson, R. Paoletti & G. Weber, Eds. pp. 269–273. Raven Press, New York, N.Y.

19. MUSLINER, T. A., E. C. CHURCH, P. N. HERBERT, M. J. KINGSTON & R. S. SHULMAN. 1977. Lipoprotein lipase cofactor activity of a carboxyl-terminal peptide of apolipoprotein C-II. Proc. Natl. Acad. Sci. USA **74:**5358–5362.

20. MUSLINER, T. A., P. N. HERBERT & E. C. CHURCH. 1979. Activation of lipoprotein lipase by native and acylated peptides of apolipoprotein C-II. Biochim. Biophys. Acta **573:**501–509.

21. SPARROW, J. T. & A. M. GOTTO, JR. 1978. Synthetic fragments of apolipoprotein C-II: Phospholipid binding studies. Circulation **58:**11–77.

22. SMITH, L. C. 1972. Hydrolysis of glycerol tri[1-^{14}C]-octanoate and glyceryl tri[1-^{14}C]-oleate monolayers by postheparin lipolytic activity. J. Lipid Res. **13:**769–776.

23. KINNUNEN, P. K. J. 1977. Purification of bovine lipoprotein lipase with the aid of detergent. Med. Biol. **55:**187–191.

24. CHOU, P. Y. & G. D. FASMAN. 1978. Empirical predictions of protein conformation. Ann. Rev. Biochem. **47:**251–276.

25. CHOU, P. Y. & G. D. FASMAN. 1978. Prediction of the secondary structure of proteins from their amino acid sequence. *In* Advances in Enzymology, A. Meister, Ed. pp. 45–148. John Wiley & Sons, New York, N.Y.

26. CATAPANO, A. L., P. K. J. KINNUNEN, A. M. GOTTO, JR., L. C. SMITH & J. T. SPARROW. Unpublished experiments.

DISCUSSION OF THE PAPER

DR. D. STEINBERG: Those few slides hide an awful lot of work. I presume that you are waiting for the primary structure of lipoprotein lipase so that you can finish the job. Maybe you can speculate a little bit on what the relationship may be between substrate and its hydrolysis on the one hand, and the change in the configuration of the lipase on the other hand.

DR. L. C. SMITH: As you say, we need the primary structure of the enzyme, which I understand is what Richard Jackson is going to provide us with one of these days. I envision these two proteins to be coplanar at the interface where they interact with each other laterally at the surface. The residues that appear between 50 and 65 seem to be involved in hydrogen bonding with the enzyme. Beyond that I do not know what changes are produced on the lipase.

DR. M. C. PHILLIPS: My question follows on from that. I would be interested to know how to do the LpL assay. What is the physical state of the substrate? Does the cofactor facilitate the penetration of LpL well into the surface, or does it have to be involved in some sort of proton transfer first?

DR. SMITH: We do not have any direct information on that at this point. We have used three or four different assay systems. The present results were obtained with surface monolayers that contain only triglycerides. The order of addition of materials in the system does not seem to make much difference. It takes usually ten minutes for the activator to interact with the surface. Questions regarding penetration really have to be answered by kinetic experiments which are contemplated.

DR. PHILLIPS: Do you normally get the same kind of results when you take a triolein emulsion for example?

DR. SMITH: You get the same pattern of activation. I do not believe I would compare the kinetics obtained in the emulsion system, where we have no idea of what the surface area of the substrate is, with those found in the monolayer.

DR. S. EISENBERG: I wonder if I can push the last question a little bit further. There are some reports with other modes of activation by apoC-II. Could you comment a little bit more on these other possibilities?

DR. SMITH: I really cannot give that much insight on that.

DR. R. L. JACKSON: Do you have any evidence that apoC-II or any of the fragments that you refer to might interact with lipoprotein lipase?

DR. SMITH: Not yet.

DR. JACKSON: We have continued our studies along these lines. It has been very difficult for us to show that you can actually isolate a complex of apoC-II and the milk enzyme.

DR. SMITH: I think that the exact mode of association of the peptide in solution requires further studies at very low protein concentrations.

DR. JACKSON: We have used 20 μg/ml solutions of apoC-II, which in my mind is a pretty low concentration. Yet we have been unable to demonstrate an actual complex between this apoprotein and the enzyme.

DR. SMITH: Have you done a sedimentation equilibrium study?

DR. JACKSON: No, we have not done that yet.

DR. R. J. HAVEL: The VLDL of the Toronto study missing apoC-II is a very nice reagent. One of the questions that can be answered with it is the amount of apoC-II required in VLDL to produce an optimal substrate for the enzyme. You have an opportunity, here, to add varying amounts to apoC-II and carefully study the product, so to get some insight into this important question.

DR. SMITH: We have looked at this question in one set of experiments and the maximum amount of apoC-II that gives activation is comparable to the amount of apoC-II that one finds in normal VLDL.

DR. J. T. SPARROW: In response to Dr. Eisenberg's question, we have sent these peptides to Tom Olivecrona, and he finds essentially the same activation that Louis Smith has presented here this afternoon.

IN VITRO EFFECTS OF LECITHIN:CHOLESTEROL ACYLTRANSFERASE ON APOLIPOPROTEIN DISTRIBUTION IN FAMILIAL LECITHIN:CHOLESTEROL ACYLTRANSFERASE DEFICIENCY *

John A. Glomset, Carolyn D. Mitchell, Weiling C. King,
Kenneth A. Applegate, Trudy Forte, Kaare R. Norum, and
Egil Gjone

*Howard Hughes Medical Institute Laboratory
Departments of Medicine and Biochemistry
and Regional Primate Research Center
University of Washington
Seattle, Washington 98195*

*Donner Research Laboratory
University of California
Berkeley, California 94720*

*Institute for Nutrition Research
and Medical Department A
Rikshospitalet
University of Oslo
Oslo, Norway*

INTRODUCTION

In recent incubation experiments with plasma from patients afflicted with familial lecithin:cholesterol acyltransferase (LCAT) deficiency,[1] we observed several changes that seemed of potential physiologic significance. First, reaction with partially purified LCAT converted the high-density lipoproteins (HDL) from a highly heterogeneous mixture of disc-shaped particles and small globular particles to material that resembled normal HDL. Second, the cholesteryl esters formed mainly accumulated in very-low-density (VLDL) and low-density lipoproteins (LDL), rather than in HDL. Third, measurements by immunoassay demonstrated an increase in content of apolipoprotein A-I (apoA-I) in HDL and a decrease in content of this apolipoprotein in the protein fraction of $d > 1.21$ g/ml. Finally, visual estimates of apolipoproteins separated by disc gel electrophoresis suggested an increase in content of apolipoprotein E (apoE) in VLDL, a decrease in content of this apolipoprotein in HDL, and generally opposite changes in the distribution of C apolipoproteins (apoC).

The changes in content of VLDL cholesteryl ester and apolipoproteins were of particular interest. They seemed to provide clues concerning the normal molecular relation between VLDL and HDL; and we imagined that a mechanism for increasing the content of apoE in VLDL might influence the fate of

* This investigation was supported by the Howard Hughes Medical Institute, by Grants HL10642, AG00299, RR00166, and HL18574 from the United States National Institutes of Health, by the Anders Jahre Foundation, and by the Norwegian Research Council for Science and the Humanities.

these lipoproteins *in vivo*. We therefore decided to perform an additional series of experiments designed to verify the changes in apolipoprotein distribution observed in our initial experiments, to provide further information concerning the mechanisms involved in the transfer of apoE, and to estimate the rate of transfer of apoE as an aid toward evaluating the possible significance of this transfer *in vivo*. Results of these experiments are described below.

MATERIALS AND METHODS

Subjects

Three Scandinavian female patients, M.R., A.A., and D.J., described previously,[2-5] were studied. Normal controls were females residing in Seattle.

Preparations

Plasma was prepared[6] from subjects who had fasted overnight. Lipoproteins were fractionated by preparative ultracentrifugation,[6] and a subfraction of HDL, rich in apoE, was prepared as described elsewhere.[7]

Triglyceride-rich particles (TRP) were isolated from a triglyceride emulsion generously supplied by AB Vitrum, Stockholm. Both the procedure for isolating the TRP and the general properties of the TRP will be described in another report.[8] The specific TRP used in the present study contained unesterified cholesterol (UC); the molar ratio of UC to phospholipid (PL) was 0.19:1.00.

Partially purified LCAT was prepared using a combination of ultracentrifugal flotation, affinity chromatography on HDL sepharose, chromatography on hydroxyl apatite, and chromatography on DEAE cellulose, as described elsewhere.[1, 9] The preparations were 2300- to 4000-fold purified, and contained traces of albumin and apoA-I, but no apoE.

Analyses

Analyses of intact HDL by electron microscopy and gradient gel electrophoresis were performed as described elsewhere.[7] Quantitative analyses of apolipoproteins were done by densitometry of urea gels and/or SDS gels, as described previously.[7] The method of Kane *et al.*[10] was employed for all apolipoproteins measured in the first experiment. In subsequent experiments this method was used only for apoC-II and apoC-III, while apoC-I and apoE were quantitated using SDS gels. Lipid analyses were performed as in previous studies.[6]

Incubations

All incubations were performed at pH 7.4 and at 37° C, either in 0.154 M NaCl, 0.001 M EDTA, 0.02% NaN_3, or in 0.154 M NaCl, 0.001 M EDTA, 0.01 M Tris-HCl. In rate experiments, the LCAT reaction was terminated by adding *N*-ethylmaleimide (NEM) to a final concentration of 10 mM. Lipoprotein fractions were reisolated after incubation by preparative ultracentrifuga-tion [6] in a 60 Ti rotor of an L2-65B preparative ultracentrifuge (Beckman Instruments, Palo Alto, Calif.). TRP were recovered from the incubation mixtures by centrifuging for 60 min at 20,000 rpm in an SW 27 rotor of the L2-65B preparative ultracentrifuge, using a discontinuous sucrose gradient.[8] The TRP were washed twice by recentrifugation under the same conditions before being analyzed.

RESULTS

We began this investigation by asking two principal questions: (1) can effects of LCAT on the distribution of apoE and apoC among the patients' lipoproteins be confirmed using quantitative techniques, and (2) if so, what are the lipoprotein requirements for these effects? To approach these questions, we fractionated the plasma of patient M.R. into VLDL, LDL, and proteins of $d > 1.063$ g/ml ("$d>1.063$"), and then recombined the fractions as follows in proportions similar to those present in the native plasma.

Mixture 1:	$d>1.063$ + LDL + VLDL
Mixture 2:	$d>1.063$ + VLDL
Mixture 3:	$d>1.063$ + LDL
Mixture 4:	$d>1.063$ + buffer.

We incubated each mixture for 24 hr in the presence or absence of partially purified LCAT, isolated fractions corresponding to VLDL, LDL_1, LDL_2, and HDL, and then analyzed the content of cholesterol and apolipoproteins in the individual fractions. In the case of mixture 1, we found that incubation with LCAT caused a 28% overall decrease in content of UC and an accompanying, nearly threefold increase in content of cholesteryl ester (CE) (TABLE 1). As in previous incubation experiments with the same patients' plasma,[1] the change in UC was largely associated with the HDL and LDL_2, whereas most of the CE formed was recovered in the LDL_2. The amount of UC in the VLDL decreased by nearly one-fourth, but the recovery of TMU-insoluble protein in the VLDL decreased by the same proportion, apparently because the VLDL were partially converted to LDL_1 (TABLE 1). Though the content of UC rela-tive to TMU-insoluble protein in the remaining VLDL did not change, that of CE relative to TMU-insoluble protein increased more than twofold.

Upon analyzing the apolipoprotein content of the fractions isolated from mixture 1, we found evidence for enzyme-dependent changes in the distribution of both apoE and apoC (TABLE 2). The content of apoE relative to TMU-insoluble protein was fourfold to fivefold higher in the VLDL that had been exposed to LCAT than in the control VLDL; and substantial changes in content of apoE also were seen in the LDL_1 and LDL_2. The increased content of this apolipoprotein in lipoproteins of $d < 1.063$ g/ml seemed to have occurred at the expense of HDL since visual estimates of apolipoprotein patterns obtained by disc gel electrophoresis (not shown) revealed an enzyme-dependent decrease in the content of apoE in this fraction. (This experiment was done at a time when only the method of Kane [10] was available for quantitation of apoE; this method does not permit measurement of apoE in the presence of large amounts of apoA-I.)

TABLE 1

EXPERIMENT 1: EFFECT OF INCUBATION WITH LCAT ON LIPOPROTEIN LIPIDS (PATIENT M.R.) *

Incubation Mixture	VLDL		LDL$_1$		LDL$_2$		HDL	
	UC	CE	UC	CE	UC	CE	UC	CE
	(nmoles/ml incubation mixture)							
1. VLDL+LDL+d>1.063								
−LCAT	189	93	86	29	1395	105	336	13
+LCAT	144	169	107	101	1063	341	118	79
2. VLDL+d>1.063								
−LCAT	163	86	14	4	115	13	341	9
+LCAT	132	188	27	29	93	79	93	105
3. LDL+d>1.063								
−LCAT	23	10	65	25	1443	112	342	13
+LCAT	14	14	76	75	1092	437	158	106
4. d>1.063								
−LCAT	n.d.	n.d.	n.d.	n.d.	119	19	336	17
+LCAT	n.d.	n.d.	n.d.	n.d.	86	98	109	193

* UC, unesterified cholesterol; CE, cholesteryl ester; n.d., not detectable; d>1.063, proteins of d>1.063 g/ml.

TABLE 2

EXPERIMENT 1: EFFECTS OF LCAT ON THE DISTRIBUTION OF APOLIPOPROTEINS AMONG LIPOPROTEINS ISOLATED FROM MIXTURE 1 *

Reisolated Lipoproteins After Incubation ±LCAT	"B"	E	Apolipoproteins				
			C-I	C-II	C-III$_1$	C-III$_2$	
			(μg amino acyl mass/ml incubation mixture ±SD)				
VLDL							
−LCAT	39.3	3.33±0.38	9.84±0.75	4.23±0.34	5.11±0.36	5.72±0.70	
+LCAT	30.2	13.14±1.83	5.57±1.17	1.81±0.17	1.98±0.23	2.11±0.37	
		$p=0.0002$	$p=0.0003$	$p < 0.0001$	$p < 0.0001$	$p < 0.0001$	
LDL$_1$							
−LCAT	29	4.27±0.53	6.05±1.07	2.36±0.32	3.23±0.41	4.22±0.54	
+LCAT	38	11.79±1.59	7.32±0.43	2.14±0.15	2.32±0.18	3.23±0.28	
		$p=0.0002$	n.s.	n.s.	$p=0.005$	$p=0.01$	
LDL$_2$							
−LCAT	226	15.29±3.54	18.86±3.26	2.83±0.26	4.75±0.47	4.88±0.63	
+LCAT	227	23.92±4.56	13.33±1.28	3.60±0.64	6.46±1.17	6.56±1.27	
		$p=0.011$	$p=0.016$	n.s.	$p=0.028$	$p=0.039$	
HDL							
−LCAT	n.m.	n.m.	13.81±2.57	3.35±0.44	4.99±0.93	4.66±0.97	
+LCAT	n.m.	n.m.	27.70±3.78	6.06±0.87	7.31±1.24	7.43±1.78	
			$p=0.01$	$p=0.02$	n.s.	n.s.	

* All TMU-soluble apolipoproteins in this experiment were measured by the method of Kane [10] using standards generously provided by him; n.m., not measured; n.s., not significant, $p > 0.05$.

TABLE 3

EXPERIMENT 1: EFFECTS OF LCAT ON THE DISTRIBUTION OF APOLIPOPROTEINS AMONG LIPOPROTEINS ISOLATED FROM MIXTURE 2 *

Reisolated Lipoproteins After Incubation ±LCAT	"B"	Apolipoproteins				
		E	C-I	C-II	C-III$_1$	C-III$_2$
		(μg amino acyl mass/ml incubation mixture ±SD)				
VLDL						
−LCAT	39.3	2.65±0.28	8.36±0.83	3.31±0.49	3.97±0.58	4.49±0.67
+LCAT	26.6	15.39±1.35	3.37±0.44	1.47±0.12	1.56±0.11	1.72±0.06
		$p=0.0002$	$p=0.0002$	$p=0.004$	$p=0.003$	$p=0.004$
LDL$_1$						
−LCAT	9.07	0.98±0.09	0.66±0.09	0.23±0.03	0.28±0.03	0.32±0.06
+LCAT	8.00	2.13±0.05	0.80±0.17	0.24±0.02	0.38±0.11	0.40±0.07
		$p<0.0001$	n.s.	n.s.	n.s.	n.s.
LDL$_2$						
−LCAT	24.98	7.06±1.08	1.41±0.46	0.32±0.07	0.52±0.16	0.62±0.23
+LCAT	29.69	20.64±3.37	3.62±0.90	1.10±0.19	2.52±0.28	2.56±0.51
		$p=0.0004$	$p=0.003$	$p=0.0003$	$p<0.0001$	$p=0.0004$
HDL						
−LCAT	n.m.	n.m.	22.51±4.72	3.09±0.45	4.56±0.91	5.26±0.68
+LCAT	n.m.	n.m.	28.14±7.09	5.10±0.92	5.90±1.21	7.34±1.09
			n.s.	$p=0.005$	n.s.	$p=0.009$

* All TMU-soluble apolipoproteins measured as indicated in TABLE 2; n.m., not measured; n.s., not significant, $p > 0.05$.

The enzyme-dependent changes in distribution of apoC were generally opposite to the changes in distribution of apoE. The contents of individual apoC, relative to TMU-insoluble protein, were 28% to 49% lower in the VLDL that had been incubated in the presence of LCAT than in the control of VLDL; and similar though less impressive changes in apoC-II and apoC-III were evident in the LDL_1. In contrast, the contents of apoC-II and apoC-III in LDL_2 and the contents of each of the apoC in HDL were higher after incubation with LCAT than in the controls. (Note that the total recovery of apoC in the combined lipoprotein fractions of $d < 1.25$ g/ml was not affected by the presence of LCAT.) We conclude that incubation with partially purified LCAT causes marked changes in the quantitative distribution of both apoE and apoC in the plasma of patients afflicted with familial LCAT deficiency.

Analysis of the lipoproteins isolated from mixtures 2–4 provided information concerning the lipoprotein requirements for these enzyme-dependent effects. Changes in distribution of VLDL apolipoproteins occurred in the presence or absence of LDL (compare TABLES 2 & 3); and similar changes in distribution of LDL_1 apolipoproteins (not shown) occurred in the presence or absence of VLDL. There was, however, no increase in content of apoE in material of $d < 1.019$ g/ml, unless VLDL or LDL_1 was present in the original incubation mixture (not shown). This suggests that the enzyme-dependent redistribution of apoE depends on transfer of apoE from HDL to pre-existing lipoproteins of $d < 1.019$ g/ml rather than on a change in flotation properties of apoE-rich HDL.

To obtain further information concerning the requirements for the LCAT-dependent redistribution of apoE, we sought to determine whether artificially prepared TRP can substitute for VLDL as acceptors of apoE. To answer this question, we performed a second experiment using HDL, and proteins of $d > 1.25$ g/ml ("$d>1.25$") prepared from the plasma of patient M.R. These fractions were mixed with the same patient's VLDL or with TRP as follows:

$$\text{Mixture 1:} \quad \text{VLDL} + \text{HDL} + d>1.25$$
$$\text{Mixture 2:} \quad \text{TRP} + \text{HDL} + d>1.25.$$

We incubated each mixture for 24 hr with or without partially purified LCAT, and then isolated fractions corresponding to VLDL and HDL by preparative ultracentrifugation. Upon analyzing the fractions isolated from mixture 1, we obtained results compatible with those found in experiment 1. Incubation with LCAT decreased the content of UC, primarily in the HDL, and increased the content of CE, primarily in the VLDL (TABLE 4). In addition, analysis of the VLDL demonstrated an enzyme-dependent increase in content of apoE and a concomitant decrease in content of apoC, whereas analysis of the HDL showed opposite changes in the apolipoproteins (TABLE 5).

Analysis of the fractions isolated from mixture 2 (TABLE 4) revealed changes in content of CE similar to those observed in the fractions of mixture 1. Furthermore, there was an *enzyme-dependent* increase in content of apoE in the TRP similar to that seen in the case of the VLDL. (Note that about 70% of the original apoE was recovered in the combined lipoprotein fractions of the two mixtures incubated without LCAT, but that less apoE was recovered after incubation in the presence of LCAT.) We conclude that TRP effectively accept both CE and apoE and that the transfer of these substances requires prior action of LCAT on patient $d>1.063$, but does not require the presence of apoB in the acceptor.

To identify the donor of apoE among the patients' plasma $d>1.063$, we performed a third experiment, using material from patient A.A. We subfractionated her HDL by affinity chromatography on heparin-agarose [7] and by gel filtration on Sephadex G 200 to prepare (1) disc-shaped HDL, rich in apoE (apoE-HDL), (2) disc-shaped HDL, containing apoA-I and apoA-II, but no apoE, and (3) small spherical HDL containing apoA-I. We mixed each subfraction with TRP, LCAT, and $d>1.25$, incubated the mixtures up to 24 hr, and analyzed the contents of CE and apoE in the reisolated TRP (results not shown). Whereas formation and transfer of CE occurred in all instances, transfer of apoE occurred only in the mixture containing apoE-HDL. No transfer of apoE occurred in a fourth mixture, which contained TRP, LCAT, and $d>1.25$ but no HDL.

To examine enzyme-dependent effects on the apoE-HDL that might be related to transfer of apoE, we performed a fourth experiment, again using

TABLE 4

EXPERIMENT 2: EFFECTS OF INCUBATION WITH LCAT ON LIPIDS OF TRIGLYCERIDE-RICH PARTICLES (TRP) AS COMPARED WITH VLDL OF PATIENT M.R.

	VLDL or TRP			HDL		
	UC	CE	TG	UC	CE	TG
Incubation Mixture	(nmoles/ml incubation mixture)					
1. VLDL+HDL+$d>1.21$ *						
−LCAT	254	97	320	236	4	10
+LCAT	221	324	301	53	77	40
2. TRP+HDL+$d>1.21$						
−LCAT	104	16	348	122	0.1	8
+LCAT	61	239	448	33	49	29

* Proteins of $d > 1.21$ g/ml.

material prepared from the plasma of patient A.A. We incubated her apoE-HDL with $d>1.25$ and TRP as follows:

Mixture 1:   apoE-HDL + $d>1.25$ + TRP; incubation for 22 hr ± LCAT
Mixture 2:   apoE-HDL + $d>1.25$; incubation for 22 hr ± LCAT
Mixture 3:   apoE-HDL + $d>1.25$; incubation for 22 hr ± LCAT, then 22 hr + TRP +NEM

We then reisolated the TRP and a second fraction containing the remainder of the lipoproteins of $d > 1.006$ g/ml (largely HDL), analyzed the lipid and apolipoprotein content of both fractions, and examined the HDL by electron microscopy and gradient gel electrophoresis. The TRP isolated from mixtures 1 and 3 showed enzyme-dependent increases in content of both CE and apoE (TABLE 6), though the change in apoE in the TRP isolated from mixture 3 was less than half that in the TRP isolated from mixture 1. No apoE was detected in the fraction corresponding to TRP isolated from mixture 2. Analyses of the reisolated HDL, however, revealed enzyme-dependent decrements

TABLE 5

EXPERIMENT 2: EFFECTS OF INCUBATION WITH LCAT ON APOLIPOPROTEINS OF TRP AS COMPARED WITH VLDL OF PATIENT M.R.

Incubation Mixture	VLDL or TRP Apolipoproteins					HDL Apolipoproteins						
	E	C-I	C-II	C-III$_1$	C-III$_2$	A-I	A-II	E	C-I	C-II	C-III$_1$	C-III$_2$
	(μg amino acyl mass/ml incubation mixture)											
1. VLDL+HDL+d>1.21 *												
−LCAT	15.9	2.42	2.59	2.19	2.62	45.8	7.0	31.5	0.91	0.55	1.00	1.06
+LCAT	31.0	1.58	1.17	1.09	1.34	68.3	12.8	8.9	2.18	1.54	2.00	1.99
2. TRP+HDL+d>1.21												
−LCAT	0.6	0.70	0.31	0.36	0.27	53.5	7.3	39.3	0.58	0.34	0.92	0.93
+LCAT	10.9	0.60	0.45	0.50	0.74	90.7	9.2	10.3	1.09	0.43	0.84	0.73

* Proteins of d>1.21 g/ml.

in content of apoE in all three mixtures (TABLE 7). Since the absolute decrements in all cases exceeded by several-fold the absolute increments in content of apoE in the TRP, incubation with LCAT clearly led to a net loss of apoE from HDL whether an acceptor was present or not. Moreover, after incubation with LCAT, apoE remaining in or released from the HDL was able to bind to TRP during a subsequent incubation performed in the absence of enzyme activity.

Further analyses of the HDL revealed several enzyme-dependent changes that might have influenced the redistribution of apoE. In addition to the changes in lipid content, there was an LCAT-dependent increment in the con-

TABLE 6

EXPERIMENT 4: REISOLATED TRP AFTER INCUBATION WITH
APOLIPOPROTEIN E-HDL±LCAT

Incubation Mixture	UC	CE	PL	ApoE
				(μg amino acyl mass/ml incubation mixture)
	(nmoles/ml incubation mixture)			
1. ApoE-HDL+d>1.25+TRP				
−LCAT	622	72	618	0
+LCAT	287	1245	616	317
2. ApoE-HDL+d>1.25				
−LCAT	0	36	10	0
+LCAT	0	41	12	0
3. ApoE-HDL+d>1.25±LCAT; then TRP and NEM added after 22 hr				
−LCAT *	622	67	750	44
+LCAT *	355	1760	808	172

* LCAT present or absent during first 22 hr incubation, i.e., before addition of N-ethylmaleimide.

tent of apoA-I (TABLE 7). Furthermore, the disc-shaped HDL were converted to spherical particles (not shown). Finally, the HDL changed in size as revealed by electron microscopy (FIGURE 1) and gradient gel electrophoresis (FIGURE 2). This change in size appeared to depend on the formation of CE by the LCAT reaction and on the transfer of CE from HDL to TRP. Which one or combination of these changes most directly promoted the redistribution of apoE between the HDL and TRP remains, however, to be established.

To study the rate of transfer of apoE from HDL to TRP, we performed an experiment with the plasma of patient D.J. We prepared d>1.063 by ultracentrifugal flotation, dialyzed it against saline-EDTA-azide, and then incubated it with TRP for periods ranging from 0.5 to 24 hr. After the incubation we added NEM to block further LCAT activity, and then separately isolated and analyzed the TRP and HDL. Analysis of the rate of formation of CE in the incubated mixtures (FIGURE 3) showed rapid formation within the first hour, followed by a gradual slowing of the reaction. The amount of CE recovered in HDL likewise increased rapidly at first and then plateaued at about 2 hr. The rate of transfer of newly formed CE to TRP was slower, but remained essentially linear for about 4 hr and then gradually decreased. The rate of transfer of apoE to TRP was still slower, and appeared to remain linear for the entire 24-hr incubation period.

We examined the effects of incubation with LCAT on the distribution of HDL by gradient gel electrophoresis (FIGURE 4). Detectable, enzyme-dependent changes occurred within 0.5 to 1 hr. Further incubation led to the formation of two subpopulations that migrated in positions corresponding to normal

TABLE 7

EXPERIMENT 4: REISOLATED HDL AFTER INCUBATION±LCAT±TRP

	UC	CE	PC	ApoE	ApoA-I
				(μg amino acyl mass/ml	
Incubation Mixture	(nmoles/incubation mixture)			incubation mixture)	
1. ApoE-HDL+d>1.25+TRP					
−LCAT	1410	83	2190	1181	206
+LCAT	290	253	1190	337	605
2. ApoE-HDL+d>1.25					
−LCAT	1743	94	2000	1194	85
+LCAT	610	1738	1034	498	746
3. ApoE-HDL+d>1.25±LCAT; then TRP and NEM added after 22 hr					
−LCAT *	1077	101	2158	947	191
+LCAT *	229	152	1210	317	557

* LCAT present or absent during first 22 hr incubation, i.e., before addition of NEM.

HDL_2 and HDL_3. Maximal expression of these subpopulations was seen at 4 hr, after which a more monodisperse population of intermediate size appeared.

Since approximately 4 hr of incubation with LCAT were required to generate a distribution of HDL similar to that present in normal plasma, it seemed possible that the rate of transfer of apoE observed in this experiment might be considerably slower than that which might occur in normal subjects *in vivo*. Thus, if disc-shaped HDL, rich in apoE, are normally secreted into human plasma, they must mix with circulating HDL that have already reacted extensively with LCAT. This would be a situation quite different from that initially occurring in our *in vitro* experiments with plasma from LCAT-deficient patients. We therefore performed a sixth experiment, designed to approach more closely the conditions presumed to exist *in vivo*. In this experiment, we incubated TRP and normal plasma d>1.063 with or without apoE-HDL from patient

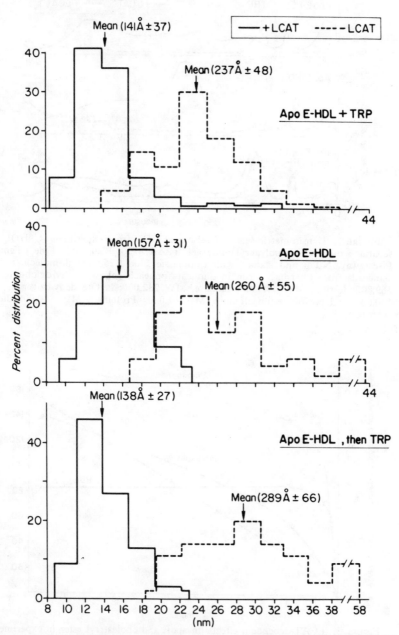

FIGURE 1. Size distribution of reisolated HDL after 22 hr incubation ± LCAT (experiment 4). Diameters were determined from electron micrographs of negatively stained particles; 100–200 particles were measured in each sample.

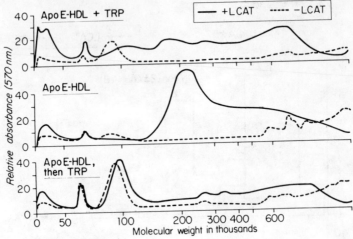

FIGURE 2. Densitometric scans of reisolated HDL from experiment 4. HDL were separated on gradient polyacrylamide gels (PAA 4/30, Pharmacia Fine Chemicals, Piscataway, N.J.), and stained with Coomassie Blue R250. High-molecular-weight standards from Pharmacia, run in duplicate on each gel, were thyroglobulin, MW 669,000; ferritin, MW 440,000; catalase, MW 232,000; lactate dehydrogenase, MW 140,000; and bovine serum albumin, MW 67,000. Proteins > MW 800,000 did not enter the gel.

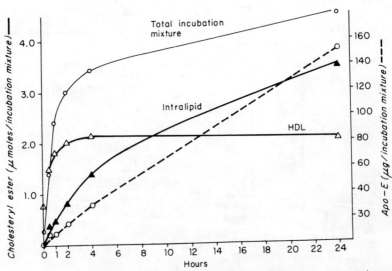

FIGURE 3. LCAT-dependent effects on apoE and cholesteryl ester in experiment 5. Plasma proteins of $d > 1.063$ g/ml from patient D.J. were incubated with TRP and LCAT. Shown are the rate of formation of cholesteryl ester, the rates of accumulation of cholesteryl ester in TRP (▲—▲) and HDL (△—△), and the rate of transfer of apoE to TRP (○---○).

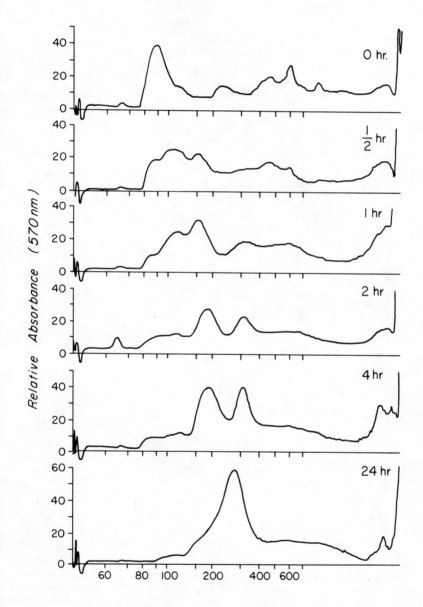

Molecular weight in thousands

FIGURE 4. LCAT-dependent effects on the distribution of HDL in experiment 5. Shown are densitometric traces of reisolated HDL electrophoresed on precast polyacrylamide gradient gels as described in FIGURE 2.

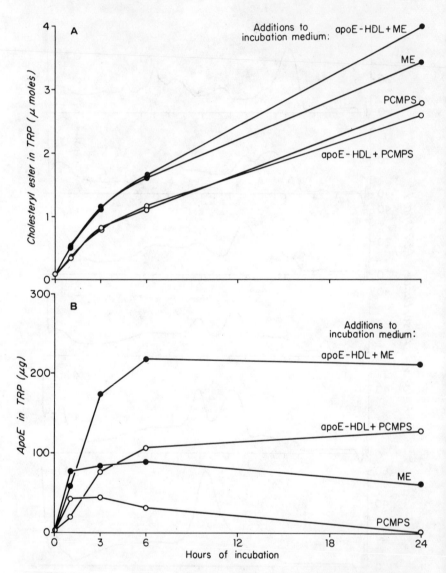

FIGURE 5. (A) Transfer of cholesteryl ester to TRP during incubation of normal plasma proteins of $d > 1.063$ g/ml $\pm$ apoE-HDL (experiment 6). Amount of cholesterol esterified in the total mixtures during 24 hr: normal proteins+apoE-HDL+mercaptoethanol (ME), 5.99 μmoles; normal proteins+ME, 5.51 μmoles; normal proteins+apoE-HDL+p-chloromercuriphenylsulfonate (PCMPS), 0.24 μmoles; normal proteins+PCMPS, 1.29 μmoles. (B) Transfer of apoE to TRP in the same experiment.

A.A. in the presence of 2 mM *p*-chloromercuriphenylsulfonate (PCMPS) or 10 mM mercaptoethanol (ME). After incubating the mixtures for 1 to 24 hr, we isolated the TRP and determined the content of CE and apoE. We found (FIGURE 5A) a relatively rapid initial accumulation of CE that seemed unaffected by the presence of added apoE-HDL but that was somewhat greater in the presence of ME than in that of PCMPS. In addition, there was a relatively rapid transfer of apoE to the TRP in all cases, maximum accumulation being reached within 6 hr (FIGURE 5B). In contrast to the rate of transfer of CE, the rate of transfer of apoE greatly depended on both the presence of added apoE-HDL, and the presence of ME as opposed to PCMPS. We conclude from these experiments that transfer of apoE occurs independently of transfer of CE; and that the rate of transfer of apoE may be affected by the interaction of apoE-HDL with both LCAT and other HDL.

DISCUSSION

The results of this investigation confirm and extend our previous impression [1] that incubation with LCAT alters the distribution of apoE and apoC in the plasma of patients afflicted with familial LCAT deficiency. The content of apoE clearly decreases in lipoproteins of $d > 1.019$ g/ml and increases in lipoproteins of $d < 1.019$ g/ml, while opposite changes occur in the content of apoC. Though the mechanisms that underlie these shifts remain to be fully clarified, the following conclusions about the redistribution of apoE seem justified. First, the source of the apoE that redistributes to VLDL and LDL_1 is clearly the "apoE-HDL." Second, these HDL are relatively stable unless incubated with LCAT. Third, action of LCAT converts the disc-shaped apoE-HDL to spherical lipoproteins that have a decreased affinity for apoE and an increased affinity for apoA-I. Fourth, these lipoproteins maintain a relatively high density compared with VLDL or LDL_1, i.e., they are not caused to float like the apoE-rich "HDL-C" of $d < 1.019$ g/ml described by Mahley and coworkers.[11] Finally, apoE that dissociates from the apoE-HDL becomes available for transfer to acceptors such as VLDL, LDL_1, or TRP. Why the action of LCAT promotes dissociation of apoE from the HDL is a critical question that remains to be answered. We suggest that attention be directed toward the effects of changing disc-shaped HDL to spherical HDL on the affinity of HDL for apoE and apoA-I.

The metabolic significance of the LCAT-dependent shifts in distribution of apoE and apoC is not completely clear. Since the patients' native VLDL contain abnormally high amounts of apoC-I and apoE, and abnormally low amounts of apoC-II and apoC-III,[12] the *in vitro* effects of the LCAT reaction in most cases exacerbate rather than ameliorate existing abnormalities in the distribution of VLDL apolipoproteins. The net result is to increase the content of apoE in the patients' VLDL to a level similar to that found for the total apoE in the VLDL of patients who have dysbetalipoproteinemia.[13] The failure of LCAT to reverse the abnormalities in the patients' native VLDL suggests that these abnormalities depend only indirectly on the LCAT deficiency. They deserve attention, however, since they may be related to the abnormality in cholesterol transport that clearly accompanies the disease.[14]

We currently speculate that the patients' apoE-HDL may be of hepatic origin, since Hamilton and colleagues [15, 16] have observed very similar HDL in rat liver perfusates. We assume that disc-shaped, apoE-HDL are secreted by the normal human liver, and that LCAT normally promotes the transfer of apoE from these HDL to VLDL and LDL_1. However, since the VLDL of LCAT-deficient patients are rich in apoE, other mechanisms for providing apoE to VLDL must exist also. Furthermore, the content of apoE in normal VLDL appears to be remarkably constant, despite changes in lipoprotein size associated with the removal of triglyceride.[12] A continuous, normal, LCAT-dependent transfer of apoE from apoE-HDL to VLDL would therefore have to be balanced by mechanisms that continuously remove apoE from VLDL as well.

Summary

Action of LCAT on the plasma of patients afflicted with familial LCAT deficiency shifts the distribution of C apolipoproteins from lipoproteins of $d < 1.019$ g/ml to lipoproteins of $d > 1.109$ g/ml, and causes an opposite shift in the distribution of apolipoprotein E. The altered distribution of apolipoprotein E appears to depend primarily on enzyme-related effects on HDL. Loss of apolipoprotein E from HDL occurs as cholesteryl esters are formed and transfer to other lipoproteins; disc-shaped HDL, rich in apolipoprotein E, are converted into spherical particles; and the population of HDL as a whole is converted first into particles the size of HDL_2 and HDL_3 and then into intermediate-sized particles. Transfer of apolipoprotein E to artificially prepared, triglyceride-rich particles occurs at a nearly linear rate that is slower than the rates of formation and transfer of cholesteryl esters or the rate of formation of "HDL_2" and "HDL_3." Transfer of apolipoprotein E is faster, however, when the patients' disc-shaped HDL are incubated with triglyceride-rich particles in the presence of normal plasma lipoproteins of $d > 1.063$ g/ml. Since the disc-shaped HDL, rich in apolipoprotein E, resemble particles reported to be released from perfused rat livers, they may be nascent lipoproteins of hepatic origin. If so, it appears that action of LCAT on these lipoproteins may be one of the factors that regulates the content of apolipoprotein E in VLDL.

References

1. NORUM, K. R., J. A. GLOMSET, A. V. NICHOLS, T. FORTE, J. J. ALBERS, W. C. KING, C. D. MITCHELL, K. R. APPLEGATE, E. L. GONG, V. CABANA & E. GJONE. 1975. Plasma lipoproteins in familial lecithin:cholesterol acyltransferase deficiency: Effects of incubation with lecithin:cholesterol acyltransferase *in vitro.* Scand. J. Clin. Lab. Invest. 35 (Suppl. 142):31–55.
2. NORUM, K. R. & E. GJONE. 1967. Familial lecithin:cholesterol acyltransferase deficiency. Biochemical study of a new inborn error of metabolism. Scand. J. Clin. Lab. Invest. 20:231–243.
3. GJONE, E. & K. R. NORUM. 1968. Familial serum cholesterol ester deficiency. Clinical study of a patient with a new syndrome. Acta Med. Scand. 183:107–112.
4. NORUM, K. R., S. BØRSTING & I. GRUNDT. 1970. Familial lecithin:cholesterol acyltransferase deficiency. Study of two new patients and their close relatives. Acta Med. Scand. 188:323–326.
5. GJONE, E., A. J. SKARBOVIK, J. P. BLOMHOFF & P. TEISBERG. 1974. Familial lecithin:cholesterol acyltransferase deficiency. Report of a third Norwegian

family with two afflicted members. Scand. J. Clin. Lab. Invest. **33** (Suppl. 137):101–105.

6. GLOMSET, J. A., K. R. NORUM & W. KING. 1970. Plasma lipoproteins in familial lecithin:cholesterol acyltransferase deficiency: Lipid composition and reactivity *in vitro*. J. Clin. Invest. **49**:1827–1837.

7. MITCHELL, C. D., W. C. KING, T. FORTE, J. A. GLOMSET, K. R. NORUM & E. GJONE. 1980. Characterization of high density lipoproteins, rich in apolipoprotein E, in familial lecithin:cholesterol acyltransferase deficiency. J. Lipid Res. In press.

8. ERKELENS, D. W., C. CHEN, C. D. MITCHELL & J. A. GLOMSET. Interaction of apolipoproteins with artificially prepared triglyceride-rich particles. To be published.

9. AKANUMA, Y. & J. GLOMSET. 1968. A method for studying the interaction between lecithin:cholesterol acyltransferase and high density lipoproteins. Biochem. Biophys. Res. Commun. **32**:639–643.

10. KANE, J. P. 1973. A rapid electrophoretic technique for identification of subunit species of apolipoproteins in serum lipoproteins. Anal. Biochem. **53**:350–364.

11. MAHLEY, R. W. 1978. Alterations in plasma lipoproteins induced by cholesterol feeding in animals including man. *In* Disturbances in Lipid and Lipoprotein Metabolism. J. M. Dietschy, A. M. Gotto & J. A. Ontko, Eds. pp. 181–197. American Physiological Society, Bethesda, Md.

12. GLOMSET, J. A., T. FORTE, K. R. NORUM, W. C. KING, K. R. APPLEGATE, C. D. MITCHELL & E. GJONE. 1980. Abnormal distribution of very low density lipoprotein apoproteins in familial lecithin:cholesterol acyltransferase deficiency. J. Lipid Res. In press.

13. HAVEL, R. J. & J. P. KANE. 1973. Primary dysbetalipoproteinemia: Predominance of a specific apoprotein species in triglyceride-rich lipoproteins. Proc. Natl. Acad. Sci. USA **70**:2015–2019.

14. GLOMSET, J. A., K. R. NORUM, A. V. NICHOLS, W. C. KING, C. D. MITCHELL, K. R. APPLEGATE, E. L. GONG & E. GJONE. 1975. Plasma lipoproteins in familial lecithin:cholesterol deficiency: Effects of dietary manipulation. Scand. J. Clin. Lab. Invest. **35** (Suppl. 142):3–30.

15. HAMILTON, R. L., M. C. WILLIAMS, C. J. FIELDING & R. J. HAVEL. 1976. Discoidal bilayer structure of nascent high density lipoproteins from perfused rat liver. J. Clin. Invest. **58**:667–680.

16. FELKER, T. E., M. FAINARU, R. L. HAMILTON & R. J. HAVEL. 1977. Secretion of the arginine-rich and A-I lipoproteins by the isolated perfused rat liver. J. Lipid Res. **18**:465–473.

DISCUSSION OF THE PAPER

QUESTION: The composition of HDL which you used has a relatively high proportion of free cholesterols and it would not be expected to be a very active substrate for LCAT. It is rather surprising that the ratio should be that high. Have you compared this activity to other reference substrates?

DR. GLOMSET: In familial LCAT deficiency, free cholesterol accumulates in all lipoproteins. With reference to the discs, I compared their reactivity with LCAT with that of other fractions of the same patient's HDL, and the apoE-rich discs seemed to react as well as the other fractions including the very small HDL, 57 Å in diameter, which contain only apoA-I. Why in these patients the reaction should stop after two hours as abruptly as it did is another question that needs to be looked at further.

DR. R. L. JACKSON: I wonder whether you have done any experiments in which a fixed amount of triglyceride-rich particles were incubated in increasing amounts with HDL. In one experiment in which we studied the distribution of apoC-II between HDL and VLDL, we found that apoC-II distributes more towards HDL than VLDL. At the same time we found the transfer of non-apoC-II protein to VLDL. Do you think that this could be apoE?

DR. GLOMSET: ApoE certainly can transfer from normal HDL to triglyceride-rich particles, but there is another possibility as well. We have incubated normal HDL, as you did, in increasing concentrations with triglyceride-rich particles, and have found transfer of apoA-I at very low concentrations of HDL. As the concentration of HDL increased, transfer of apoA-I decreased, however, and there was an increased transfer of apoC. So it may be apoA-I that is transferring and not apoE. The point that I want to make is that transfer of apoE does not occur from the disks, which are very, very stable. This is in contrast to normal HDL which have been circulating for a while, and are not as stable as the disks. I think that evidence from several labs indicates that apoE comes off these lipoproteins very easily. So I think that LCAT alters the structure of discs and thereby alters their affinity for apoE. How exactly this occurs will remain for wiser investigators to determine. An additional interesting question is why incubation with LCAT should cause loss of apoE from the HDL but uptake of apoA-I.

COMMENT: We have done experiments in Melbourne, Australia, showing that a large amount of LDL cholesterol ester is probably derived from HDL. I wonder whether VLDL E apoprotein might come from HDL with the HDL cholesterol.

DR. GLOMSET: I do not think that apoE is involved necessarily in the cholesterol ester transport. I think that the cholesterol transport is dependent on the cholesterol ester transfer protein. We have done incubation experiments like the ones I reported with other subfractions of the patients HDL, with the plasma proteins of density greater than 1.25. Under those conditions we get formation of cholesterol esters and transfer of cholesterol esters, as well as extensive transfer of the triglyceride-rich particle, but no transfer of apoE.

DR. A. M. SCANU: My question is again related to ratio between lecithin and free cholesterol in your discoidal particles. We have been working with vesicles where this ratio appears of importance for LCAT activity. My question is, do disks have such a relatively strict requirement? Would the difference in curvature be a factor?

DR. GLOMSET: These are very interesting possibilities. Another possibility is suggested by Chris Fielding's recent work emphasizing the potential importance of a very reactive particle that appears to be a complex of LCAT, cholesterol ester exchange protein, and apoA-I. This complex is said not to contain much lipid and to transfer cholesterol ester to other lipoproteins as soon as it has been formed. Even though our results might be interpreted to suggest that the disks were reacting directly with the enzyme, we have not really proved that. We do not know what else is present in our mixtures. In addition to these disks, there is surely apoA-I in the 1.21 g/ml bottom as well as other unidentified components.

Dr. STEINBERG: Can I ask you if you have performed experiments using LCAT and a triglyceride-rich particle to see whether apoA-I is transferred?

Dr. GLOMSET: ApoA-I does not transfer under those conditions. I think that apoA-I transfers whenever the content of free cholesterol on the acceptor lipoprotein is low. One thing about these patients' plasma is that in addition to whatever you isolate in terms of disks, you also have some lipoprotein as well as lots of free cholesterol, and phosphatidylcholine. Unless you get rid of these components, the LCAT action persists causing a redistribution of lipid. In some of our experiments, there is virtually no change in phospholipid or in free cholesterol in HDL for example. As long as that occurs then, you do not get transfer of apoA-I.

IDENTIFICATION OF THE LIPID BINDING SITE OF THE PHOSPHATIDYLCHOLINE EXCHANGE PROTEIN WITH A PHOTOSENSITIVE NITRENE AND CARBENE PRECURSOR OF PHOSPHATIDYLCHOLINE

K. W. A. Wirtz, P. Moonen, and L. L. M. van Deenen

Department of Biochemistry
University of Utrecht
5308-TB Utrecht, The Netherlands

R. Radhakrishnan and H. G. Khorana

Departments of Biology and Chemistry
Massachusetts Institute of Technology
Cambridge, Massachusetts 02139

Lipid–protein structures like biological membranes and serum lipoproteins derive their stability and identity to a large extent from the unique properties of the aqueous medium.[1,2] These structures have an apolar core in common, yet are characterized by a heterogeneous mixture of chemically distinct lipids and proteins. To understand the mode by which these structures function, insight into the spatial organization of lipids and proteins is required. Specifically, this demands the identification of the intrinsic proteins, the delineation of the protein segments that are embedded in the apolar core, and the analysis of the lipids in contact with these hydrophobic protein segments.

In an attempt to elucidate this architectural puzzle by labeling the intrinsic membrane proteins from within the bilayer, Gitler and coworkers [3-6] developed lipophilic photosensitive reagents that dissolve into the apolar core of natural membranes. In sarcoplasmic reticulum membranes and erythrocytes, use of 1-azido-5-[^{125}I]iodonaphthalene has demonstrated that the photogenerated nitrene derivative coupled covalently to the intrinsic proteins.[4] In membranes containing (Na$^+$,K$^+$)ATPase, coupling of this nitrene derivative occurred predominantly to a membrane-embedded fragment of this sodium pump protein.[5] In erythrocytes approximately half of the coupling products consisted of the trypsin-insoluble, trans-membrane segment of glycophorin.[6] Incorporation of 1-azido-4-iodo-[^{3}H]benzene into human erythrocyte membranes has confirmed that the photogenerated nitrene covalently couples to the intramembranous region of glycophorin.[7,8]

These studies suggest that the lipophilic, *in situ* generated arylnitrenes are useful tools to identify the intrinsic membrane proteins and their segments in contact with the lipid bilayer. Bayley and Knowles,[9] however, have argued against the use of arylnitrenes whose relatively long lifetime and electrophilic character may prevent the desired indiscriminate labeling of the intramembranous protein segments. These disadvantages can be overcome by the use of the more reactive carbenes, derived photochemically from diazirines as lipophilic labeling reagents.[10] In contrast to phenylnitrene, the photogenerated carbenes of phenyldiazirine and adamantyl-diazirine dissolved into the bilayer of phospholipid vesicles, are sufficiently reactive to insert into the carbon–hydrogen bonds of saturated fatty acids.[9,10]

To probe systematically the intramembranous protein segment along its length through the membrane, it is required that the photogenerated reagent occupy within the lipid bilayer a fixed position relative to the protein. To satisfy this condition nitrene and carbene precursors have been attached to fatty acids at specific positions in the chain.[11-13] Fatty acids substituted with azido groups and 4-azido-2-nitrophenoxy groups are incorporated biosynthetically into the phospholipids of *Eschericia coli*[14] and eukaryotic cell lines in tissue culture.[12, 15, 16] Photolysis-induced cross-linking of these fatty acid derivatives to the adjacent proteins allows the analysis of the topographical arrangement of phospholipids and proteins in the membranes of these organisms. For example, recently it was demonstrated that irradiation of vesicular stomatitis virus containing 16-azido-[9,10-^{3}H$_2$]palmitic acid in its envelope lipids, covalently linked the photogenerated nitrene exclusively to the membrane-embedded spike protein.[16] In addition, irradiation of reconstituted high-density lipoprotein particles containing phosphatidylcholine with photosensitive azido fatty acids, coupled phosphatidylcholine covalently to apolipoproteins A-I and A-II.[17] At present, however, there remains doubt whether the coupling of the aliphatic azides occurs by a primary insertion reaction of the photogenerated nitrene. Nitrenes generated from the aliphatic or aromatic azido groups in phospholipids failed to form cross-links by insertion into carbon–hydrogen bonds of a second fatty acyl chain.[18] This type of primary insertion has been detected on photolysis of phospholipids containing the carbene precursor moieties, β-trifluoro-α-diazopropionoxy and *m*-diazirinophenoxy, in the ω-positions of fatty acyl chains at the glycerol-*sn*-2 position.[18]

The present paper describes the use of photosensitive phosphatidylcholine in an effort to determine the lipid binding site of the phosphatidylcholine exchange protein from bovine liver. It will become evident that this protein provides a good model to address the problems now emerging in the use of photolabeled lipids.

Phosphatidlycholine Exchange Protein (PC-PLEP)

PC-PLEP is one of a series of proteins that catalyze the transfer of phospholipids between membranes. This protein acts as a specific carrier of phosphatidylcholine (PC) between membranes.[19] Though less specific, proteins for the transfer of phosphatidylinositol, phosphatidylethanolamine, and sphingomyelin have also been isolated.[20-22] It appears that at the interface PC-PLEP exposes a binding site that interacts specifically with the polar head group of PC.[23] Thus, transfer is inhibited or abolished when (a) the distance between phosphorus and quaternary nitrogen is decreased or increased and (b) a methyl group on the quaternary nitrogen is removed or substituted by an ethyl or propyl group. Alterations about the glycerol backbone and in the apolar moiety of PC have less of an effect on the interaction with the protein.

PC-PLEP has a molecular weight of 28,000 based on sodium dodecyl sulfate (SDS)-polyacrylamide slab gel electrophoresis and the primary structure (manuscript in preparation). Its amino acid composition, presented in TABLE 1, indicates that of the 237 amino acid residues, 37% belong to the polar residues (Lys, His, Arg, Glx, Asx) and 40% to the apolar residues (Trp, Ile, Leu, Met, Tyr, Pro, Phe, Val). It has an average hydrophobicity of 1338 calories per mole residue, which is rather high relative to its molecular weight.[24, 25] It

TABLE 1

AMINO ACID COMPOSITION OF PC-PLEP

Amino Acid	Moles/Mole Protein	Amino Acid	Moles/Mole Protein
Asx	20	Met	5
Thr	6	Ile	7
Ser	12	Leu	18
Glx	35	Tyr	17
Pro	12	Phe	9
Gly	16	Lys	20
Ala	17	His	3
Val	22	Arg	10
Cys	4	Trp	4

contains two disulfide bridges and has a blocked amino-terminus consisting of an acetyl-methionine residue. Circular dichroism measurements indicate its α-helix content to be 10% at neutral pH but less at lower pH.[26]

As a carrier PC-PLEP forms a one-to-one molar complex with PC. As indicated in FIGURE 1, PC in the complex is assumed to be well shielded from the medium since it is not accessible to hydrolytic cleavage by phospholipases A_2, C, and D.[27] Phosphatidylcholine can be extracted by detergents, e.g.,

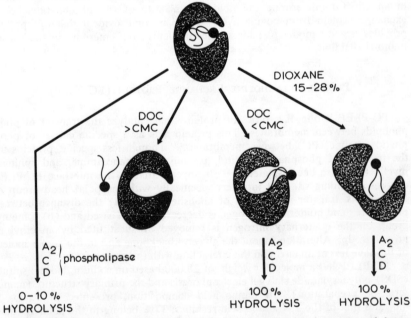

FIGURE 1. Localization of PC in PC-PLEP in the absence and presence of deoxycholate (DOC) and dioxane, and its accessibility to the hydrolytic action of phospholipases A_2, C, and D.[27] CMC is critical micelle concentration.

deoxycholate, above the critical micelle concentration. It is enzymatically hydrolysed upon addition of deoxycholate and dioxane at concentrations at which delipidation of PC-PLEP does not occur. We presume that these agents enhance the accessibility of PC either by its displacement on the protein (deoxycholate) or by induction of conformational change (dioxane).

Additional evidence that PC may be buried in the exchange protein accrues from experiments on the incorporation of 2-acyl spin-labeled PC into the protein. Electron spin resonance spectroscopy demonstrated that the spectra of the spin-labeled PC-PLEP complex were typical of a strongly immobilized probe and were unaffected by the presence of ascorbate.[28, 29] This indicates that the protein protects the nitroxide group against reduction by ascorbate.

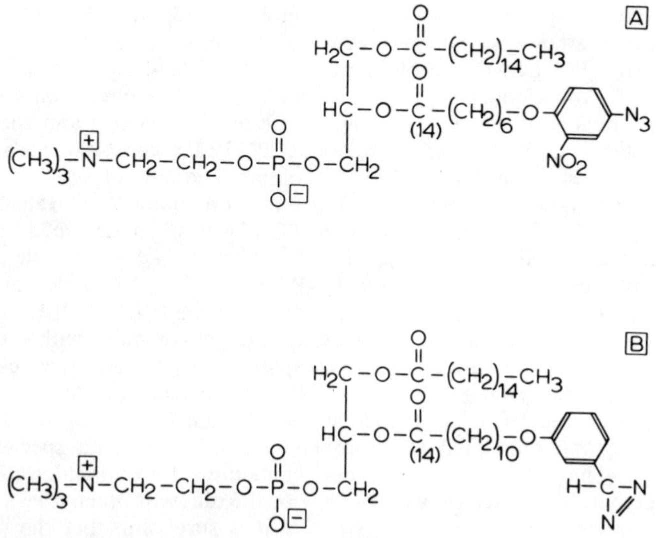

FIGURE 2. Chemical structure of 1-palmitoyl-2(7-(4-azido-2-nitrophenoxy) [1-^{14}C] heptanoyl)-*sn*-glycero-3-phosphocholine (A) and 1-palmitoyl-2(11-m-diazirinophenoxy) [1-^{14}C] undecanoyl)-*sn*-glycero-3-phosphocholine (B).

PHOTOSENSITIVE PHOSPHATIDYLCHOLINE

To advance our knowledge of the lipid binding site, in the present study, two photosensitive phosphatidylcholine derivatives have been used. Their chemical structures are shown in FIGURE 2. Thus, one contains at the 2-position the nitrene precursor 7-(4-azido-2-nitrophenoxy)[1-^{14}C]heptanoic acid (NAP-[^{14}C]PC), and the second contains the carbene precursor 11-(*m*-diazirinophe-noxy)[1-^{14}C]undecanoic acid (diazirino-[^{14}C]PC). The bulky azidonitrophe-noxy and diazirinophenoxy group have been attached to the ω-position of the 2-fatty acyl chain to obtain a configuration that resembles PC with an aliphatic fatty acyl chain. Photolysis of a sonicated suspension of diazirino-PC and characterization of the cross-linking products demonstrated carbene insertion into the C–H bonds of the 1-palmitoyl chain.[18] NAP-[^{14}C]PC and diazirino-

[^{14}C]PC have been synthesized as described previously.[11, 13, 30] The carboxyl group of the 2-fatty acyl chain was made highly radioactive to facilitate the detection of the cross-linked products. NAP-[^{14}C]PC (λ_{max} 365 nm, ϵ 5000) and diazirino-[^{14}C]PC (λ_{max} 340 nm, ϵ 250) can be photoactivated at wavelengths where proteins do not absorb, thus limiting radiation damage.

PHOTOSENSITIVE PC-EXCHANGE PROTEIN COMPLEX

Incubation of PC-PLEP with vesicles of both NAP-[^{14}C]PC and diazirino-[^{14}C]PC resulted in the incorporation of photolabeled PC (TABLE 2). Incorporation occurs by the exchange of the endogenous PC molecule bound to the protein, with a PC molecule present in the outer monolayer of the vesicles.[19, 31] As for both phospholipids, PC-PLEP contained approximately 45% of the radioactivity that one would have expected at complete equilibration of the photosensitive PC between protein and vesicles. This equilibrium value is determined by the amount of protein-bound PC, the amount of photosensitive [^{14}C]PC in the vesicle outer monolayer (an estimated 65%), and the specific activity of the [^{14}C]PC.[31] The photolabeled PC-PLEP complex was separated from the vesicles on a Biogel A-0.5m column and photolysed with a high pressure mercury lamp employing a 340 nm cut-off filter.[30] Covalent linking of NAP-[^{14}C]PC and diazirino-[^{14}C]PC to PC-PLEP was determined by disruption of the photolysed complex with SDS followed by SDS-polyacrylamide slab gel electrophoresis. The gels for the NAP-[^{14}C]PC-PLEP complex are shown in FIGURE 3 and are identical to those for the diazirino-[^{14}C]PC-PLEP complex. After fixing and staining all the ^{14}C-label on the gel coincides with the protein band (FIGURE 3B); disruption of the complex prior to photolysis releases all ^{14}C-label from the protein (FIGURE 3A). The extent of cross-linking was calculated from the ^{14}C-label applied to the gel and that recovered from the protein band, and amounted to approximately 30% for both species of PC (TABLE 2). The nature of the products containing the remainder (70%) of the radioactivity is not yet known. In view of the different reactivities of photo-generated aryl carbenes and nitrenes,[9, 10, 18] it is surprising that the phenoxy-

TABLE 2

INCORPORATION AND CROSS-LINKING OF NAP-[^{14}C]PC AND DIAZIRINO-[^{14}C]PC
TO PC-PLEP *

Incubation Mixture			After Incubation		
Protein (nmol)	Photolabeled PC	Amount of Radioactivity (cpm)	Radioactivity Incorporated into PC-PLEP (cpm)	Radioactivity Cross-Linked (cpm)	Extent of Cross-Linking (%)
110	NAP-[^{14}C]PC	3.2×10^6	6.5×10^4	2.2×10^4	30
110	Diazirino-[^{14}C]PC	3.0×10^6	7.4×10^5	2.0×10^5	27

* Vesicles of NAP-[^{14}C]PC (2 μmol PC; sp act 0.74 mCi/mmol) and diazirino-[^{14}C] PC (0.03 μmol PC; sp act 50 mCi/mmol) were prepared and incubated with PC-PLEP (110 nmol) as previously described.[30]

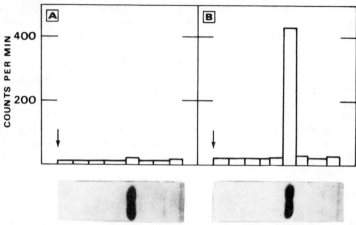

FIGURE 3. Sodium dodecyl sulfate (SDS)-polyacrylamide gel electrophoresis of the NAP-[^{14}C] PC-PLEP complex. Sample contained 30 μg of protein. After staining gel was sliced and ^{14}C-radioactivity determined. (A) Nonphotolysed complex. (B) Photolysed complex.

carbene moiety on the undecanoyl chain and the nitrophenoxy-nitrene moiety on the heptanoyl chain covalently couple to PC-PLEP to the same extent. This suggests that the 2-fatty acyl chains of both PC-derivates have a comparable orientation in the binding site, which determines the efficacy of cross-linking. From the incorporation of NAP-[^{14}C]PC and diazirino-[^{14}C]PC into PC-PLEP and the extent of coupling (TABLE 2), it can be estimated that 10% and 2% of the PC-PLEP, respectively, contain covalently linked PC.

IDENTIFICATION OF THE PEPTIDE(S) CROSS-LINKED TO PHOSPHATIDYLCHOLINE

Photolysis of NAP-[^{14}C]PC-PLEP and diazirino-[^{14}C]PC-PLEP give rise to PLEP-NH-nitrophenoxy[^{14}C]PC and PLEP-CH$_2$-phenoxy-[^{14}C]PC, respectively (FIGURE 4). To determine the site of coupling, the protein moiety of the photolysed complexes was reduced, carboxymethylated, and citraconylated and then digested by *Staphylococcus aureus* protease.[30] The peptides were isolated by column chromatography after the ester bonds of the covalently coupled -NH-nitrophenoxy[^{14}C]PC and -CH$_2$-phenoxy[^{14}C]PC were hydrolysed (0.1N NaOH; 15 min; 40°). Hydrolysis reduces the hydrophobicity of the ^{14}C-labeled peptide and therefore promotes "cochromatography" of the ^{14}C-labeled peptide with the unlabeled "parent" peptide. Results show that both -NH-nitrophenoxy[1-^{14}C]heptanoic acid and -CH$_2$-phenoxy[1-^{14}C]undecanoic acid were coupled to the same *Staphylococcus* protease peptide. This peptide with lysine as *N*-terminal residue consists of an estimated 65 amino acid residues, and its amino acid sequence has been partially elucidated (FIGURE 5). It contains three arginine residues at positions 6, 13, and 22 (Arg$_6$, Arg$_{13}$, Arg$_{22}$). Since the lysine residues are citraconylated, digestion by trypsin gives the four peptides T$_1$, T$_2$, T$_3$, and T$_4$ expected from cleavages at Arg$_6$, Arg$_{13}$, and Arg$_{22}$. Because of inherent chymotryptic activity, prolonged tryptic digestion converts peptide T_4 completely into its subpeptides T_{4a}, T_{4b}, and T_{4c}. Digestion of the protease peptide by clostripain—a proteolytic enzyme that specifically cleaves Arg-X bonds [32]—gives exclusively the peptides T_1, T_2, T_3, and T_4.

The protease peptide (FIGURE 5) containing covalently coupled -NH-nitrophenoxy[1-^{14}C]heptanoic acid has been digested by trypsin for a brief period (20 min; 37°) and the peptides isolated by molecular sieve chromatography (FIGURE 6). The ^{14}C-label was mainly concentrated in fractions A and D; fraction A contained the peptides T_4 (43 residues) and T_{4c} (35 residues) and fraction D the small peptides T_{4a} and T_{4b}. A prolonged tryptic digestion (3 hr; 37°) of PC-PLEP containing cross-linked -NH-nitrophenoxy [^{14}C]PC concentrated the ^{14}C label virtually completely into fraction D. This chromato-

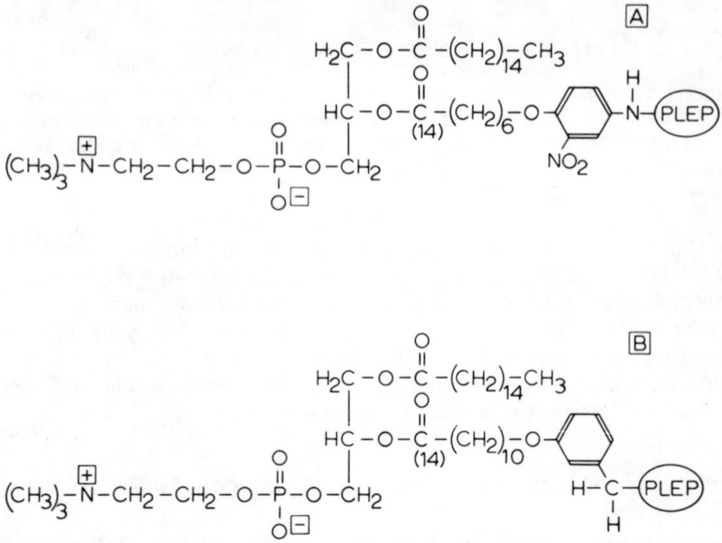

FIGURE 4. Chemical structures of the crosslinked products of PC-PLEP and the photogenerated nitrene from NAP-[^{14}C]PC (A) and the photogenerated carbene from diazirino-[^{14}C]PC (B).

graphic behavior strongly suggests that the photogenerated nitrene has coupled to the peptide segment T_{4a-b} whose sequence has previously been shown to be -Gly-Ser-Lys-Val-Phe-Met-Tyr-Tyr.[30]

A similar series of degradations has been performed on the protease peptide (FIGURE 5) containing covalently linked -CH$_2$-phenoxy[1-^{14}C]undecanoic acid by clostripain. After digestion (3 hr; 37°) chromatography of the peptide mixture showed that all the ^{14}C-label coincided with the peptides present in fractions 26–31 (FIGURE 7; cf. fraction A of FIGURE 6). Dansyl end group analysis indicated that T_4 (N-terminal residue Gly) was the major peptide. Incomplete cleavage of the Arg_{22}-Gly_{23} bond, which was relatively resistant to clostripain digestion, accounted for a slightly larger peptide T_{3-4} (N-terminal residue Leu). Prolonged tryptic digestion (3 hr; 37°) of PC-PLEP containing cross-linked -CH$_2$-phenoxy[^{14}C]PC followed by isolation of the ^{14}C-labeled

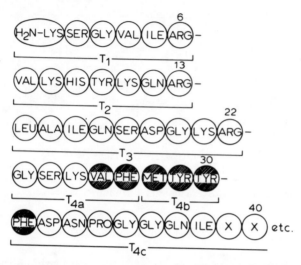

FIGURE 5. Partial amino acid sequence of the *Staphylococcus* protease peptide cross-linked to -NH-nitrophenoxy [1-¹⁴C] heptanoic acid and -CH₂-phenoxy [1-¹⁴C] undecanoic acid. T_4 equals $T_{4a-4b-4c}$. The crosshatched circles indicate the amino acid residues in the lipid binding site of PC-PLEP.

peptide, indicated that -CH₂-phenoxy[1-¹⁴C]undecanoic acid was coupled to one peptide with glycine as N-terminal residue. The chromatographic behavior of this peptide resembled that of peptide segment T_{4a-b}. Purity of the peptide was confirmed by thin-layer chromatography as demonstrated by the radioactive scan shown in FIGURE 8. These results provide strong evidence that the photo-generated carbene has also inserted into the T_{4a-b} segment of the protease peptide.

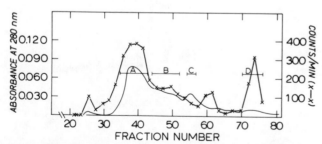

FIGURE 6. Gel filtration profile of the tryptic digest of the *Staphylococcus* protease peptide containing cross-linked -NH-nitrophenoxy[1-¹⁴C]heptanoic acid. Digest was applied to a column of Sephadex G-50 fine (100×0.85 cm) and eluted with 0.1 M $(NH_4)HCO_3$ (pH 8.5). Fractions of 0.8 ml were collected. A, B, C, and D indicate the pooled fractions.

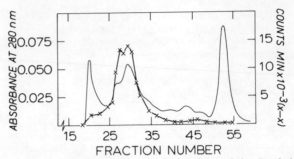

FIGURE 7. Gel filtration profile of the clostripain digest of the *Staphylococcus* protease peptide containing cross-linked -CH₂-phenoxy[1-¹⁴C]undecanoic acid. For conditions, see legend to FIGURE 6. Fractions of 1.05 ml were collected.

THE LIPID BINDING SITE

It appears that photolysis of NAP-[¹⁴C]PC and diazirino-[¹⁴C]PC as part of the PC-PLEP complex, cross-links both species to the same peptide segment. Accordingly, the binding site appears to severely restrict the freedom of motion of the PC-ligands to the extent that the photo-generated nitrene and carbene at the 2-fatty-acyl chain occupy fixed positions relative to the amino acids in the binding site. This agrees with the observation that, upon incorporation into PC-PLEP, PC spin-labeled with nitroxide groups at various positions along the 2-fatty-acyl chain, gives electron spin resonance spectra characteristic of a strongly immobilized probe.[28, 29]

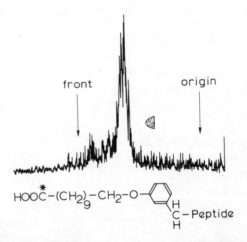

FIGURE 8. Radioscan of peptide (T$_{4a}$ or T$_{4a-b}$) containing cross-linked -CH₂-phenoxy [1-¹⁴C]undecanoic acid. Thin-layer chromatography on cellulose (Polygram cel 400, Macherey-Nagel) with butanol:pyridine:acetic acid:water (75:50:15:60, vol/vol) as developing solvent. The ¹⁴C-labeled peptide runs ahead of the unlabeled "parent" peptide. The parent peptide is indicated by the stained spot.

The site(s) of cross-linking of the -NH-nitrophenoxy[1-^{14}C] heptanoyl and -CH$_2$-phenoxy[1-^{14}C] undecanoyl chain awaits further chemical analysis of the labeled peptide. Manual Edman degradation of peptide T$_4$ containing the cross-linked -CH$_2$-phenoxy[1-^{14}C]undecanoic acid moiety, has failed to release the ^{14}C-label. This possibly reflects insertion of the carbene into a bond of the peptide crucial to the course of the Edman degradation. All evidence, however, indicates that the bulk of radioactivity was linked to the peptide segment Gly-Ser-Lys-Val-Phe-Met-Tyr-Tyr- (residues 23–30, T$_{4a-b}$), containing part of the extremely hydrophobic cluster of amino acids -Val-Phe-Met-Tyr-Tyr-Phe- (residues 26–31). This hexapeptide has an average hydrophobicity of 2440 calories per mole residue compared to 1338 calories for the total protein. Since both the photogenerated nitrene and carbene derivative of PC have cross-linked to the same peptide region, we propose that this hydrophobic hexapeptide constitutes part of the lipid binding site of PC-PLEP.

An analysis of the secondary structure of the binding site according to the method of Chou and Fasman [33, 34] predicts a β-sheet structure for the hexapeptide -Val-Phe-Met-Tyr-Tyr-Phe- (TABLE 3). According to this analysis the

TABLE 3

PREDICTIVE ANALYSIS OF CONFORMATIONAL FEATURES IN THE BINDING SITE OF PC-PLEP *

Peptide Segment	[P$_\alpha$]	[P$_\beta$]	[P$_t$]	Conformation
21–24	0.80	0.79	1.31	β turn
26–31	0.97	1.41	0.82	β sheet
33–36	0.60	0.72	1.65	β turn

* [P$_\alpha$], [P$_\beta$], and [P$_t$] are the average conformational potential for the peptide to be in the α helix, β sheet, and β turn conformation, respectively.[33]

tetrapeptides on either side of the hexapeptide (residues 21–24, 33–36, respectively) would form β turns. A hexapeptide in β-sheet structure has an estimated length of 14 Å (B. Dijkstra, personal communication). This suggests that the binding site has the proper dimensions to accommodate the 2-fatty acyl chain of naturally occurring PC. The binding site of the 1-fatty acyl chain of PC is at present totally unknown, but use of PC with photolabeled 1-fatty acyl chains may elucidate the amino acid residues contributing to this site.

CONCLUSION

This paper describes the successful use of NAP-[^{14}C]PC and diazirino-[^{14}C]PC in the elucidation of the lipid binding site of PC-PLEP. A number of general remarks can be made:

1. Azidonitrophenoxy and diazirinophenoxy groups attached at the ω-position of the 2-fatty acyl chain do not impair the incorporation of PC into PC-PLEP. It is to be expected that by its mode of action as a carrier PC-PLEP

will be a very useful tool to transfer these photosensitive species of PC from "donor" vesicles to both natural and reconstituted membranes.

2. Photolysis of NAP-[^{14}C]PC-PLEP and diazirino-[^{14}C]PC-PLEP complexes cross-links both species of PC to the same peptide segment. This makes PC-PLEP a good model to analyze and compare the cross-linked products of the photogenerated nitrene and carbene derivates.

3. This paper presents proof that photolabeling can be a very powerful tool in the detection of hydrophobic lipid binding sites on proteins.

REFERENCES

1. SINGER, S. J. 1971. The molecular organization of biological membranes. *In* Structure and Function of Biological Membranes. L. I. Rothfield, Ed. pp. 145–222. Academic Press, New York, N.Y.
2. TANFORD, C . 1978. Science **200:**1012–1018.
3. KLIP, A. & C. GITLER. 1974. Biochem. Biophys. Res. Commun. **60:**1155–1162.
4. BERCOVICI, T. & C. GITLER. 1978. Biochemistry **17:**1484–1489.
5. KARLISH, S. J. D., P. L. JORGENSEN & C. GITLER. 1977. Nature **269:**715–717.
6. KAHANE, I. & C. GITLER. 1978. Science **201:**351–352.
7. WELLS, E. & J. B. C. FINDLAY. 1979. Biochem. J. **179:**257–264.
8. WELLS, E. & J. B. C. FINDLAY. 1979. Biochem. J. **179:**265–272.
9. BAYLEY, H. & J. R. KNOWLES. 1978. Biochemistry **17:**2414–2419.
10. BAYLEY, H. & J. R. KNOWLES. 1978. Biochemistry **17:**2420–2423.
11. CHAKRABARTI, P. & H. G. KHORANA. 1975. Biochemistry **14:**5021–5033.
12. STOFFEL, W., K. SALM & U. KÖRKEMEIER. 1976. Hoppe-Seyler's Z. Physiol. Chem. **357:**917–924.
13. GUPTA, C. M., R. RADHAKRISHNAN & H. G. KHORANA. 1977. Proc. Natl. Acad. Sci. USA **74:**4315–4319.
14. GREENBERG, G. R., P. CHAKRABARTI & H. G. KHORANA. 1976. Proc. Natl. Acad. Sci. USA **73:**86–90.
15. FRANCHI, A. & G. AILHAUD. 1977. Biochimie. **59:**813–817.
16. STOFFEL, W., C. SCHREIBER & H. SCHEEFERS. 1978. Hoppe-Seyler's Physiol. Chem. **359:**923–931.
17. STOFFEL, W. & P. METZ. 1979. Hoppe-Seyler's Z. Physiol. Chem. **360:**197–206.
18. GUPTA, G. M., R. RADHAKRISHNAN, G. E. GERBER, W. L. OLSEN, S. C. QUAY & H. G. KHORANA. 1979. Proc. Natl. Acad. Sci. USA **76:**2595–2599.
19. DEMEL, R. A., K. W. A. WIRTZ, H. H. KAMP, W. S. M. GEURTS VAN KESSEL & L .L. M. VAN DEENEN. 1973. Nature New Biol. **246:**102–105.
20. HELMKAMP, G. M., M. S. HARVEY, K. W. A. WIRTZ & L. L. M. VAN DEENEN. 1974. J. Biol. Chem. **249:**6382–6389.
21. BLOJ, B. & D. B. ZILVERSMIT. 1977. J. Biol. Chem. **252:**1613–1619.
22. DYATLOVITSKAYA, E. V., N. G. TIMOFEEVA & L. D. BERGELSON. 1978. Eur. J. Biochem. **82:**463–471.
23. KAMP, H. H., K. W. A. WIRTZ, P. R. BAER, A. J. SLOTBOOM, A. F. ROSENTHAL, F. PALTAUF & L. L. M. VAN DEENEN. 1977. Biochemistry **16:**1310–1316.
24. BIGELOW, C. C. 1967. J. Theoret. Biol. **16:**187–211.
25. MANAVALAN, P. & P. K. PONNUSWAMY. 1978. Nature **275:**673–674.
26. WIRTZ, K. W. A. & P. MOONEN. 1977. Eur. J. Biochem. **77:**437–443.
27. KAMP, H. H., E. D. SPRENGERS, J. WESTERMAN, K. W. A. WIRTZ & L. L. M. VAN DEENEN. 1975. Biochim. Biophys. Acta **398:**415–423.
28. DEVAUX, P. F., P. MOONEN, A. BIENVENUE & K. W. A. WIRTZ. 1977. Proc. Natl. Acad. Sci. USA **74:**1807–1810.
29. MACHIDA, K. & S. I. OHNISHI. 1978. Biochim. Biophys. Acta **507:**156–164.
30. MOONEN, P., H. P. HAAGSMAN, L. L. M. VAN DEENEN & K. W. A. WIRTZ. 1979. Eur. J. Biochem. **99:**439–445.

31. KAMP, H. H., K. W. A. WIRTZ & L. L. M. VAN DEENEN. 1975. Biochim. Biophys. Acta **398:**401–414.
32. GILLES, A. M., J. M. IMHOFF & B. KEIL. 1979. J. Biol. Chem. **254:**1462–1468.
33. CHOU, P. Y. & G. D. FASMAN. 1974. Biochemistry **13:**211–222.
34. CHOU, P. Y. & G. D. FASMAN. 1974. Biochemistry **13:**222–245.

DISCUSSION OF THE PAPER

DR. F. R. LANDSBERGER: If you take your model at face value, you have half a basket, and the other half is exposed. To protect your phospholipid lipase digestion you need a lid on the basket. Could your photo-activatable phospholipids link to this lid.

DR. K. W. A. WIRTZ: You talk about a lid. I am not really sure if it is possible for the site to be rather close to the surface. The transfer protein at the interface may undergo conformational changes by which it exposes its lipid molecule; but we have no evidence for conformational change at least not from the present studies.

DR. LANDSBERGER: I do not mean a lid in the literal sense. Just something else to cover up that surface. Otherwise the lipase will get to it presumably.

DR. WIRTZ: Again from the prediction analysis we have some interesting hexapeptide regions in this protein and perhaps those structures are involved in forming the complete binding site.

DR. R. L. JACKSON: There is also the uncertainty of the influence of the interaction between the phospholipid and your exchange protein on bonds that the enzyme is trying to hide. So it is not a matter of accessibility, but it is also a matter of shape of the substrate.

DR. B. SHEN: Do you know the stereospecificity of your binding protein. I assume that the lipid you synthesize is a DL mixture.

DR. WIRTZ: It is an L. We have been looking at whether or not the conformation of the lipid molecule is important to the interaction. We have found that particular changes introduced into the polar region affect the interaction with the protein.

DR. JACKSON: How was your specificity with respect to the polar head group? Have you extended the model out at the ends to see whether or not it could accommodate a polar head group?

DR. J. A. HUNTER: I was wondering if you have information on the binding constant of the phospholipid to the exchange protein. Also I wonder whether you could care to speculate a little bit on the mechanism of the exchange; what you imagine occurs at the new lipid surface, when there is an exchange.

DR. WIRTZ: What happens at the interface, we really do not know, but some disturbance must occur. For example, as molecules are pushed away the dielectric constant at the interface has changed. When that happens of course the major force that keeps little molecules in place is affected. At the moment I should be as vague as this.

DR. HUNTER: You do think that there must be some configurational change in the protein?

DR. WIRTZ: Based on our results we have to assume that a conformational change does occur.

LDL–CELL INTERACTION *IN VIVO* AND *IN VITRO* *

Daniel Steinberg

Division of Metabolic Disease
Department of Medicine
University of California at San Diego
La Jolla, California 92093

INTRODUCTION

Until quite recently it was thought that the degradation of plasma low-density lipoprotein (LDL) must be an exclusively hepatic process. The role of LDL in atherogenesis and in the formation of xanthomata was recognized as evidence of extrahepatic LDL catabolism, but these were regarded as extreme departures from the norm, possibly relevant only in pathologic states. This view had to give way when it was shown, by studies in hepatectomized animals, that the periphery has a very large capacity for LDL degradation even at normal LDL levels.[1, 2] The seminal studies of Goldstein, Brown, and coworkers [3, 4] first established the nature and functioning of the high-affinity, specific LDL receptor in fibroblasts. A number of other cell types of extrahepatic origin have also been shown to have a functional LDL receptor.[5-7] The concordance between inherited deficiencies in LDL receptor number in cells from patients with familial hypercholesterolemia, on the one hand, and elevation of steady-state plasma LDL levels, on the other, makes a rather convincing case for the functional importance of the receptor. Uptake of LDL via the high-affinity receptor is associated with a decrease in endogenous cholesterol biosynthesis, an increase in cholesterol esterification, and a down-regulation of the number of cell-surface LDL receptors.[4] Thus all of the elements needed for a regulated system of delivery of cholesterol to cells are present. Some evidence that such regulation is operative in experimental animals *in vivo* has been provided.[8, 9]

Thus the LDL in plasma may represent a potentially valuable vehicle for cholesterol transport under physiologic conditions while being a potentially catastrophic vehicle for cholesterol transport in relation to atherogenesis. This paper is concerned with some recent studies on the specificity of the LDL–receptor interaction and with the relative importance of different tissues in LDL uptake under physiologic conditions *in vivo*.

DETERMINANTS OF LDL RECOGNITION BY RECEPTOR

The specificity of the interaction between LDL and the plasma membrane probably rests largely on recognition of the apoprotein. The work of Mahley and Innerarity shows that both apoB and apoE are recognized, the latter with higher affinity than the former.[10, 11] Studies from our laboratory show that one can extract the nonpolar lipids from LDL almost quantitatively without

* This work was supported by Research Grant HL-14197, awarded by the National Heart, Lung, and Blood Institute.

significantly affecting its interaction with the cell membrane.[12] Thus, the non-polar core lipids evidently play a minor role at most in maintaining the apoprotein in the configuration recognized by the receptor. The size and shape of the LDL after extraction of lipids was grossly altered, suggesting that size and shape are not critical. Little or none of the phospholipid was removed by the extraction procedure used and so it is presumably the apoprotein–phospholipid interaction that confers the required specific protein configuration.

Conversely, modification of the apoprotein can and does abolish LDL recognition by the receptor. Studies by Mahley and coworkers [13, 14] and studies by Goldstein and coworkers [15] show that blocking of the amino groups on the apoprotein, either apoprotein B or apoprotein E, almost completely abolishes specific binding and uptake. These studies again strongly suggest that LDL–cell interaction depends predominantly if not exclusively on apoprotein–membrane interaction.

At low concentrations of LDL most of the uptake and degradation occurs by the specific, high-affinity mechanism but at higher concentrations a significant fraction of LDL metabolism occurs by low-affinity processes.[3, 16–18] Little is known about the relationship between molecular structure and the low-affinity uptake process. Since the predominant mode of uptake in patients with familial hypercholesterolemia is uptake by low-affinity mechanisms, it would be of interest to know to what extent such uptake is sensitive to molecular modifications of LDL. We have shown previously that the uptake of LDL by fibroblasts of patients with homozygous familial hypercholesterolemia (i.e., low-affinity uptake) is markedly *increased* when the LDL is first digested with trypsin.[19] Other molecular modifications markedly reduce uptake by way of the specific LDL receptor,[20] and the significance of this is under active investigation.

Species Specificity

Another way of examining the specificity of LDL-cell interaction is to compare the metabolism of LDL from different species. Studies in our laboratory by Dr. Christian A. Drevon, Mr. Alan D. Attie, and Ms. Sharon H. Pangburn have been concerned with comparisons of rat and human LDL metabolism in rat and in human skin fibroblasts. Several significant differences were apparent that demonstrate some degree of species specificity of the LDL receptor. For example, the binding of human [125I]LDL to human fibroblasts was considerably greater than that of human [125I]LDL to rat fibroblasts. Rates of degradation were also much greater in human cells. Whereas human LDL potently suppressed 3-hydroxy-3-methylglutarylcoenzyme A reductase activity in human cells, it had only small effects in rat cells. Sensitivity to stimulation of cellular cholesterol esterification by human LDL was also greater in human cells. Finally, prior incubation of the human cells in lipoprotein-deficient serum for 24 hours markedly increased their subsequent ability to degrade human [125I]LDL, in agreement with the previous studies of Goldstein and Brown,[4] whereas human LDL degradation by rat cells was not affected. These studies imply a significant difference in the configuration of the LDL receptors of human and rat fibroblasts. Some of the findings also imply a much smaller total number of receptors in rat fibroblasts.

In collaboration with Ms. Sharon H. Pangburn and Dr. David B. Weinstein, we have examined the issue of species specificity in metabolism of LDL by cultured rat hepatocytes. Homologous (rat) LDL was degraded more rapidly than heterologous (human) LDL. Furthermore, the rate of degradation of *human* LDL was essentially linear as a function of concentration up to 100 µg LDL protein/ml whereas the relationship was curvilinear for rat LDL, i.e., the slope was greater at lower concentrations of LDL. Further studies are needed to determine the physiologic significance of these findings but they suggest the presence in rat hepatocytes of a receptor recognizing homologous LDL but not recognizing heterologous LDL (or at least not with equal affinity).

Sites of LDL Uptake and Degradation *in Vivo*

Studies of cells in culture can provide a wealth of information regarding the qualitative mechanisms involved in lipoprotein uptake. However, it is unlikely that they can provide a reliable index of how these cells behave *in vivo*, in the quite different environment of the intact organ. As an example, let us consider the rates at which various cell types in culture have been found to degrade LDL. The rates are so remarkably high that if one extrapolates from them (assuming comparable rates per unit mass of tissue *in vivo*), one calculates a total capacity for LDL degradation that far exceeds the rates of LDL degradation actually observed in the intact animal! [22] We know that the number of LDL receptors is very much a function of the growth status of the cells, of prior exposure to lipoproteins and undoubtedly of many other variables as well. The only way to be certain about the relative importance of different tissues *in vivo* is to carry out studies *in vivo*. Unfortunately, the usual methods are seldom applicable in the study of LDL or other plasma proteins. Because most of these proteins have fairly long half-lives, the arteriovenous differences are generally too small to allow reliable measurement of uptake. When one uses iodinated proteins the degradation products do not accumulate in the tissue but exit very rapidly and are excreted with little delay. Thus it is not possible to assess the importance of a tissue in LDL degradation by measuring how much radioactivity is found there at time intervals after injection of LDL. Nor can the accumulation of *intact* LDL be used as an index of the importance of a tissue in degradation. In fact, one might even tend to find *higher* concentrations of undegraded LDL in tissues in which degradation occurs more *slowly*.

In collaboration with Dr. Ray C. Pittman, Ms. Simone R. Green, Mr. Alan D. Attie, and Dr. Thomas E. Carew, we have recently devised and validated a method that should be applicable to determination of tissue sites of degradation of any plasma protein.[23-25] The approach is based on the fact that sucrose is degraded very slowly if at all by lysosomal hydrolases. Once sucrose enters the lysosome it remains trapped there, leaking at less than 10% per day, according to studies in cultured cells. We argued that if we could covalently link sucrose to a plasma protein of interest, it would enter the cells and be transported to the lysosomes with the protein. The protein moiety would then be hydrolyzed rapidly by the acidic lysosomal proteases but the sucrose would remain behind undigested. Then, knowing the specific radioactivity of the protein and the total amount of radioactivity from radioactive sucrose accumulating in the cell or tissue, one could calculate the total amount of protein taken in and degraded. It should be noted that if there is some extralysosomal degradation, the ^{14}C-labeled degradation products may also be retained or they may leak out of the cell. The validity of this approach was first demonstrated using cultured skin fibroblasts and showing that degradation of LDL (estimated as I have just described it) agreed very well with estimates based on degradation of iodinated LDL measured in the conventional way.[24] The validity of the method *in vivo* was first tested in rats using asialofetuin, a protein known to be rapidly and almost exclusively removed by the liver. Using [14C-sucrose]asialofetuin, we found 88% of the injected dose in the liver 1 hour after injection. Rats sacrificed 24 hours after the injection still showed retention of most of the sucrose 14C in the liver although a part of it had by then appeared in the bile. The latter finding may be of interest with respect to the lysosomal contribution to biliary excretion products.

The method was then applied to the study of LDL degradation in intact swine.[25] The fractional rate of removal of [14C-sucrose]LDL was indistinguishable from that of [125I]LDL, suggesting that the cells responsible for at least the major part of LDL degradation do not distinguish sucrose-derivatized LDL from native (iodinated) LDL. Animals were killed and tissue concentrations of degradation products determined at 24 or 48 hours. Accumulated degradation products were related to the total amount of plasma LDL degraded over the 24- or 48-hour interval, the latter being determined from analysis of the concurrently measured plasma decay curve. The results at 24 and at 48 hours were similar, tending further to validate the underlying assumptions.

Just under 40% of total body LDL degradation was accounted for by the liver. By digesting a piece of the liver with collagenase and separating nonparenchymal cells from parenchymal cells, it was shown that the latter accounted for over 90% of the total accumulated hepatic sucrose 14C. The result shows that under physiologic conditions little or no LDL degradation occurs in nonparenchymal cells. It is well known that denatured plasma proteins (e.g., albumin) are preferentially degraded in nonparenchymal cells. Conceivably, then, some chemical modifications of LDL might cause it to be rapidly removed by nonparenchymal cells. Our results in swine, however, suggest this is not a physiologically significant mechanism although it may come into play under pathologic conditions.

The degradation of LDL in extrahepatic tissues was, in sum, comparable to that in the liver. Total recovery of 14C degradation products corresponded to about 80% of the calculated amount of [14C-sucrose]LDL degraded and 36% was accounted for in the extrahepatic tissues examined. Adipose tissue made the largest contribution (4%–6%) and muscle, intestine, skin, and lungs were next in importance.

Another way of examining the results is to express uptake per gram of tissue, a kind of "LDL-uptake specific activity." In these terms the adrenal gland was by far the most active tissue, 3- to 5-fold more active than the liver. The possibility that the adrenal can utilize plasma cholesterol as a precursor for steroidogenesis has long been recognized. From our data we could calculate the amount of LDL cholesterol delivered daily to the pig adrenal under "physiologic" conditions. The quotation marks are used because our animals were restrained in slings, had had several indwelling catheters placed, and were much attended to over the 24 to 48 hours of these studies. We calculate that the uptake of LDL cholesterol was 1.4 mg/g per day. The maximum rate of steroidogenesis by the isolated swine adrenal under ACTH stimulation has been reported to be 1.2 mg/g per day.[26] In other words, LDL could potentially supply all of the precursor cholesterol for steroidogenesis. Of course the adrenal can also synthesize cholesterol *de novo* and probably both endogenous and exogenous cholesterol contribute to steroidogenesis. Studies of bovine adrenal cells in culture have shown that availability of LDL can be rate-limiting for steroidogenesis.[27] Maximal ACTH-induced steroidogensis was only possible in the presence of LDL and ACTH was shown to increase the number of LDL receptors. Thus, basal steroid hormone production may be supported primarily or exclusively by endogenous cholesterol synthesis but stress-induced increases may depend predominantly on uptake of cholesterol in LDL.

DETERMINANTS OF TISSUE SITES OF LDL DEGRADATION

The relative and absolute contribution of various tissues to LDL degradation *in vivo* will depend on a number of factors. The key proximate factors will be: (1) The concentration of LDL in the fluid immediately available to the cell surface. (2) The rate of binding and internalization of LDL at that concentration. Each of these in turn will depend upon a number of secondary determinants.

The concentration of LDL in the extravascular, extracellular fluid is not known with certainty. Reichl *et al.*[28] have examined human foot lymph and estimate LDL concentrations there to be about 10% those in plasma, both in normal subjects and in patients with familial hypercholesterolemia. How closely this approximates the value in the fluid immediately bathing the cells is uncertain. Nor is it known how much variation there may be from one organ to another. In organs characterized by a fenestrated capillary endothelium the concentration may be much higher. The parenchymal cells in the liver, for example, are presumably exposed to LDL at the full concentration found in plasma. Thus, liver cells may be taking up LDL from a pool ten times more concentrated than that available to muscle or adipose cells. Even at a constant plasma level of LDL, the extravascular level may vary depending on all the factors regulating movement from plasma to extracellular space (blood pressure, blood flow, capillary permeability, transendothelial cell transport rate, etc.).

Despite all of these ancillary variables that could potentially influence tissue sites of LDL degradation, it is remarkable that there appears to be a fairly good correlation between receptor density and rate of LDL uptake *in vivo*. Kovanen *et al.*[29] have measured the density of receptors on isolated plasma membrane fractions prepared from a variety of bovine tissues. Comparison of the ranking of tissues by this criterion with observed *in vivo* activity of the corresponding tissues of the pig in our *in vivo* studies shows a roughly similar rank order. The concordance between LDL receptor density and *in vivo* activity in LDL uptake lends strong support to the importance of the receptor as a primary determinant of LDL uptake.

CONCLUSION

The "LDL receptor" is now recognized to be, more properly, an apoprotein B–apoprotein E receptor. Lipoproteins other than LDL *are* recognized and can to some extent compete with LDL for uptake if they also contain apoprotein B. If they contain apoprotein E they may be even more effective than LDL in competing for binding to the receptor. The ability of HDL to compete with LDL for binding and uptake, for example, probably reflects the presence of apoprotein E in subsets of lipoprotein molecules in the HDL density class. The size, shape, and lipid composition of the lipoproteins are probably minor determinants of lipoprotein binding and uptake.

Whereas there is a good deal of immunologic cross-reactivity between LDL molecules from different animal species, there is evidence that the LDL receptor is sufficiently specific to distinguish them to some extent. Heterologous lipoproteins may interact with the receptor and yield qualitatively similar responses. However, there are instances in which the quantitative differences are so marked as to appear to be qualitative. It would be best, whenever possible, to study LDL-receptor interactions only in homologous systems.

The ^{14}C-sucrose labeling method has provided for the first time a means of quantifying the contributions of various tissues to the degradation of LDL (and of other plasma proteins) *in vivo*. The results confirm the significant participation of the extrahepatic tissues in LDL degradation but show also that the liver plays a major role. In swine the adrenal gland is the most active tissue in LDL uptake (per unit wet weight), supporting the concept that *exogenous* cholesterol, derived from plasma LDL, is an important source of the cholesterol used for steroidogenesis. In general, the rate of uptake of LDL *in vivo* correlates well with the density of LDL receptors on plasma membranes. However, the concordance is not absolute and this probably reflects the many additional relevant parameters that either control the concentration of LDL in the extravascular space or that regulate the number of receptors actually expressed under *in vivo* conditions.

REFERENCES

1. SNIDERMAN, A. D., T. E. CAREW, J. G. CHANDLER & D. STEINBERG. 1974. Science **183:**526–528.
2. STEINBERG, D., T. E. CAREW, J. G. CHANDLER & A. D. SNIDERMAN. 1974. *In* Regulation of Hepatic Metabolism. F. Lundquist & N. Tygstrup, Eds. pp. 144–156. Munksgaard, Copenhagen.
3. GOLDSTEIN, J. L. & M. S. BROWN. 1974. J. Biol. Chem. **249:**5153–5162.
4. GOLDSTEIN, J. L. & M. S. BROWN. 1977. Ann. Rev. Biochem. **46:**897–930.
5. HO, Y. K., M. S. BROWN, H. J. KAYDEN & J. L. GOLDSTEIN. 1976. J. Exp. Med. **144:**444–455.
6. GOLDSTEIN, J. L. & M. S. BROWN. 1975. Arch. Pathol. **99:**181–184.
7. WEINSTEIN, D. B., T. E. CAREW & D. STEINBERG. 1976. Biochim. Biophys. Acta **424:**404–421.
8. ANDERSON, J. M. & J. M. DIETSCHY. 1977. J. Biol. Chem. **252:**3652–3659.
9. BALASUBRAMANIAM, S., J. L. GOLDSTEIN, J. R. FAUST, G. Y. BRUNSCHEDE & M. S. BROWN. 1977. J. Biol. Chem. **252:**1771–1779.
10. MAHLEY, R. W. & T. L. INNERARITY. 1977. J. Biol. Chem. **252:**3980–3986.
11. INNERARITY, T. L. & R. W. MAHLEY. 1978. Biochemistry **17:**1440–1447.
12. STEINBERG, D., P. J. NESTEL, D. B. WEINSTEIN, M. REMAUT-DESMETH & C. M. CHANG. 1978. Biochim. Biophys. Acta **528:**199–212.
13. MAHLEY, R. W., T. L. INNERARITY, R. E. PITAS, K. H. WEISGRABER, J. H. BROWN & E. GROSS. 1977. J. Biol. Chem. **252:**7279–7287.
14. WEISGRABER, K. H., T. L. INNERARITY & R. W. MAHLEY. 1978. J. Biol. Chem. **253:**6289–6295.
15. GOLDSTEIN, J. L., S. K. BASU, G. Y. BRUNSCHEDE & M. S. BROWN. 1976. Cell **7:** 85–95.

16. STEIN, O., D. B. WEINSTEIN, Y. STEIN & D. STEINBERG. 1976. Proc. Natl. Acad. Sci. USA **73**:14–18.
17. MILLER, N. E., D. B. WEINSTEIN & D. STEINBERG. 1977. J. Lipid Res. **18**:438–450.
18. KOSCHINSKY, T., T. E. CAREW & D. STEINBERG. 1977. J. Lipid Res. **18**:451–458.
19. CAREW, T. E., M. J. CHAPMAN, S. GOLDSTEIN & D. STEINBERG. 1978. Biochim. Biophys. Acta **529**:171–175.
20. MAHLEY, R. W. & T. L. INNERARITY. 1978. Adv. Exp. Med. Biol. **109**:99–127.
21. DREVON, C. A., A. D. ATTIE, S. H. PANGBURN & D. STEINBERG. Submitted for publication.
22. STEINBERG, D. 1978. *In* Drugs, Lipid Metabolism, and Atherosclerosis. D. Kritchevsky, R. Paoletti & W. L. Holmes, Eds. pp. 3–27. Plenum Publishing Corp., New York, N.Y.
23. PITTMAN, R. & D. STEINBERG. 1978. Biochem. Biophys. Res. Commun. **81**:1254–1259.
24. PITTMAN, R. C., S. R. GREEN, A. D. ATTIE & D. STEINBERG. 1979. J. Biol. Chem. **254**:6876–6879.
25. PITTMAN, R. C., A. D. ATTIE, T. E. CAREW & D. STEINBERG. 1979. Proc. Natl. Acad. Sci. USA **76**:5345–5349.
26. DVORAK, M. 1972. Endocrinology **54**:473–481.
27. KOVANEN, P., J. R. FAUST, M. S. BROWN & J. L. GOLDSTEIN. 1979. Endocrinology **104**:599–609.
28. REICHL, D., L. A. SIMONE, N. B. MYANT, J. J. PFLUG & G. L. MILLS. 1973. Clin. Sci. Mol. Med. **45**:313–329.
29. KOVANEN, P., S. K. BASU, J. L. GOLDSTEIN & M. S. BROWN. 1979. Endocrinology **104**:610–616.

DISCUSSION OF THE PAPER

DR. S. EISENBERG: I was surprised to see that you had almost the same activity in the spleen and in the liver. Are you confident in those numbers?

DR. D. STEINBERG: Well, that was true in the rat. It was not true in the pig. I only showed you one "representative" study. They say the best experiment is a representative experiment. Actually it is not true in this instance. It is a randomly chosen experiment, so it is not necessarily representative. The activity of the spleen being at least relatively high, raises in our mind the question of whether the reticuloendothelial system might in fact be involved. I think that the relatively high activity of the lymph node fits this notion. However, the thing that speaks against it is that the Kupffer cells in the liver seem to participate only to a minimum extent. Maybe there are reasons for that, I am no hepatologist.

DR. EISENBERG: Could they reflect, say, the activity by lymphocytes or other cells that would be present in the spleen and in lymph nodes, but not in the liver?

DR. STEINBERG: Yes. It could be. Both of those have leukocytes and they do not behave the same way as macrophages or other RE cells.

DR. R. J. HAVEL: It has occurred to a number of us, and you too, I am sure, that active tissues that synthesize new cells, provide new membrane-like products and cholesterol. I noticed that the gut and the small intestine were fairly high on the list of activity. The question is, does the spleen from the rat manufacture blood cells?

DR. STEINBERG: You are right; you would expect that the tissues or the cells that are duplicating rapidly are also those with a most active uptake.

DR. A. R. TALL: In relation to the sucrose-LDL studies, in terms of actual radioactivity in tissues, what sort of recoveries are you actually dealing with? How much was precipitated by TCA and what was the validation of that method?

DR. STEINBERG: The validation was provided in a number of ways: first, in fibroblast cultures where we could compare rates of degradation for both methods and control them. In fact, if you use TCA you do carry down some of the degradation products and that is true in tissues as well. That is why we turned to gel filtration columns to separate the intact LDL from all degradation products, whatever their size. There are partially degraded peptide fragments in all of these preparations and some of those (perhaps to a greater extent in the case of the sucrose tag) are precipitated by 10% TCA. They have a molecular weight of 1,000 to 2,000 and some higher. The counts in the tissues vary tremendously of course; when you are talking about the muscle they are probably as low as any other place, but even there we carry out counts from a couple of grams of tissues. We know the background well enough to know when the results are reliable.

DR. A. M. SCANU: Dr. Steinberg, how many molecules of sucrose did you employ? Does it make any difference in your results?

DR. STEINBERG: I am glad you asked the question. In our earlier experiments we "overderivatized" and the product did not behave normally. I think this is probably because we covered too many amino groups. So we limited the reaction to one micromole of the activated sucrose for each 30 milligrams of LDL protein. In doing so we obtained about 20% efficiency of labeling, which is something like 1 mole of sucrose per 50 or 100,000 grams of protein.

DR. SCANU: We have been trying your method and we felt it very crucial to establish the number of molecules labeled by this procedure.

DR. STEINBERG: I agree with you entirely. You have to find a suitable marker. For that reason we are trying to develop a higher radioactivity marker other than sucrose. We have been trying some D-peptides, which do not get hydrolyzed in the lysosomes. Unfortunately, they seem to leak out from the lysosomes more rapidly than sucrose.

COMMENT: I am interested in the stoichiometry of the sucrose to LDL because we do not know about the relationship between receptors of liver as opposed to other tissues. I just wonder whether the fact that there is sucrose in LDL may influence the way this lipoprotein is taken up by the liver and other tissues.

DR. STEINBERG: A very good point. The only way one is ever certain about this issue is to do the experiments at one level of labeling moles and then two to five times as high. If you get the same answer you are okay. That has not been done yet, and I think it should be done.

DR. J. T. GWYNN (University of North Carolina, Chapel Hill, N.C.): Given the accumulation of the sucrose upon LDL uptake in the adrenals, could you estimate the delivery of cholesterol and compare it to steroid production.

DR. STEINBERG: We have done that in pig adrenals and found an excellent agreement. In other words the amount of cholesterol delivered by LDL *in vivo* would be enough to provide cholesterol for the maximum rate of steroidogenesis.

DR. GWYNN: How about the rat?

DR. STEINBERG: We have not done those studies.

DR. GWYNN: I think that the rat is of a particular interest in light of the presumed interaction of their adrenals with HDL.

DR. STEINBERG: Agreed.

DR. GWYNN: We recently described in rat adrenals a receptor for HDL; it is not pronase sensitive as the receptor described for swine and hepatic homogenates as well.

ALTERATIONS IN METABOLIC ACTIVITY OF PLASMA LIPOPROTEINS FOLLOWING SELECTIVE CHEMICAL MODIFICATION OF THE APOPROTEINS

Robert W. Mahley, Thomas L. Innerarity, and
Karl H. Weisgraber

Gladstone Foundation Laboratories for Cardiovascular Disease
University of California, San Francisco
San Francisco, California 94140

INTRODUCTION

Identification of the sites within the body and elucidation of the mechanisms responsible for the uptake and catabolism of the plasma lipoproteins and their cholesterol remain important questions which need to be studied. Control of lipoprotein catabolism has important implications for lipid metabolism and atherogenesis. It is now established that different cell types (fibroblasts, leukocytes, hepatocytes, adrenal cortical cells, and others) are capable of interacting with specific plasma lipoproteins. In studying these processes, our attention has been focused on the protein moieties of the lipoproteins as the determinants responsible for the interaction with cells.

These studies have relied on the use of various plasma lipoproteins which have specific lipid and apoprotein constituents. Low-density lipoproteins (LDL) from various species, including man, contain almost exclusively the B apoprotein. Another useful class of lipoproteins with a lipid composition and particle size similar to those of LDL has been identified in the plasma of various animals. These lipoproteins, which are related to high-density lipoproteins (HDL), are referred to as HDL_1 and HDL_c in control and cholesterol-fed dogs, rats, and swine, respectively.[1-5] The HDL_1 and HDL_c occur, in part, in the low-density range, but are distinctly different from LDL in that they lack the B apoprotein. They contain the E and A-I apoproteins or exclusively the E apoprotein, the latter is referred to as apoE HDL_c. Such lipoproteins are present in human plasma, and their concentration appears to increase after cholesterol feeding.[6, 7] The role of specific apoproteins has been studied by comparing the metabolism, *in vitro* and *in vivo*, of these particular lipoproteins, including LDL containing the B apoprotein, HDL_c containing exclusively the E apoprotein (apoE HDL_c), and HDL containing primarily the A-I (or A-I and A-II) apoprotein without the E apoprotein. Selective chemical modification of lysine and arginine residues of these lipoproteins has been used to probe the nature of lipoprotein cell interactions *in vitro* in cultured cells and *in vivo* in various animals after intravenous injection.

CELL SURFACE INTERACTION *in Vitro*

It has been established that the recognition site on lipoproteins responsible for their binding to the cell surface receptors of cultured fibroblasts and arterial

265

smooth muscle cells resides with specific apoproteins.[8-11] Both the B apoprotein of low-density lipoproteins (LDL) and the E apoprotein of certain high-density lipoproteins (HDL₁, HDL$_c$) react with the same receptors on the cell surface.[8, 12] High-density lipoproteins that lack the E apoprotein do not bind to the cell surface receptors.[8, 12] The modification of a limited number of arginine and lysine residues prevents these lipoproteins from reacting with the apoB, E receptor sites.[13, 14]

Arginine residues are selectively modified with 1,2-cyclohexanedione by a mild procedure which does not otherwise significantly alter the physical or chemical properties of the LDL or HDL$_c$.[13] The lysine residues are modified by acetoacetylation and reductive methylation.[14] Both procedures are selective and mild. An important difference between the two procedures used for lysine modification is that acetoacetylation neutralizes the positive charge on the ε-amino group, whereas reductive methylation does not alter the charge.

Since modification of the arginine or lysine residues abolished the ability of LDL and HDL$_c$ to react with the cell surface receptors, it was postulated that if these modified lipoproteins were injected intravenously, they would be removed slowly from the plasma. This would demonstrate that the modification had interfered with receptor-mediated uptake *in vivo*. However, as will be described, several unexpected results were obtained, which may ultimately provide information related to the sites and mechanisms involved in lipoprotein catabolism. The effects of selective chemical modification of the lysine and arginine residues on the metabolism of LDL and HDL$_c$ in dogs, rats, or monkeys are summarized in the discussion to follow (see References 15–17 for details of both the methodology and results).

EFFECTS OF CHEMICAL MODIFICATION ON LDL METABOLISM *in Vivo*

When acetoacetylated [^{125}I]LDL are injected into dogs, they are rapidly removed from the plasma. As shown in FIGURE 1, approximately 90% of the injected dose is removed within 4 min. For control [^{125}I]LDL, 50% of the injected dose is still in the plasma after approximately 6 hr. We had no indication that the acetoacetylation of the LDL had denatured these lipoproteins. Furthermore, after reversal of the acetoacetylation, the LDL are cleared from the plasma at a rate identical to that of the untreated LDL (FIGURE 1). These results have been repeated in numerous studies with dogs using both canine and human LDL [16] and with rats using rat and human LDL.[15] Identical results are obtained when 30% to 60% of the total lysine residues are modified by acetoacetylation. The only property of the modified LDL that is altered is an increase in the electrophoretic mobility, indicative of the neutralization of the positive charge on the lysine residues.

It is possible to correlate the accelerated removal of the acetoacetylated LDL from the plasma (left, FIGURE 2) with the appearance of the acetoacetylated LDL in the liver (right, FIGURE 2). At 10 min, when 90% to 95% of the modified LDL is removed from the plasma, approximately 90% of the total injected dose is accounted for in the liver.[16] In other studies using the isolated perfused rat liver, it has been shown that the acetoacetylated LDL taken up by the liver appears in the Kupffer cells.[15] The acetoacetylated LDL are catabolized, as indicated by the appearance of degradation products in the plasma (FIGURE 2).

Furthermore, it has been shown that the acetoacetylated LDL are taken up and degraded by cultured peritoneal macrophages.[16] As shown in FIGURE 3, approximately 10-fold more acetoacetylated LDL than normal LDL are degraded by macrophages. Normal LDL are only very minimally degraded. These data are in agreement with the recent studies reported by Goldstein *et al.*,[18] who demonstrated that peritoneal macrophages are capable of taking up and degrading acetylated LDL. They presented evidence that indicates that

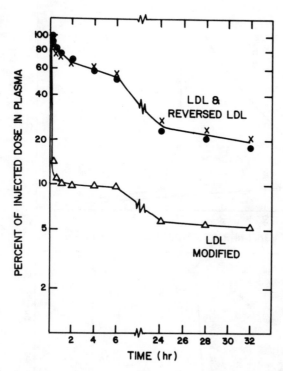

FIGURE 1. Percent of the total injected dose of control canine [^{125}I]LDL (●), acetoacetylated [^{125}I]LDL (△) that had 56% of the lysine residues modified, and acetoacetylated-reversed [^{125}I]LDL (X) remaining in the canine plasma. One mg of lipoprotein protein was injected into each dog. (From Mahley *et al.*[16] By permission of the *Journal of Clinical Investigation.*)

macrophages have receptor sites for the acetylated LDL but not for normal LDL.

One can ask the question as to whether such a mechanism for clearance ever occurs in nature. Do modifications such as these trigger the removal of LDL normally? Whether such a mechanism is ever operative in nature, and whether it might account for the clearance of LDL through a scavenger cell pathway, remains to be determined. It does appear, however, that the alteration in the positive charge on LDL may be involved in the accelerated clearance of the acetoacetylated LDL because, as will be shown, modification of LDL by

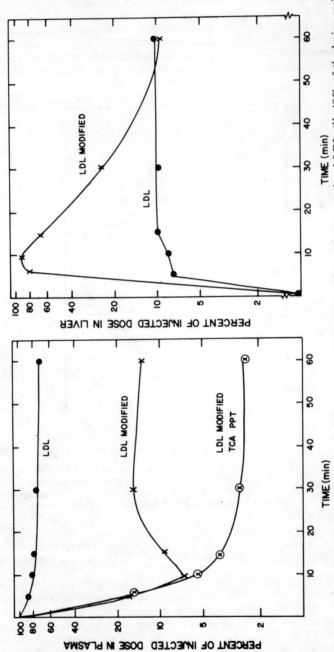

FIGURE 2. Percent of the total injected dose of human control [125I]LDL (●) and acetoacetylated LDL (X, 48% of the lysine residues modified) that remained in the plasma (left) and that appeared in the liver (right). With control LDL, >98% of the activity remaining in the plasma was TCA precipitable. With modified LDL, a significant fraction of the plasma radioactivity after 5 min was not TCA precipitable; data replotted on the basis of injected dose remaining in the plasma that was TCA precipitable (⊗). One mg of lipoprotein protein was injected. (From Mahley et al.[16] By permission of the Journal of Clinical Investigation.)

reductive methylation, which does not modify the charge on lysine, does not stimulate the Kupffer cell-mediated uptake.

When methylated LDL are injected into whole animals, their clearance is retarded.[17] These results are in agreement with our postulate that a modification which prevents cell surface receptor binding *in vitro* might interfere with receptor mediated uptake *in vivo*. The reductively methylated LDL do not trigger the Kupffer cell or macrophage removal process. As shown in FIGURE 4, reductively methylated rat [^{125}I]LDL remains in the plasma longer than the control [^{131}I]LDL injected into rats.[17] The half-life ($t_{1/2}$) of the methylated and control LDL in the plasma is 7 hr and 4.7 hr, respectively. The fractional catabolic rate (FCR) for the methylated LDL is 0.133 as compared to an FCR of 0.256 for control LDL. In this study, rat LDL are obtained by Geon-Pevikon

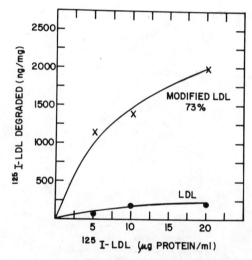

FIGURE 3. Degradation of canine LDL by canine peritoneal macrophages. Control [^{125}I]LDL (●) were compared with acetoacetylated [^{125}I]LDL (X, 73% of the lysine residues modified). (From Mahley *et al.*[16] By permission of the *Journal of Clinical Investigation*.)

block electrophoresis of the $d = 1.02–1.063$ ultracentrifugal fraction. Previously, we have shown that LDL, uncontaminated by HDL$_1$ and the E apoprotein, can be prepared by this procedure.[5]

Similar results are obtained using human LDL injected into the rat. The rate of clearance for methylated human LDL is approximately one-half that observed for control LDL. If the postulate is correct that methylation has interfered with a specific receptor mediated process as occurs in the *in vitro* studies, then one can conclude from the *in vivo* data that 50% of the clearance of LDL in the rat occurs by this receptor mediated uptake process.[17]

These observations are not unique to the rat. When control and methylated human LDL are injected into Rhesus monkeys, the clearance of the methylated

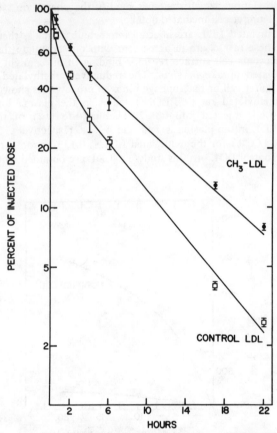

FIGURE 4. Percent of the total injected dose of control rat [^{131}I]LDL (□) and reductively methylated rat [^{125}I]LDL (CH$_3$-LDL, ●) that remained in the plasma vs time after intravenous injection into rats. The mean ± SD (bar) represents values obtained in 3 rats by dual isotope counting at each time point. The reductively methylated LDL had 95% of the lysine residues modified. Each rat received 20 µg of control and methylated LDL protein. (After Mahley et al.[17])

LDL is retarded (FIGURE 5). As in the rat, the FCR for control LDL (0.115) is approximately twice that of the modified LDL (0.055) suggesting that receptor mediated uptake may account for 50% of the LDL clearance.[17]

Thus, acetoacetylation of the B apoprotein of LDL, which neutralizes the charge on the lysine residues, accelerates the plasma clearance of these lipoproteins. The acetoacetylation of LDL triggers the scavenger cell system (particularly the Kupffer cells), which rapidly removes the circulating LDL.[15, 16] However, with reductive methylation of LDL, the plasma clearance is retarded.[17] Presumably, methylation blocks a receptor-mediated uptake process, which is lysine dependent. Furthermore, modification of approximately 50% of the arginine residues of LDL by treatment with 1,2-cyclohexanedione also retards the plasma clearance of LDL.[17] However, care must be taken using the cyclohexanedione modification since this modification is reversible at 37° C in serum. Reductive methylation of lysine residues is not reversible.[17] To our knowledge, the results obtained with methylated and cyclohexanedione-treated LDL represent the first time a chemical modification has been shown to prolong the circulation time of any plasma protein.

EFFECTS OF CHEMICAL MODIFICATION ON HDL$_c$ METABOLISM *in Vivo*

The effects of selective chemical modification of the lysine residues of apoE HDL$_c$ on their metabolism has also been investigated. As discussed

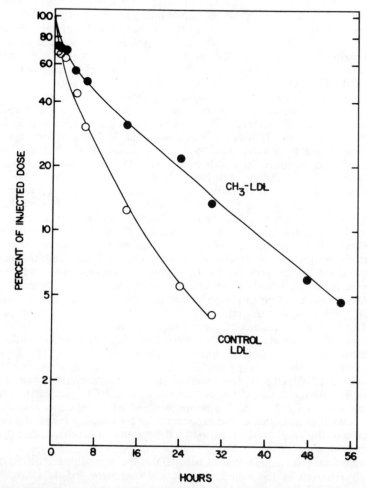

FIGURE 5. Percent of the total injected dose of control human [^{131}I]LDL (◯) and methylated human [^{125}I]LDL (CH₃-LDL, ●) that remained in the plasma of a Rhesus monkey after 500 μg of each lipoprotein had been simultaneously injected. The methylated LDL had 90% of the total lysine residues modified. (After Mahley *et al.*[17])

previously, modification of the lysine residues of apoE HDL_c prevents their interaction with the receptors of fibroblasts *in vitro*,[14] and, as will be shown, acetoacetylation or methylation of canine apoE HDL_c retards their clearance from the plasma of dogs [16] or rats.[15] As shown in FIGURE 6A, the clearance of the acetoacetylated HDL_c from the plasma is markedly decreased. The most dramatic effects can be seen within the first few minutes after injection. Within 5 min after the injection, more than 50% of the native apoE HDL_c is cleared from the plasma, but less than 20% of the acetoacetylated apoE HDL_c is removed. It is noteworthy that the rate of clearance of the native apoE HDL_c is extremely rapid ($>$50% of the injected dose removed in 5 min) (FIGURE 6A).

The liver is responsible for the rapid, acute clearance of the native apoE HDL_c from the plasma.[15, 16] As shown in FIGURE 7 for a representative experiment conducted in the dog, by 20 min after injection, when 60% of the injected dose of native HDL_c is cleared from the plasma, 40% of the injected dose can be accounted for in the liver (i.e., two-thirds of the amount cleared from the plasma in 20 min is present in the liver). The acetoacetylated apoE HDL_c is cleared much less rapidly, and approximately 10% of the injected dose appears in the liver (FIGURE 7). Therefore, the liver appears to be the site responsible for the acute uptake of native apoE HDL_c. Acetoacetylation of the lysine residues interferes with the hepatic uptake process. The native apoE HDL_c is catabolized and excreted ($\sim$10% of the injected dose is accounted for in the urine within 2 hr). It has now been shown that the hepatic parenchymal cells are responsible for greater than 95% of the uptake of the native HDL_c (unpublished data obtained in collaboration with Dr. Bette Sherrill, Southwestern Medical Center, Dallas, Texas).

It should be pointed out that after the first hour the rates of removal of the native and modified apoE HDL_c are similar (FIGURE 7). This may be related to a redistribution or exchange of the labeled E apoprotein among the various apoE-containing lipoproteins in the plasma. Once redistribution occurs after the acute phase, then the rate of removal would depend on the actual class of lipoprotein with which the label is associated. On the other hand, this may be accounted for by the presence of an inhibitor, which associates with the HDL_c in the plasma and masks or interferes with the rapid uptake process.

Consideration was given to the possibility that the rapid removal of native apoE HDL_c within the first few minutes of injection could be due to the absence of an HDL_c pool in the plasma of normal dogs. Therefore, native [^{131}I]HDL_c and ^{125}I-labeled acetoacetylated HDL_c were injected simultaneously into a hypercholesterolemic dog and the rate of clearance measured.[16] The rapid, acute clearance of the native [^{131}I]HDL_c and the retarded clearance of the acetoacetylated [^{125}I]HDL_c is also observed in the hypercholesterolemic dog (FIGURE 6B). Within 5 min, 50% of the native apoE HDL_c is cleared from the plasma while only 20% of the acetoacetylated apoE HDL_c is removed. However, with respect to the second exponential of the dieaway curve, the rate of clearance of the apoE HDL_c is slower in the hypercholesterolemic dog than in the control dog.

To summarize the results obtained with HDL_c, the unmodified apoE HDL_c are rapidly removed by the liver in normal and cholesterol-fed dogs. Acetoacetylation of 30% or more of the lysine residues of apoE HDL_c interferes with the removal, which suggests that the apoE may be involved in the hepatic recognition of these lipoproteins and that the recognition process may be a

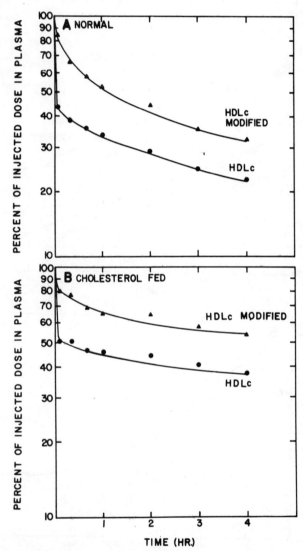

FIGURE 6. Percent of the total injected dose of native [131I]apoE HDL$_c$ (●) and acetoacetylated [125I]apoE HDL$_c$ (▲) that remained in the plasma of a normolipidemic (A) or a hypercholesterolemic (B) dog. The native 131I-HDL$_c$ (100 cpm/ng of protein) and the acetoacetylated [125I]HDL$_c$ (166 cpm/ng of protein) were injected simultaneously into each dog (0.4 mg of each lipoprotein based on protein). (From Mahley *et al.*[16] By permission of the *Journal of Clinical Investigation*.)

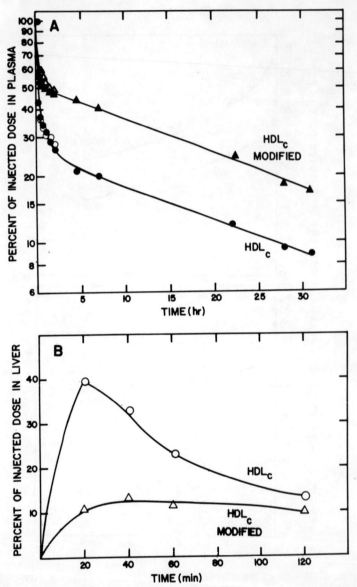

FIGURE 7. Percent of the total injected dose of control [¹²⁵I]apoE HDL꜀ (●) and acetoacetylated [¹²⁵I]apoE HDL꜀ (▲, 60% of the lysine residues modified) which remained in the plasma with time in hours (A) and which appeared in the liver in minutes (B). Additional data from 2 separate dogs which received either control [¹²⁵I]apoE HDL꜀ (○) or acetoacetylated [¹²⁵I]apoE HDL꜀ (△); 400 µg of lipoprotein protein was injected. (From Mahley *et al.*[16] By permission of the *Journal of Clinical Investigation*.)

TABLE 1

EFFECTS OF SELECTIVE CHEMICAL MODIFICATION OF LYSINE AND ARGININE RESIDUES

	Residue Modified	In Vitro		In Vivo	
		Fibroblast Interaction *	Macrophage Uptake	Plasma Clearance ($t_{1/2}$)	General Comments
LDL					
Control	—	Yes (apoB)	No	(5–8 hr) †	Uptake by various tissues (? liver)
Acetoacetylated	Lysine	Blocked	Yes	Accelerated (~5 min)	Kupffer cell uptake triggered
Methylated	Lysine	Blocked	No	Retarded (10–16 hr)	Peripheral cell uptake blocked
Cyclohexanedione	Arginine	Blocked	No	Retarded	
HDLc					
Control	—	Yes (apoE)	No	Rapid	Hepatocyte uptake involved
Acetoacetylated	Lysine	Blocked	No	Retarded	Hepatocyte uptake blocked
Methylated	Lysine	Blocked	No	Retarded	

* Ability of the lipoprotein to bind with high affinity to the cell surface receptors of cultured human fibroblasts via the apoB of LDL or the apoE of HDLc.[8, 13, 14]

† Range of results obtained with rat, canine, or human lipoproteins when injected intravenously into rats, dogs, or monkeys.[15–17]

lysine-dependent system blocked by modification of the lysine residues. It is suggested from these data that the hepatocyte has an apoE receptor.[15, 16]

CONCLUSIONS

The effects of the selective chemical modification of LDL and HDL_c on the metabolism of these lipoproteins by fibroblasts and macrophages *in vitro* and on their metabolism after intravenous injection *in vivo* are summarized in TABLE 1.

Chemically Modified LDL. Acetoacetylation triggers an extremely rapid clearance of LDL from the plasma by the hepatic Kupffer cells.[15, 16] By contrast, reductive methylation of the lysine of LDL retards the plasma clearance.[17] In addition, cyclohexanedione modification of arginine residues of LDL results in a retardation in plasma clearance. The use of methylated LDL may provide an estimate of receptor-mediated uptake of LDL *in vivo*. In the Rhesus monkey and the rat, our data indicate that approximately 50% of the clearance of LDL is receptor mediated.[17] This is in agreement with the 66% estimated by Brown and Goldstein [19] to be cleared by the receptor pathway.

Chemically Modified HDL_c. Modification of the lysine residues inhibits the hepatic parenchymal cells from clearing HDL_c from the plasma.[15, 16] By contrast, the native apoE HDL_c are rapidly removed from the plasma and may represent one of the reverse cholesterol transport vehicles. Our data indicate that hepatic parenchymal cells take up native apoE HDL_c, and that the process may be mediated by a hepatocyte receptor for apoE in the dog and rat.[15, 16] The existence of an apoE receptor in the rat liver was suggested by the data presented at this conference by Havel *et al.*[20]

The use of selective chemical modification of various amino acid residues of plasma apolipoproteins appears to be a useful procedure with which to probe the pathways involved in lipoprotein metabolism. Such modifications should provide useful information on various aspects of lipoprotein structure–function.

REFERENCES

1. MAHLEY, R. W. 1978. Alterations in plasma lipoproteins induced by cholesterol feeding in animals including man. *In* Disturbances in Lipid and Lipoprotein Metabolism. J. M. Dietschy, A. M. Gotto, Jr. & J. A. Ontko, Eds. pp. 181–197. American Physiological Society, Bethesda, Md.
2. MAHLEY, R. W., T. L. INNERARITY, K. H. WEISGRABER & D. L. FRY. 1977. Canine hyperlipoproteinemia and atherosclerosis. Accumulation of lipid by aortic medial cells *in vivo* and *in vitro*. Am. J. Pathol. 87:205–225.
3. MAHLEY, R. W., K. H. WEISGRABER, T. INNERARITY, H. B. BREWER, JR. & G. ASSMANN. 1975. Swine lipoproteins and atherosclerosis. Changes in the plasma lipoproteins and apoproteins induced by cholesterol feeding. Biochemistry 14:2817–2823.
4. MAHLEY, R. W. & K. S. HOLCOMBE. 1977. Alterations of the plasma lipoproteins and apoproteins following cholesterol feeding in the rat. J. Lipid Res. 18:314–324.
5. WEISGRABER, K. H., R. W. MAHLEY & G. ASSMANN. 1977. The rat arginine-rich apoprotein and its redistribution following injection of iodinated lipoproteins into normal and hypercholesterolemic rats. Atherosclerosis 28:121–140.
6. WEISGRABER, K. H. & R. W. MAHLEY. 1978. Apoprotein (E-A-II) complex of

human plasma lipoproteins. I. Characterization of this mixed disulfide and its identification in a high density lipoprotein subfraction. J. Biol. Chem. **253:** 6281–6288.

7. MAHLEY, R. W., T. L. INNERARITY, T. P. BERSOT, A. LIPSON & S. MARGOLIS. 1978. Alterations in human high-density lipoproteins, with or without increased plasma-cholesterol, induced by diets high in cholesterol. Lancet (2):807–809.

8. MAHLEY, R. W. & T. L. INNERARITY. 1978. Properties of lipoproteins responsible for high affinity binding to cell surface receptors of fibroblasts and smooth muscle cells. *In* Drugs, Lipid Metabolism, and Atherosclerosis. D. Kritchevsky, R. Paoletti & W. L. Holmes, Eds. pp. 99–127. Plenum Publishing Corp., New York, N.Y.

9. BERSOT, T. P., R. W. MAHLEY, M. S. BROWN & J. L. GOLDSTEIN. 1976. Interaction of swine lipoproteins with the low density lipoprotein receptor in human fibroblasts. J. Biol. Chem. **251:**2395–2398.

10. INNERARITY, T. L. & R. W. MAHLEY. 1978. Enhanced binding by cultured human fibroblasts of apo-E-containing lipoproteins as compared with low density lipoproteins. Biochemistry **17:**1440–1447.

11. PITAS, R. E., T. L. INNERARITY, K. S. ARNOLD & R. W. MAHLEY. 1979. Rate and equilibrium constants for binding of apo-E HDL$_c$ (a cholesterol-induced lipoprotein) and low density lipoproteins to human fibroblasts: Evidence for multiple receptor binding of apo-E HDL$_c$. Proc. Natl. Acad. Sci. USA **76:** 2311–2315.

12. INNERARITY, T. L., R. W. MAHLEY, K. H. WEISGRABER & T. P. BERSOT. 1978. Apoprotein (E–A-II) complex of human plasma lipoproteins. II. Receptor binding activity of a high density lipoprotein subfraction modulated by the apo(E–A-II) complex. J. Biol. Chem. **253:**6289–6295.

13. MAHLEY, R. W., T. L. INNERARITY, R. E. PITAS, K. H. WEISGRABER, J. H. BROWN & E. GROSS. 1977. Inhibition of lipoprotein binding to cell surface receptors of fibroblasts following selective modification of arginyl residues in arginine-rich and B apoproteins. J. Biol. Chem. **252:**7279–7287.

14. WEISGRABER, K. H., T. L. INNERARITY & R. W. MAHLEY. 1978. Role of the lysine residues of plasma lipoproteins in high affinity binding to cell surface receptors on human fibroblasts. J. Biol. Chem. **253:**9053–9062.

15. MAHLEY, R. W., K. H. WEISGRABER, T. L. INNERARITY & H. G. WINDMUELLER. 1979. Accelerated clearance of low-density and high-density lipoproteins and retarded clearance of E apoprotein-containing lipoproteins from the plasma of rats after modification of lysine residues. Proc. Natl. Acad. Sci. USA **76:** 1746–1750.

16. MAHLEY, R. W., T. L. INNERARITY, K. H. WEISGRABER & S. Y. OH. 1979. Altered metabolism (*in vivo* and *in vitro*) of plasma lipoproteins after selective chemical modification of lysine residues of the apoproteins. J. Clin. Invest. **64:**743–750.

17. MAHLEY, R. W., K. H. WEISGRABER, G. W. MELCHIOR, T. L. INNERARITY & K. S. HOLCOMBE. 1979. Inhibition of receptor-mediated clearance of lysine- and arginine-modified lipoproteins from the plasma of rats and monkeys. Proc. Natl. Acad. Sci. USA **77:**225–229.

18. GOLDSTEIN, J. L., Y. K. HO, S. K. BASU & M. S. BROWN. 1979. A binding site on macrophages that mediates the uptake and degradation of acetylated low density lipoprotein, producing massive cholesterol deposition. Proc. Natl. Acad. Sci. USA **76:**333–337.

19. BROWN, M. S. & J. L. GOLDSTEIN. 1979. Familial hypercholesterolemia: Model for genetic receptor disease. The Harvey Lectures (1977–1978) **73:**163–201.

20. HAVEL, R. J. 1980. Biosynthesis and metabolism. Ann. N.Y. Acad. Sci. This volume.

DISCUSSION OF THE PAPER

DR. D. STEINBERG: Thank you very much for the interesting data, Dr. Mahley. I think this field is coming of age where you can talk about apoE, HDL_C and its interactions with apoCs and string along these observations which people not in the field think are very mysterious. Then you know you have got maturity in the field!

DR. H. L. SEGAL: I would like to come back to this observation of the extremely rapid clearance of HDL, modified HDL, in which about 50% is taken up by a process of a couple of orders of magnitude more rapid than the remainder of the clearance. This is a tracer dose, is it not?

DR. R. W. MAHLEY: That is correct; but let me qualify it. It depends upon the animal that receives it. We inject about 0.5 mg of apoE HDL_C into a control or a cholesterol-fed animal. That is a very large amount for a control dog, but a small amount for a cholesterol-fed animal.

DR. SEGAL: And you got similar results?

DR. MAHLEY: Yes.

DR. SEGAL: Well, is there a competition for uptake between the iodinated and the noniodionated material? If I can also pose that question to Dr. Steinberg, I am not sure that you said that in the isolated cell study there was a competition between native and derivatized molecules. Is that the case?

DR. MAHLEY: In our case we are unable to do those experiments *in vivo* because we cannot obtain that much of the apoE HDL_C. We are doing studies now in the isolated rat liver (1980. J. Biol. Chem. **255**:1804–1807). It appears that the apoE HDL_C are taken up by the chylomicron remnant mechanism in the perfused system mediated by the presence of the E apoprotein. The remnants do compete with HDL_C for that uptake process.

DR. SEGAL: I am just concerned whether the labeling process might have produced a population of partially denatured molecules, which are most rapidly taken up and which would be excluded from competition experiments.

DR. MAHLEY: Well, in response to that, the modified apoE HDLC, which has gone through more extensive handling, is taken up much less rapidly during the acute phase.

DR. S. EISENBERG: If I am reading correctly between the slides, you mentioned that apoE HDL_C disappears in two phases. One explanation is that the injected protein interacted with apoC or other plasma components inducing a retardation of its clearance.

DR. MAHLEY: That may be entirely correct. That is all I can say. I really thought that we were going to be able to show that the change in the slope was due to rapid exchange, which I assumed to be occurring. But I was unable to really prove extensively that apoE of the apoE HDL_C particle exchanges very rapidly. In fact, it does appear that the exchange does not occur very rapidly. So I am left with the inhibitor hypothesis. We are doing studies in this direction.

DR. J. A. K. HARMONY (*Indiana University, Bloomington, Ind.*): Are the inhibitors the C proteins?

DR. MAHLEY: I do not know.

DR. HARMONY: You have a good system for testing the role of apoB versus apoE in regard to the uptake of lipoproteins by the various tissues. Have you started such studies by changing the apoprotein composition of your lipoproteins and then repeating your studies?

DR. MAHLEY: Well, we have tried those studies but we have been unable to add detectable amounts of apoE in LDL.

COMMENT: I am having difficulty getting it off.

DR. MAHLEY: You can isolate LDL containing apoE. But if you take LDL without any E, and tried to add this apoprotein you are unable to detect it in the re-isolates of LDL.

DR. STEINBERG: With regard to the apparently mysterious way in which acetylation and acetoacetylation cause a difference in cell uptake, is this not just due to change in charge?

DR. MAHLEY: All of the data right now do not really fit the interpretation of change in charge. In the case of apoE HDLC, when its electrophoretic mobility is modified just as much as LDL, it gives totally different results.

DR. STEINBERG: I am suggesting that that sort of pseudo-peptide bond that you create when you acetylate the lipoprotein is what is recognized by the macrophage receptors.

DR. R. J. HAVEL: Yesterday we presented data indicating that the addition of C apoproteins to VLDL obtained from perfused rat livers markedly inhibits the clearance of those lipoproteins by the cells. Previously we have shown that one can add apoE to rat chylomicrons. We can increase the content by a factor of 10 simply by adding an apoE-containing lipoprotein in the presence of the bottom fraction. We have now done this with chylomicrons from estrogen-treated rats. These chylomicrons might not contain apoE, because this apoprotein is made, as I mentioned yesterday, in the liver, and only to a minor extent if at all in the gut. In fact, what we get are lymph chylomicrons containing apoB, apoA-I, and apoIV, but essentially no apoE as indicated by radioimmunoassay techniques and very little apoC. Now if we add purified apoE (rat) to those particles it will be as in the normal case, namely, small chylomicrons are picked up very avidly. Those modified chylomicrons now behave identically to chylomicrons remnants as they are taken up by the rat liver with an AV difference in the circulation of at least 30% or 40%. This material is cleared more rapidly than that from those rats that were not treated with apoE. So, under these circumstances one can get apoE to stick to something and modify its behavior.

DR. MAHLEY: These are really very interesting findings. Now maybe we can start looking at ratios of apoproteins as determinants for directing fat metabolism.

COMMENT: Both of you, Dr. Steinberg and Dr. Mahley, have used a term receptor for the modified lipoproteins with respect to the macrophage uptake from the liver. It seems to me that when you modify the protein you produce a very nonspecific type of responsiveness by the cell that recognizes just it from the other materials. In addition, when you make a modification you may induce protein–protein interactions in the serum. There may be a rather nonspecific type of interaction with gamma globulins, for example, and these can rise to complexes that the macrophage will recognize.

DR. STEINBERG: With respect to aggregates, at least as determined by the parameters of electrophoretic mobility and negative staining by electron microscopy, we do not see gross aggregates. Whether or not there are some microaggregates, I cannot respond to, but gross aggregates I do not believe are present. The studies that Brown and Goldstein did were with isolated macrophages and there were no interactions in the serum. There is no strong basis for talking about a specific receptor, only that there is a biphasic curve of uptake depending upon concentration.

DR. D. M. SMALL: I have two questions. One of them refers to your plasma decay curve, in which you show an acute phase of uptake but a slower decay. Have you considered whether the effect of your acetylacetylation has inhibited the normal extent by which apoE reacts with cells, and thus caused a slower acute uptake. The second question relates to something that you mentioned and elaborated upon; you have studied the decay curve of HDL_C apoE, in hypocholesterolemic dogs. What was the approximate decay rate of apoE?

DR. MAHLEY: In regard to the second question, the acute phase was identical in both animals, namely, cholesterol fed and normals. After that acute phase, the slower phase was different in the cholesterol-fed animals; the rate was about half that which occurred in the controls. With respect to your first question, whether or not the acetoacetylation changed the exchange rate, I really do not know. The one thing that may have some bearing on this is that the acetoacetylated apoE forms a complex with DMPC disks just as well as unmodified apoE. I do not know that this has direct bearing.

GENERAL DISCUSSION

D. Steinberg, *Moderator*

Division of Metabolic Disease
Department of Medicine
University of California at San Diego
La Jolla, California 92093

DR. D. M. SMALL: Dr. Mahley, if what you said is correct, that the dieaway curves of those first 5 or 10 minutes are identical for the hypocholesterolemic and the normal animals, is it not true that the hypocholesterolemic animal has much more lipoproteins?

DR. MAHLEY: That is correct.

DR. SMALL: Would that not indicate that what Dr. Eisenberg has suggested may in fact be the case. That is, when you isolate the HDL$_C$ you lose the protection from uptake by the liver. Otherwise, with a larger pool you expect somewhat a delay.

DR. MAHLEY: Well, I think that this is correct unless the reservoir is big, but we cannot say anything about it.

DR. SMALL: I do not understand your answer. It could easily mean that the half-life of that component is very rapid, even in the dogs that have a higher concentration of it.

DR. MAHLEY: Well if you had it down to seconds, you should see some difference.

DR. SMALL: It depends on how fast it is generating, does it not? If it is generating rapidly, the fractional catabolic rate may be independent of the concentration of that HDL$_C$ pool, which is what I am suggesting.

DR. R. L. HARRIS (*University of Texas, Dallas, Texas*): I would like to make a comment that might be of interest to Dr. Glomset and his studies in familial LCAT deficiency. We have recently characterized some abnormal lipoprotein that may prove useful in the study of lipoprotein metabolism and LCAT. In severely burned patients, we made two interesting observations regarding the anemia that is associated with thermal injury. Firstly, there is an abnormal morphology of the red cells of burned patients. This can be induced by incubation of the normal cells with plasma of burned subjects and corrected by placing the abnormal cells into normal plasma. Secondly, there is around 60% to 70% reduction of the survival of the chromium-labeled red blood cells transfused into burned patients as compared to controls.

From these observations we began studying the plasma lipids. The burned patients have a two- to threefold increase in triglycerides and 50% reductions in cholesterol, and phospholipids due to the formation of cholesterol esters in HDL. The phospholipid distribution was compatible with that found in familial LCAT deficiency in that there was an increase in the percentage of phosphatidylcholine with a decrease in sphingomyelin. Finally, we found a 50% reduction in LCAT activity in the plasma in some of those patients. We feel that

281

the burned patients may have an intermediately severe type of LCAT deficiency, which may explain the anemia and may serve as a useful model for the study of lipoprotein metabolism *in vivo*.

DR. GLOMSET: I think it was a very interesting observation. As I mentioned one problem when the distribution of HDLs is altered is carefully determining the very fast initial rates of the LCAT reaction, which remains to be done yet in these burned patients.

DR. R. BLUMENTHAL (*National Institutes of Health, Bethesda, Md.*): The technique that Dr. Wirtz described seems to be extremely powerful to characterize protein interactions. My question is has it been applied to other membranes or other proteins?

DR. K. W. A. WIRTZ: Yes. It has been possible to reconstitute lipid–protein systems, although hard data have not yet been published. The evidence is that indeed you can couple the PC molecules to the membrane proteins. I think that those lipid molecules would also be very powerful tools to determine how the apolipoproteins are embedded in the core of the lipoproteins. One study has been published by Stoffel, with regard to apoA-I and apoA-II in HDL. I think it is just the beginning of what should prove to be a very exciting area.

DR. A. R. TALL: In that little pocket or basket are two tyrosines and a phenylalanine?

DR. WIRTZ: Two phenylalanines.

DR. TALL: It seems to me that one should be able to demonstrate the changes in the motion of those residues by absorption in the UV region.

DR. WIRTZ: The problem with this particular protein is that you have to look at high and low concentrations. Generally, the concentrations needed to do this kind of spectroscopy are generally where the proteins tend to aggregate.

DR. TALL: What sort of concentration?

DR. WIRTZ: You are talking about concentrations of below 100 mg per ml.

DR. TALL: You should be able to do it around a 100 mg per ml.

DR. WIRTZ: There will be a borderline of significance.

DR. H. G. ROSE (*VA Medical Center, Bronx, N.Y.*): I would like to ask Dr. Glomset this question. There have been at least three pretenders for a cholesterol ester transferor exchange protein. The first one was apoE, because of studies in LCAT deficiencies that showed that this protein transfers simultaneously with cholesteryl esters. Now Dr. Fielding has some evidence that apoD is involved in the transfer of cholesteryl esters. Then, Don Zilversmit has evidence that it is not an apoprotein that is involved. Could you please clarify this issue?

DR. J. A. GLOMSET: Maybe Richard Havel may have something to say about the work by Dr. Fielding. I think that like many other situations a lot depends on what incubation system is used in measuring the activity. We had evidence a long time ago, that radioactive cholesteryl esters transfer from HDL to LDL. On the other hand, if you take patients with LCAT deficiency there is very little cholesteryl ester in their lipoprotein, mainly triglycerides. If I recall, a five-fold increase in the cholesterol ester content occurs if you incubate

LDL with the patients HDL and LCAT. But, I think that much of that net transfer-exchange business depends on how much of a core of lipid there is in the acceptor protein. If you have normal LDL, full to capacity with cholesteryl esters, one very interesting problem which is of course related to the structure of LDL is to determine where there are constraints on this exchange process imposed by apoB and the net size of the molecules. In other words, it may make a difference if one is dealing with a lipoprotein when the core is terribly rich in cholesterol ester from a lipoprotein like LDL, which has a core with a certain amount of triglycerides in it. Depending upon the saturation you may have an exchange or a transfer.

DR. STEINBERG: I think that you, Dr. Glomset, have enlarged the list of possibilities for Dr. Rose to think about. Dr. Havel, do you want to try addressing yourself to this issue?

DR. HAVEL: Because of the lateness of the hour, not very much. ApoE is just a hypothesis. There were never data. For apoD there are solid data and those studies by the Fieldings are published. What happened under their conditions is that there is an equimolar reciprocal movement between cholesteryl ester and triglycerides, on one hand between HDL and VLDL, and on the other hand between HDL and LDL, nothing between VLDL and LDL, all of these under the particular conditions of their experiments. I simply endorse what John said, there may be in some cases very rapid movements of one polar lipid reciprocated by another with only relatively small net transfers. Under some circumstances, for instance, in the LCAT deficient plasma, one may get a very substantial movement or a net movement of nonpolar lipids from one particle to another. I think that apoE protein has been shown very clearly to have the potential for net transfer of cholesterol ester produced by LCAT. A net movement can also be effectuated by apoD, regardless of its mechanism.

X-RAY AND NEUTRON SCATTERING STUDIES OF
PLASMA LIPOPROTEINS *

David Atkinson, Donald M. Small, and G. Graham Shipley

Biophysics Division
Departments of Medicine and Biochemistry
Boston University School of Medicine
Boston, Massachusetts 02118

INTRODUCTION

A detailed knowledge of the organization of the plasma lipoproteins at a molecular level is necessary for a basic understanding of the principles governing lipoprotein assembly, interconversion and interactions, and the role of lipoproteins in the regulation of lipid metabolism. In the spectrum of plasma lipoproteins, varying from large emulsion particles (chylomicrons) to the compositionally better defined high-density class, low-density (LDL) and high-density (HDL) lipoproteins have been the most extensively studied.

Our present concepts of lipoprotein structure are derived from a wide variety of experimental methodologies ranging from physical to biochemical (for recent reviews see References 1 & 2). However, this report will be concerned primarily with the details of lipoprotein molecular architecture obtained from the use of the structure probing techniques of x-ray and neutron small-angle scattering.[6-11] In the first section, we review the details of current models for the structure of native lipoproteins with particular emphasis on the molecular arrangement of the neutral lipid core. We describe studies on a range of normal and abnormal lipoproteins, and by comparing structural information from this range of lipoprotein particles, some general principles of lipoprotein molecular organization are suggested.

For high-density lipoproteins the techniques of delipidation to give water soluble apoproteins[3] and the recombination of either the total apoprotein or the constituent apoproteins (A-I, A-II, and C peptides) with polar phospholipids or mixtures of phospholipids and neutral lipids[4, 5] provide an opportunity for detailed study of the interaction and structures formed between the apoproteins and various lipid classes. The second section describes some recent studies on recombinant systems formed from HDL apoproteins and dimyristoyl phosphatidylcholine. These studies utilizing neutron scattering were specifically designed to probe the location of the apoproteins on the recombinant particles.

THE STRUCTURE OF NATIVE PLASMA LIPOPROTEINS.

Plasma lipoproteins (HDL, LDL) are usually described as quasispherical "emulsion-like" particles consisting of a neutral lipid (cholesterol ester, triglyceride) core surface-stabilized by phospholipids and specific apolipoproteins.

* This work was supported by U.S. Public Health Service Grants HL 18673 and HL 13262 and Training Grant HL 07291.

However, as first demonstrated by Deckelbaum *et al.*[12] using differential scanning calorimetry, LDL undergoes a thermally induced structural transition over the temperature range 20°–40° C. This thermal transition corresponds in temperature and enthalpy to the liquid crystalline smectic-to-disorder transition

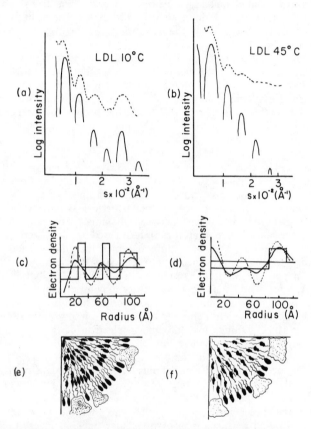

FIGURE 1. Small angle x-ray scattering curves (a, b), radial electron density distributions (c, d), and schematic models of the structural organization (e, f) for normal human LDL below (10° C) and above (45° C) the thermal transition. The dashed curves in (a–d) are the experimentally determined scattering profiles and radial electron density distributions derived from the experimental data as discussed in the text. The solid curves are the calculated scattering profiles (a, b) calculated for the step distribution of electron density (c, d) corresponding to the schematic models in (e) and (f). The electron density profiles for these models derived from the calculated scattering data at the same resolution as the experimental data are shown by the solid curves in (c) and (d). The experimental details are described in REFERENCE 7.

of the isolated cholesterol esters of LDL,[12, 13] and thus reflects a thermal transition of the cholesterol esters (~1500 molecules per LDL particle) packed in the core of LDL from an ordered packing below the transition to a more disordered state above.

FIGURE 1 (a & b) shows small angle x-ray scattering profiles obtained for

LDL at temperatures below (10° C) and above (45° C) the thermal transition. The scattering profiles at both temperatures exhibit a series of well resolved subsidiary maxima at scattering angles corresponding to $S < 1/40$ Å^{-1} typical of the scattering of a quasispherical particle. Thus, the quasispherical morphology of LDL is essentially unchanged below and above the transition. However, an intense scattering maximum at $S \approx 1/36$ Å^{-1} in the scattering profile obtained at 10° C is absent from the scattering profile obtained above the thermal transition.

Isolated cholesterol esters from LDL exhibit a smectic liquid crystalline phase characterized by a single sharp x-ray diffraction maximum at 1/36 Å^{-1}.[12, 13] This sharp diffraction is not observed at higher temperatures where the cholesteric and isotropic phases are present. This parallel with the behavior of the 1/36 Å^{-1} scattering range in the scattering profile for LDL suggested that the cholesterol esters in the core of LDL may undergo a similar "smectic-like" to disordered transition.[12, 13]

FIGURE 1(c & d) shows the spherically averaged radial electron density distributions for LDL derived from the x-ray scattering curves at 10° C and 45° C. These electron density distributions were obtained by Fourier transformation of $I^{1/2}(s)$. This procedure assumes that the particle is perfectly spherically symmetric. However, for perfect spherical symmetry the minima in the scattering should go to zero between maxima. The nonzero minima observed experimentally were therefore interpolated to true zero using the positions of the maxima. This procedure assumes that the nonzero minima are due mainly to the heterogeneous particle size distribution rather than deviations from perfect spherical symmetry. The radial distribution obtained at both temperatures exhibits an electron density maximum centered at ~100 Å interpreted as the surface location of the phospholipid head groups and protein, the outer radius of the particle being ~110 Å. More importantly the distribution obtained at 10° C exhibits two maxima in electron density at ~30 Å and ~60 Å superimposed on the average low electron density of the core region. These peaks of electron density in the core region directly indicate an ordered arrangement for the core-located components. The electron density distribution obtained for LDL at 45° C shows only one low maximum in the core region at approximately 45 Å indicating that the core has a less ordered structure.

Models for the molecular packing of the cholesterol ester in the core of LDL, based on limited perturbations of molecular packing in crystalline cholesteryl myristate,[14] suggested that these core-located electron density peaks observed for LDL below the transition (10° C) are due to regions within the core where the steroid moieties of the cholesterol esters are packed in register.[17] A radial packing of the cholesterol esters, shown schematically in FIGURE 1e, in which concentric regions of the core located at radii of ~30 and ~60 Å have a high electron density (FIGURE 1c) due to closely packed steroid moieties of the cholesterol esters, adequately accounts for the observed scattering profile and the electron density distribution (FIGURE 1a & c).[7] At 45° C above the thermal transition these positional correlations between the steroid moieties are absent (FIGURE 1f). The electron density distribution of the core region is therefore more uniform, as illustrated by the model electron density profile in FIGURE 1d, resulting in a scattering profile in which the subsidiary maximum at 1/36 Å^{-1} no longer has a high relative intensity.

The lipoprotein HDL$_c$ isolated from cholesterol-fed miniature swine is a cholesterol ester-rich particle intermediate in size between LDL (~220 Å diameter) and normal HDL ($\sim$100 Å diameter).[15, 16] Differential scanning calorimetry and x-ray small angle scattering evidence indicate that the cholesterol esters in this lipoprotein can, like LDL, also undergo a cooperative thermal order-disorder transition (peak temperature 38° C).[16, 18] In contrast to the x-ray small angle scattering profile of LDL, the profile for HDL_c at 10° C (FIGURE 2a) exhibits four subsidiary maxima at larger angular spacing consistent with a particle size smaller than that of LDL. For HDL_c the fourth subsidiary maximum is centered at $1/36$ Å^{-1} and has a high relative intensity. At 45° C above the transition this maximum is absent from the scattering profile similar to the behavior observed for LDL.

FIGURE 2b illustrates the spherically averaged radial electron density distribution obtained for HDL_c at 10° C. The surface location of the protein and phospholipid polar head groups is clearly shown by the surface-located electron density peak centered at $\sim$80 Å, the outer radius of the particle being $\sim$90 Å. Again of particular importance is the *single* core-located electron density maximum centered at $\sim$40 Å, which may be contrasted with the distribution for LDL exhibiting two core located maxima.

The electron density distributions for LDL and HDL_c, however, show a striking similarity when the two profiles are compared with the surface protein/polar group peaks superimposed as shown in FIGURE 3. The core electron density maximum located $\sim$40 Å from the surface protein/polar head group peak (i.e. the peak at $\sim$60 Å in the radial electron density profile for LDL and the peak at $\sim$40 Å radius in the profile for HDL_c) is a common feature of the electron density distribution of both HDL_c and LDL at 10° C. This similarity in the electron density profiles suggests a common structural arrangement for these lipoproteins in the region of the core close to the surface-located proteins and polar phospholipids.[18]

As illustrated in the schematic model shown in FIGURE 2c, the $\sim$20 Å size difference between LDL and HDL_c can be accommodated with a similar packing for the cholesterol esters below the phase transition. The first molecular layer located at the center of the particle in LDL is removed in the model for HDL_c. Thus, whereas in the model for LDL the regions of overlapping steroid moieties are centered at $\sim$30 Å and $\sim$60 Å radii, removal of the first molecular layer gives regions of overlap centered at $\sim$10 Å and $\sim$45 Å radii (FIGURE 2b). The x-ray scattering profile and electron density distribution derived for this model are in good agreement with those obtained experimentally for HDL_c at 10° C (FIGURE 2a and b).

Thus, a direct comparison of the radial electron density profiles for HDL_c and LDL together with the model calculations suggests a common structural arrangement of the cholesterol esters in the lipoprotein core at temperatures below the phase transition. This common molecular arrangement in which the cholesterol esters are radially packed, producing molecular layers in with the steroid ring moieties in register, is probably similar in molecular arrangement and interactions to the smectic phase exhibited by isolated cholesterol esters.

Recent studies on LDL, isolated from cholesterol-fed monkeys, which are enriched in cholesterol esters giving larger lipoprotein particles with molecular weights in the range 3–7 $\times$ 10^6 daltons have extended this concept of a common molecular packing for the core located cholesterol esters.[17] X-ray scattering measurements and model calculations suggest that for LDL with a molecular weight greater than $\sim$6 $\times$ 10^6 daltons the core region or LDL can accomodate

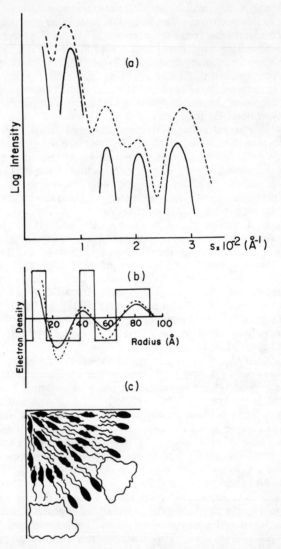

FIGURE 2. Small angle x-ray scattering curve (a), radial electron density distribution (b), and schematic model of the structural organization (c) for swine HDL$_c$ below the thermal transition (10° C). The dashed curves in (a) and (b) are the experimental scattering profile and radial electron density distribution. The solid curves are the calculated scattering profile (a) calculated for the step distribution of electron density (b) corresponding to the molecular organization in (c). The electron density profile for this model derived from the calculated scattering data at the same resolution as the experimental data is shown by the solid curve in (b). The experimental details are described in Reference 8.

an additional layer of cholesterol ester molecules producing three layered regions of in register steroid moieties in the core of the particle.

The observation that the distance between the electron density maxima due to the region of packed steroid groups juxtaposed to the surface of the lipoprotein is similar in HDL_c and LDL suggests a similar structural arrangement and interactions between the outer region of the cholesterol esters of the core and the layer of phospholipids and proteins at the surface. A similar organization may apply to the cholesterol esters of normal HDL. For normal HDL_2 and HDL_3 the particle size (80–100 Å) is insufficient for additional repeating layers of cholesterol esters necessary for an organized domain capable of undergoing thermal rearrangement. Differential scanning calorimetry shows no evidence for a thermal transition of the cholesterol esters in normal HDL.[18] For

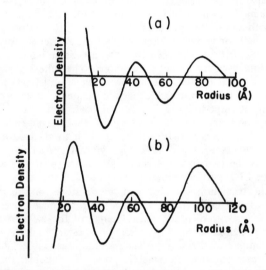

FIGURE 3. The radial electron density distributions for normal human LDL (a) and swine HDL_c (b), as illustrated in FIGURES 1 and 2, are shown with the outer electron density peaks, correspondent to the surface location of the protein and phospholipid polar head groups, superimposed.

example, x-ray scattering data for normal HDL are consistent with a spherical particle ~100 Å with a surface layer 10 Å thick containing protein and polar head groups with no indication of any structural organization of the core located cholesterol esters.[6, 9]

An orienting effect of the surface organization on the core-located cholesterol esters is likely to persist above the thermal transition. Thus, above the thermal transition these surface constraints may result in residual radial alignment of the cholesterol esters (at least of the molecules adjacent to the surface) resulting in structural arrangement resembling a nematic or cholesteric phase (i.e., alignment of molecular long axes but not layering of molecules) rather than an isotropic liquid. The transition temperature and enthalpy of the cholesterol ester transition in intact LDL and HDL_c have been shown to be similar to those observed for the smectic-cholesteric transition of the isolated cholesterol esters.[18] A structural rearrangement of this nature in which the overlapping region of the steroid moieties are removed primarily by introducing disorder parallel to the molecular long axis would average the electron density of the particle core and account for the observed changes in the x-ray scattering profiles above the thermal transition.

A recent detailed analysis of x-ray scattering data for LDL collected below and above the thermal transition together with model calculations has been reported by Luzzati and co-workers.[11] In this study an alternative arrangement has been proposed for the cholesterol ester organization in the core of LDL. The general features described above for the cholesterol ester organization at low temperature, involving separation of the steroid and hydrocarbon moieties of the cholesterol esters and the absence of this segregation at high temperatures, are also major features of this proposal. However, the regions of packed steroids are modeled as spherical elements with ~16 Å radius arranged in cubic packing within the lipoprotein core. These two alternative arrangements (spherical shells or cubic packing of spherical elements) for the packing of the cholesterol moieties in the core of LDL are each based on an individual set of assumptions used for model calculations. The spherical shell model discussed previously is based on the assumption of the quasispherical symmetry of the LDL particle, whereas the cubic packed elements described by Luzzati *et al.* represent an attempt to allow for deviations from perfect spherical symmetry. The cubic symmetry for the packing of the steroid-rich elements is made *a priori*. In fact, we note that packing of the high electron density, steroid-rich, spherical elements arranged in cubic symmetry described by Luzzati *et al.* approximates the two spherical shells located at ~30 Å and ~60 Å from the center of the LDL particle as described in the shell model.

Since the transition enthalpy and temperature for the structural transition of the cholesterol esters in LDL are similar to those observed for the liquid crystalline smectic-to-disorder phase change of the isolated esters, the assumption that the organization of the cholesterol esters in LDL at low temperature is at least similar to the smectic state seems reasonable. Although no precise molecular description of the smectic phase is available, this liquid crystalline phase is thought to be a layered structure approximately 35 Å thick. Liquid crystalline phases for cholesterol esters displaying cubic symmetry have not been observed in the bulk state.

This review has concentrated up to this point on the organization of the neutral lipid core regions of high- and low-density lipoproteins. Our current understanding of the organization of the phospholipids and specific apoproteins at the surface of these lipoproteins is less well developed.

For HDL, the major advances in describing the primary structure of the constituent apoproteins A-I, A-II, and C peptides [19-22] have led to a conceptual description of the secondary structure of the protein and its mode of interaction with the lipid components. This primary sequence information coupled with structure prediction methods [23, 24] has led to the attractive concept of amphipathic helices.[25-27] Apoprotein A-I (apoA-I), for example, is thought to have several sections of helical secondary structure 25–35 Å long, each section of helix having a polar and an apolar face ideally suited for an interfacial location at the surface of the HDL particle. The ~10–12 Å thickness of the surface region of HDL determined from x-ray scattering studies presumably reflects this localization of the electron-rich protein at the surface. However, so far there is no direct structural evidence for the existence of the amphipathic helix or its role in lipid–protein interactions.

For LDL there is even less information concerning the surface arrangement. The difficulty in isolating apoB in a soluble form has hindered its physico-characterization and even a conceptual description of the LDL surface is lacking. However, it is important to note that for both HDL and LDL the phospholipid and apoprotein constituents are *individually* insufficient to cover the available surface area of the particle. For example, the phospholipid content of HDL is sufficient to cover only approximately ⅓ of the particle surface assuming ~75 Å per molecule typical of the surface area per molecule in a phospholipid monolayer or bilayer.[28] Thus, for both HDL and LDL relatively large areas of the surface are covered by protein implying large amounts of protein–protein as well as lipid–protein contact and interaction. These details of the tertiary and quaternary protein organization are unknown. From a detailed analysis of the x-ray scattering data, Luzzati *et al.*[11] have indicated that the protein organization of the surface of LDL is noncentrosymmetric and have proposed a tetrahedral arrangement of globular protein subunits at the surface of the LDL particle. This suggestion is supported by freeze-etching electron microscopy observations.

RECOMBINANT SYSTEMS

Recombination of specific lipoprotein apoproteins with well characterized lipid systems provides a powerful methodology for investigating the interactions and structures formed by the surface constituents of plasma lipoproteins. For HDL the techniques of delipidation and recombination are well established.[5] The interaction of HDL apoproteins or the individual apoproteins with phospholipids provides a system which has been studied in detail. ApoHDL or the constituent peptides will solubilize multilamellar phospholipid dispersions. Using electron microscopy, it has been demonstrated that the resulting recombinant particle formed with dimyristoyl lecithin has a discoidal structure rather than the spherical morphology of native HDL.[27, 29] This discoidal morphology resembles that of "nascent" HDL secreted by the liver [30] and intestine.[31] Thus, these recombinant systems may also represent models for the organization of this "nascent" form of HDL.

Small-angle x-ray scattering measurements on complexes formed from porcine apoHDL and dimyristoyl lecithin demonstrated that the discoidal particle is a remnant of phospholipid bilayer solubilized and stabilized by the proposed amphipathic apolipoproteins.[32] Similar conclusions have been made by Laggner *et al.* for complexes formed from apoC-III and dimyristoyl lecithin.[33] Of interest is the fact that in the absence of the neutral lipid component the structural organization of the apoprotein/phospholipid complex is dominated by the fundamental bilayer organization of the phospholipid. The spherical morphology of native HDL is thus derived as a consequence of solubilizing the neutral lipid.[32]

Spectroscopic (NMR, ESR, fluorescence),[27, 34] electron microscopy,[29] and calorimetry [29] studies have been used extensively to investigate the molecular interactions in these recombinant particles. Two models for the molecular arrangement of the particles have been proposed from these studies, differing in the location of the apoprotein on the particle. The first model features the particle as an oblate micelle organization of phospholipid with the amphipathic helices of the apoprotein intercalated with the phospholipid head groups producing some curvature at the bilayer surface (FIGURE 4b).[27, 32] The second model suggests that the remnant phospholipid bilayer disc is solubilized by protein occupying a position at the edge of the disc, shielding the peripheral phospholipid hydrocarbon chains from the aqueous environment (FIGURE 4c).[29, 34]

We are currently using neutron small angle scattering to determine the location of the apoprotein on these discoidal recombinant particles. The com-

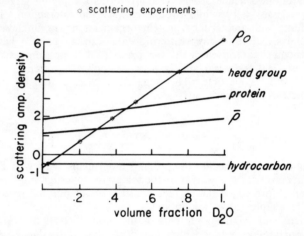

FIGURE 4. Neutron scattering length densities (units $\times 10^{-14}$ cm/Å^3) for the specifically deuterated [N-(CD$_3$)$_3$] phospholipid head groups, hydrocarbon chains, and protein in the recombinant particles formed from apoHDL and dimyristoyl lecithin, shown as a function of the D$_2$O volume fraction of the aqueous solvent (ρ_0). The small dependence of the scattering length density of the protein on solvent composition is due to hydrogen-deuterium exchange and was calculated assuming exchange of all non-carbon-bonded hydrogens in the protein. Phospholipid head groups and hydrocarbon chains have no exchangeable hydrogen atoms. $\bar{\rho}$ is the calculated mean scattering length density of the particle. The calculated value for contrast match ($\rho = 1.38 \times 10^{-14}$ cm/Å^3) corresponding to 0.3 volume fraction D$_2$O in the solvent is in agreement with the experimentally determined value. Neutron scattering measurements were made at the contrasts indicated.

plexes studied were formed from specifically deuterated N–(CD$_3$)$_3$ dimyristoyl lecithin and apo HDL at 2.5:1 weight ratio. A homogeneous population of the complexes was isolated by gel chromatography on Sepharose 4B (Pharmacia) and shown by negative staining electron microscopy to be discoidal particles ~95 Å diameter × ~50 Å. The use of the specific deuterium label in the lipid head group gives good separation of the neutron scattering length density of the head groups from that of the protein as illustrated in FIGURE 5. Neutron scattering measurements have been recorded at specific solvent H$_2$O/D$_2$O ratios that match the average scattering length density of each

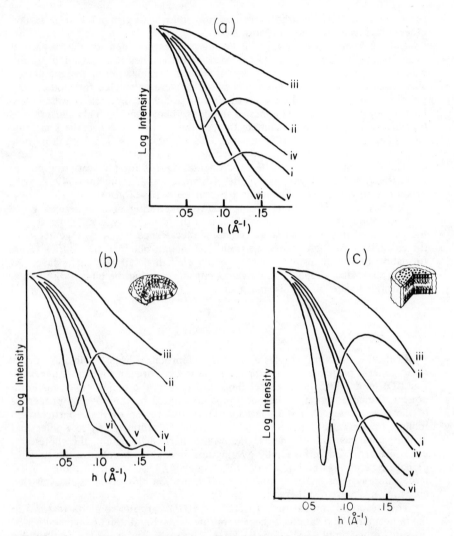

FIGURE 5. (a) Neutron scattering profiles obtained for the recombined particles formed from apoHDL and [N-(CD₃)₃] dimyristoyl lecithin as a function of solvent H₂O/D₂O composition (contrast). (b & c) Neutron scattering profiles calculated for models of the structural organization of the recombinant particle are shown schematically in the inserts. FIGURE 5b is the oblate micelle model with protein uniformly intercalated with the phospholipid head groups (dimensions ∼108 Å×∼50 Å outer shell containing head groups and protein ∼10 Å thick). FIGURE 5c is the discoidal bilayer model with protein exclusively at the periphery (dimensions 91 Å×49 Å annulus containing protein ∼10 Å thick). The experimental and calculated curves are for solvent D₂O volume fractions: i, 0.03 (−0.45×10⁻¹⁴ cm/Å³); ii, 0.20 (0.75× 10⁻¹⁴ cm/Å³); iii, 0.37 (1.90×10⁻¹⁴ cm/Å³); iv, 0.50 (2.85×10⁻¹⁴ cm/Å³); v, 0.75 (4.55×10⁻¹⁴ cm/Å³); vi, 1.00 (6.30×10⁻¹⁴ cm/Å³). The values in parentheses are the neutron scattering length densities corresponding to the H₂O/D₂O composition of the solvent.

component (i.e., hydrocarbon, protein, and lipid head groups) and at several other contrasts as indicated in FIGURE 5.

FIGURE 5 shows the neutron scattering profiles obtained for the complexes as a function of solvent H_2O/D_2O. Also shown are neutron scattering profiles calculated for the two models for the molecular organization of the complexes. The scattering profiles for the model particles were calculated for models with the dimensions given in the legend of FIGURE 5. These dimensions were calculated using the molecular volumes of the constituent phospholipids and proteins together with the chemical composition of the particle, the average scattering length density $\bar{\rho} = 1.38 \times 10^{-14}$ cm/Å^3, and radius of gyration for the particle shape $R_g = 34$ Å determined from the neutron scattering data.

The best agreement with the experimental data is for the scattering curves calculated for the bilayer disc model (diameter 91 Å, thickness 49 Å with protein occupying a surface annulus approximately 10 Å thick).

A more detailed analysis of the neutron scattering data in terms of the decomposition of the scattering profiles into the characteristic functions due to the particle shape, internal structure, and interference function, together with the calculation of the distance distribution function obtained by Fourier transformation of the intensity data will be reported in detail at a later stage. At present, these data support the above conclusion favoring the bilayer disc model with protein located at the disc periphery.

CONCLUSIONS

From the structural studies of plasma lipoproteins discussed in this review some general principles governing their molecular organization are suggested. For LDL and HDL$_c$ that have cholesterol esters as the major molecular component, the core region of the particle is dominated by the physical properties of the core-located cholesterol esters. Thus, this region of these particles exhibits a temperature dependent molecular reorganization which resembles that of the isolated core components. Below the thermal transition, the cholesterol esters are arranged with radially overlapping steroid ring moieties in a manner perhaps resembling the liquid crystalline smectic phase found for bulk cholesterol ester systems. Above the thermal transition the cholesterol ester-rich core region is more disordered.

The structural comparison of LDL and HDL$_c$ suggests common features in the molecular organization of these lipoproteins having different surface-located protein components (LDL, apoB, HDL$_c$, apoA–I, and apoE). The similar location of the first region of closely packed steroid moieties with respect to the surface-located components suggests a similar interaction of the outer layer of cholesterol esters with the protein and phospholipid at the surface. An extrapolation of the arrangement to normal HDL shows that the core of HDL is too small to accommodate an organized cholesterol ester domain capable of undergoing cooperative thermal rearrangement.

In general, information concerning the surface organization of HDL is more developed than for LDL. The concept of the amphipathic helix suggests some modes of interaction between the proteins and lipid at the surface of HDL. However, the detailed topography of the phospholipid, free cholesterol and protein, together with details of the tertiary and quaternary organization of the apoproteins at the surface of HDL and LDL remains undefined.

Current studies using neutron small angle scattering have been designed to probe the location of the apoprotein of HDL on recombinant particles formed with phospholipids. The use of isotopic substitution with deuterium in the head group of the phospholipid allows the positions of the molecular components to be probed in more detail.

These initial experiments point to the direction future structural studies must take. Recombination techniques together with compositional modification of native lipoproteins must be coupled with a combination of high accuracy x-ray and neutron scattering studies, the latter employing isotopic substitution with deuterium to highlight specific areas of the structure. This approach will undoubtedly provide a higher resolution picture of the molecular organization of plasma lipoproteins.

ACKNOWLEDGMENTS

Neutron scattering measurements were carried out at the High Flux Beam Reactor, Brookhaven National Laboratory. We gratefully acknowledge the interest and collaboration of Dr. B. P. Schoenborn. We thank Ms. Irene Miller for preparation of the manuscript.

REFERENCES

1. BRADLEY, W. A. & A. M. GOTTO. 1978. Disturbances in lipid and lipoprotein metabolism. American Physiological Soc. 111–37.
2. SMITH, L. C., H. J. POWNALL & A. M. GOTTO. 1978. Ann. Rev. Biochem. **47:** 751–77.
3. SCANU, A. M. & C. EDELSTEIN. 1971. Anal. Biochem. **44:**576.
4. SCANU, A. M., E. CUMH, T. TOGH, S. KOGA, E. STILLER & L. ALBERS. 1970. Biochemistry **9:**1327.
5. KRUSKI, A. W. & A. M. SCANU. 1974. Chem. Phys. Lipids **13:**27–48.
6. ATKINSON, D. 1975. Ph.D. Dissertation, Council for National Academic Awards, England.
7. ATKINSON, D., R. J. DECKELBAUM, D. M. SMALL & G. G. SHIPLEY. 1977. Proc. Natl. Acad. Sci. USA **74:**1042.
8. ATKINSON, D., A. R. TALL, D. M. SMALL & R. W. MAHLEY. 1978. Biochemistry **78:**3930–3933.
9. LAGGNER, P. & K. W. MULLER. 1978. Quart. Rev. Biophys. **11:**371–425.
10. STUHRMAN, H. B., A. TARDIEU, L. MATEU, C. SARDEL, V. LUZZATI, L. AGGERBECK & A. M. SCANU. 1975. Proc. Natl. Acad. Sci. USA **72:**2270.
11. LUZZATI, V., A. TARDIEU & L. AGGERBECK. 1979. J. Mol. Biol. **131:**435–473.
12. DECKELBAUM, R. J., G. G. SHIPLEY, D. M. SMALL, R. S. LEES & P. K. GEORGE. 1975. Science **190:**392.
13. DECKELBAUM, R. J., G. G. SHIPLEY & D. M. SMALL. 1976. J. Biol. Chem. **252:** 744.
14. CRAVEN, B. M. & G. T. DE TITTA. 1976. J. Chem. Soc. Perkin Trans. **2:**814.
15. MAHLEY, R. W., K. H. WEISGRABER, T. INNERARITY, H. B. BREWER & G. ASSMAN. 1975. Biochemistry **14:**2817–2823.
16. TALL, A. R., D. ATKINSON, D. M. SMALL & R. W. MAHLEY. 1978. J. Biol. Chem. **251:**7288–7293.
17. TALL, A. R., D. M. SMALL, D. ATKINSON & L. RUDEL. 1978. J. Clin. Invest. **62:** 1354–1363.
18. TALL, A. R., R. J. DECKELBAUM, D. M. SMALL & G. G. SHIPLEY. 1977. Biochim. Biophys. Acta **487:**145–153.

19. MORRISETT, J. D., R. L. JACKSON & A. M. GOTTO. 1975. Ann. Rev. Biochem. **44:**183.
20. JACKSON, R. L., J. D. MORISETT & A. M. GOTTO. 1976. Physiol. Rev. **56:**259.
21. BREWER, H. B., S. E. LUX, R. RONAN & U. M. JOHN. 1978. Proc. Natl. Acad. Sci. USA **69:**1304.
22. JACKSON, R. L., A. N. BAKER, E. B. GILLMAN & A. M. GOTTO. 1977. Proc. Natl. Acad. Sci. USA **74:**1942.
23. CHOU, P. Y. & G. D. FASMAN. 1974. Biochemistry **13:**211–222.
24. CHOU, P. Y. & G. D. FASMAN. 1974. Biochemistry **13:**222–245.
25. SEGREST, J. P., R. L. JACKSON, J. D. MORRISETT & A. M. GOTTO. 1974. FEBS Lett. **38:**247–253.
26. JACKSON, R. L., J. D. MORRISETT, A. M. GOTTO & J. P. SEGREST. 1975. Mol. Cell Biochem. **6:**43–50.
27. ANDREWS, A. L., D. ATKINSON, M. D. BARRATT, E. G. FINER, H. HAUSER, R. HENRY, R. B. LESLIE, N. L. OWENS, M. C. PHILLIPS & R. N. ROBERTSON. 1976. Eur. J. Biochem. **54:**549–563.
28. LUZZATI, V. 1968. *In* Biological Membranes, D. Chapman, Ed., pp. 71–123. Academic Press, New York, N.Y.
29. TALL, A. R., D. M. SMALL, R. J. DECKELBAUM & G. G. SHIPLEY. 1977. J. Biol. Chem. **252:**4701–4717.
30. HAMILTON, R. L., M. C. WILLIAMS & C. J. FIELDING. 1976. J. Clin. Invest. **58:**667–680.
31. GREEN, P. H. R., A. R. TALL & R. M. GLICKMAN. 1978. J. Clin. Invest. **61:**528–534.
32. ATKINSON, D., H. M. SMITH, J. DICKSON & J. P. AUSTIN. 1976. Eur. J. Biochem. **64:**541–547.
33. LAGGNER, P., A. M. GOTTO & J. D. MORRISETT. 1979. Biochemistry **18:**164–171.
34. JONAS, A., D. S. KRAJNOVICH & B. W. PATTERSON. 1977. J. Biol. Chem. **252:**2200–2205.

DISCUSSION OF THE PAPER

DR. M. C. PHILLIPS: You made a point with your model that the phospholipids were determining the structure. Do you think that the protein actually determines the size?

DR. D. ATKINSON: The protein determines the size, but the phospholipid bilayer structure determines the overall organization.

DR. PHILLIPS: Would you like to say something on how the protein determines the size and on how the size of a disc varies upon changing the hydrocarbon chains in the phospholipid?

DR. ATKINSON: Well, the popular view would be that the amphipathic helices of apoA-I are located around the disc periphery such that the apolar face of the helix is just opposed to the hydrocarbon region of the phospholipid bilayer. Then, if one has a discrete number of protein molecules adopting their conformations around the edge of the disc, one would have a palisade where the amphipathic helices wind up and down around the edge of the disc. Then, the number of protein molecules, whether two or three, will define the size of the perimeter of the disc and thus the overall size of that disc.

DR. P. LAGGNER: We have investigated together with the group in Houston similar complexes formed by apoC-III with dimyristoyl lecithin. From what we saw, there is a strong indication for a protein rim. We have done calculations on the basis of our results and came out with an ellipsoidal model. More-over, the recombinant particles seem to differ strongly. Yours is, as I under-stand, only about 90 Å in diameter and we, if I can remember correctly, had something like 170 Å. Could you comment on that?

DR. ATKINSON: I would like to say that the dimensions of 95 × 50 Å that I obtained by neutron scattering agree with those which I measured by electron microscopy on these very complexes and also agree with the dimensions which I determined by small-angle x-ray scattering within two or three Å.

One can only conclude that the difference in size between the discoidal structures formed with apoC-III and apoA-I are due to the protein. I have no concrete ideas as to what the organizational features of those two proteins are.

DR. LAGGNER: May I add a short question on apoA-I? You showed the transition going from cholesteric to nematic. Now, is there any evidence from x-rays that the nematic type is really there?

DR. ATKINSON: There is no evidence from x-ray scattering that the high temperature form resembles either a nematic or a cholesteric phase. That evidence is derived from calorimetric data.

DR. J. T. SPARROW: In comparing your model curve to the experimental curve, I presume that you tried various combinations on the assumption that there was a mixture of discoidal and oblate ellipsoid to see if such a mixture would fit your experimental curve better.

DR. ATKINSON: In an x-ray or neutron scattering study one is always measuring what one must admit is a heterogeneous population of particles of average properties. Thus the structures which one describes are equivalent in terms of their scattering to the average scattering and of the particle population examined. In answer to your question, I have not mixed those two types of particles.

DR. P. C. JOST: I am reminded of the correspondence of this model with that proposed by Dr. Small on the cholate micelles with lecithin. Do you find that the size of your disc varies upon protein ratio?

DR. ATKINSON: Dr. Tall has, in fact, done that work by electron microscopy when he was in the Boston group. He found a correlation between the size, the diameter specifically, of the discoidal particle and the protein ratio.

DR. A. M. SCANU: If I understand correctly, you have used the whole of HDL. I would be curious to know whether the apoprotein ratios in your disc were similar to those before interaction with lipids. Next question is, what would happen if you now use individual polypeptides?

DR. ATKINSON: This kind of study would be much better done with the individual polypeptides. I actually have these studies on the list of experiments to be done. So, I have no information yet.

QUESTION: What I am going to say is relevant to the last question. Dr. Stoffel has described about the same structure as yours just with apoA-I. Could you comment on that?

DR. ATKINSON: The dimensions which he derived for the apoA-I structure are somewhat different from the dimensions that I have derived, but he started off with a rather different lipid-to-protein initial ratio. I do not remember the exact ratio, a 1:1 ratio rather than a 2.5:1 ratio; and the structure that he derived, I think, is 33 Å thick, which I must admit surprises me.

I would make a comment that the model was derived from just two pieces of information, that is, the radius of gyration of the particle with 100% deuteration of the fatty acid chains and the radius of gyration with 100% hydrogen-containing fatty acid chains. I am fairly confident that one could probably derive a lot of different size models from those sets of data. You really would need much more data to be able to make a good selection of a model.

DYNAMICS OF LIPID MOTIONS IN HIGH-DENSITY LIPOPROTEIN SUBFRACTIONS HDL$_2$ AND HDL$_3$: MAGNETIC RESONANCE STUDIES

James R. Brainard, Roger D. Knapp, Josef R. Patsch,
Antonio M. Gotto, Jr., and Joel D. Morrisett *

*Departments of Medicine and Biochemistry
Baylor College of Medicine and The Methodist Hospital
Houston, Texas 77030*

*Department of Chemistry
Indiana University
Bloomington, Indiana 47401*

INTRODUCTION

Although plasma lipoproteins are often isolated as distinct particle populations, it is now clear that these different populations form a dynamic system, within which exchange, net transfer, and metabolism of lipid and protein components occur. Consequently, there is considerable interest in the possible metabolic relationships among the various lipoprotein classes and subclasses. Differences in structural features may play an important role in determining the suitability of various lipoproteins as enzyme substrates or as acceptors or donors of lipids and/or proteins for exchange to other systems within the plasma compartment. Consequently, the elucidation of the structural features of the native lipoprotein classes and subclasses is an important first step in understanding the possible role of these features in metabolic interrelationships.

One of the most intensely studied metabolic pathways is the catabolism of very-low-density lipoproteins (VLDL) and chylomicrons by the lipolytic enzyme, lipoprotein lipase. Recently, several groups have reported data that suggest a role for the high-density lipoprotein (HDL) subfractions in this pathway.[1, 2] Patsch *et al.*[3] have described the conversion of HDL$_3$ (an HDL subfraction isolated between 1.125 and 1.210 g/ml) to a particle closely resembling native HDL$_2$ (an HDL subfraction isolated between 1.063 and 1.125 g/ml) during the *in vitro* lipolysis of VLDL. During the *in vitro* lipolysis of triglyceride-rich lipoproteins, pnospholipid, cholesterol, and apoprotein constituents of the surface monolayer are transferred to HDL$_3$ resulting in a larger HDL particle. This conversion suggests a number of interesting questions about the role of HDL$_2$ and HDL$_3$ in VLDL and chylomicron metabolism, and about the relationship of the structural differences between HDL$_2$ and HDL$_3$ to their respective metabolic roles. For example, does the transfer of phospholipid, cholesterol, and apoprotein affect the lipid organization and dynamics within these particles? Do HDL$_2$ and HDL$_3$ exhibit different abilities to serve as acceptors for the surface components released by the triglyceride-rich lipo-

---

* Address correspondence to: Dr. Joel D. Morrisett, The Methodist Hospital, Mail Station A601, 6516 Bertner Blvd., Houston, TX 77030.

proteins during lipolysis? What determines the amount of surface components that may be taken up by the acceptor HDL?

There are a number of structural differences between HDL_2 and HDL_3 already established; among the most notable are density, Stokes radius and composition (TABLE 1).

Physical studies on a variety of phospholipid model and naturally occurring membranes have shown that the mobility of membrane lipid molecules is closely associated with several physical and biological properties.[4, 5] The relationship between lipid fluidity and biological functions that has been observed in membranes suggests that the dynamics of lipids within lipoproteins might also be related to their functional roles. Accordingly, we have undertaken a study of the lipid dynamics of HDL_2 and HDL_3, using two physical techniques that have found wide application in the study of membrane dynamics, spin label electron paramagnetic resonance and ^{13}C nuclear magnetic resonance.

TABLE 1

PHYSICAL PROPERTIES AND COMPOSITION OF HDL₂ AND HDL₃

	HDL_2	HDL_3
Density, g/dl *	1.063–1.125	1.125–1.21
Diameter (Å) *	70–100	40–70
Composition (% by weight) †		
Protein	41.1	54.9
Free cholesterol	3.5	0.8
Cholesteryl esters	17.1	17.4
Phospholipids	33.8	22.4
Triglycerides	4.0	4.5

* From Scanu A. M. & M. C. Ritter. 1973. Adv. Clin. Chem. **16**:111.
† Composition for pool of lipoproteins used in this study.

MATERIALS AND METHODS

Total high density lipoproteins were isolated from pooled freshly collected plasma, obtained from eight normal male donors, by ultracentrifugal flotation in KBr. The purified HDL_2 and HDL_3 subfractions were isolated by zonal ultracentrifugation using a three-step nonlinear density gradient of NaBr.[6] To further increase the homogeneity of these two populations, the center two thirds of each zonal peak was respun. HDL subfractions were dialyzed for 24 hr against 100 mM NaCl, 10 mM Na phosphate (Tris-HCl for EPR measurements), 1 mM EDTA, 1 mM NaN₃, pH 7.4, prior to use.

The doxyl † fatty acid spin probes, 5-doxylstearic acid and 12-doxylstearic

† Spin-labeled molecule containing the 4′,4′-dimethyloxazolidinyl-N-oxyl heterocyclic group.

acid (Syva, Palo Alto, Calif.), were incorporated into the lipoproteins by adding known amounts of the fatty acids in a 2% ethanol solution to a 100 × 13 mm Pyrex tube and evaporating the solvent under nitrogen. Sufficient buffered lipoprotein solution (~30 mg/ml) was then added to the test tube containing the thin film of spin label to bring the spin label concentration to ~1.5 mM. The mixture was incubated, with stirring, for 1 hr at room temperature. To incorporate cholesteryl esters of the doxyl fatty acid probes, lipoproteins were incubated at 45° C for one half hour with an aqueous dispersion of the ester. This microdispersion of the ester (0.67 mg/ml) was prepared by injection of an isopropanol solution into aqueous buffer at 60° C. Concentrations of lipoproteins and spin-labeled esters are given in the FIGURES.

EPR spectra were recorded on a Varian E-12 spectrometer operated at a microwave frequency of 9.15 GHz. The temperature of the EPR cavity was controlled by a Varian variable temperature controller and measured by a Thinc TM-401 digital thermometer.

High resolution ^{13}C-NMR spectra at 63.4 kG were obtained on a spectrometer system consisting of a Bruker superconducting solenoid, a Bruker 15 mm probe, quadrature detection, laboratory-built radio-frequency electronics and a Nicolet 1080 computer. The spectrometer was not equipped with a field-frequency lock. To insure that resonances of interest lay within the envelope of decoupling frequencies, separate spectra of the unsaturated choline-glycerol backbone, and saturated carbon regions were obtained with the ^{1}H irradiation centered respectively at 5.2, 3.7, and 1.5 ppm downfield from the proton resonance of tetramethylsilane (TMS) using coherent broad band decoupling with a clock frequency of 100 Hz. These decoupler frequencies were selected based on the proton chemical shifts reported for phospholipids and model compounds. Additionally, the selections were experimentally verified to give the minimum linewidth for the resonances studied. For ^{13}C excitation, 90° pulse widths of 13–17 μsec duration were used. Time domain spectra were accumulated in 2 × 8,192 addresses using a spectral width of 13,888 Hz. Further accumulation and data processing conditions are given in the FIGURES. The magnetic field stability was checked after data acquisition by remeasuring the ^{13}C resonance frequency of ethylene glycol. For all 63.4 kG spectra reported herein, the ^{13}C resonance frequency of ethylene glycol did not change by more than 1.1 Hz. Sample temperature was controlled by the flow rate of cooling air over the sample. The sample temperature was measured by removing the sample from the probe and quickly inserting a small thermocouple. The estimated accuracy is ±1° C.

^{13}C-NMR spectra at 23.2 kG were recorded on a Varian Associates XL–100–15 spectrometer system equipped with a Nicolet TT–100 data system, quadrature detection, and a Varian variable temperature controller. H_0 stability was maintained by an internal frequency lock on approximately 10% D$_2$O in the sample buffer. For ^{13}C excitation, 90° pulse widths of 25 μsec duration were used. Time domain spectra were accumulated in 2 × 4,096 or 2 × 8,192 addresses using a spectral width of 6,024 Hz. Additional accumulation and data processing conditions are given in the FIGURES.

EPR STUDIES OF HDL SUBFRACTIONS USING SPIN-LABELED FATTY ACIDS

Doxyl-labeled fatty acids have found wide application in the study of model and natural membranes, as well as liquid crystalline systems. Under favorable conditions, an order parameter, which is a quantitative measure of doxyl ring motion, may be calculated directly from the EPR spectrum. Although spin-labeled lipids are subject to many of the disadvantages of extrinsic probes, the sensitivity of their EPR spectra to the physical state of the environment has been well established.[8-17] Limitations of these probes have also been described.[14-17]

The 9.16 GHz EPR spectra of 5-doxylstearate (5-DS) incorporated into purified HDL_2 and HDL_3 at 37° C are shown in FIGURE 1. While both spectra are characteristic of rapid anisotropic motion of the doxyl fatty acid, comparison of the hyperfine splitting between the outer extrema indicate that the motion of 5-DS is slightly more restricted in HDL_3 populations. The estimated order parameters for 5-DS in HDL_2 and HDL_3 over the temperature range 15–65° C are compared in FIGURE 2. These order parameters were calculated from the expression [7]:

$$S_{NO} = \frac{T_{\parallel} - T_{\perp}}{T_{zz} - \frac{1}{2}(T_{xx} + T_{yy})} \cdot \frac{a'}{a} \tag{1}$$

where $T_{\parallel}$ and $T_{\perp}$ were estimated directly from the inner and outer spectral extrema; values for the hyperfine tensors and the polarity correction to the isotropic hyperfine splitting constant, a'/a, were taken from Hubbell and McConnell.[7] Errors in these order parameters originating from the uncertainty in determining the positions of the spectral extrema were estimated to be ~0.001 over most of the temperature range. Order parameters calculated from

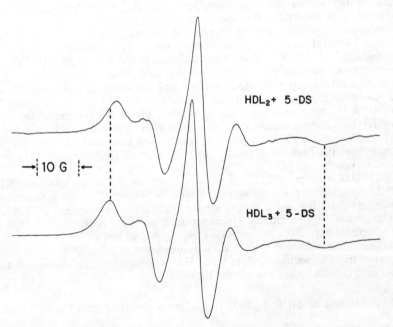

FIGURE 1. 9.1 GHz EPR spectra (39°) of 5-doxylstearate incorporated into HDL_2 and HDL_3 at ~23° C.

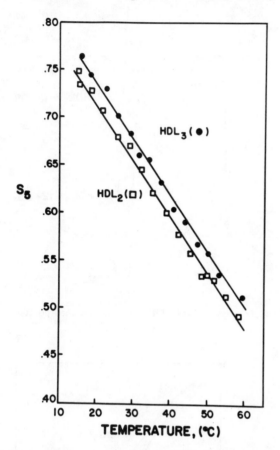

FIGURE 2. Estimated order parameters for 5-doxylstearate in HDL$_2$ and HDL$_3$ over the temperature range 15°–65° C.

EPR spectra of 5-DS incorporated into HDL$_2$ are slightly less than those for HDL$_3$ over the temperature range 15°–65° C.

In order to probe acyl chain motion further from the lipoprotein surface, another doxyl-labeled fatty acid probe, 12-doxylstearic acid (12-DS), was incorporated into HDL$_2$ and HDL$_3$. A comparison of the spectra of 12-DS in HDL$_2$ and HDL$_3$ is presented in FIGURE 3. The EPR spectra of this probe also indicate that the motion of the probe is slightly, but significantly, different in the two HDL subfractions.

The temperature dependence of the estimated order parameters calculated from the EPR spectra for the 12-DS probe in HDL$_2$ and HDL$_3$ is shown in FIGURE 4. These data indicate that the order parameter calculated for this probe in HDL$_3$ is slightly higher than in HDL$_2$.

It should be noted that the values for $T_{\parallel}$ and $T_{\perp}$ estimated directly from the EPR spectra are only approximations for the true values.[14] For systems where the degree or order is small (<0.3) or where the doxyl ring undergoes

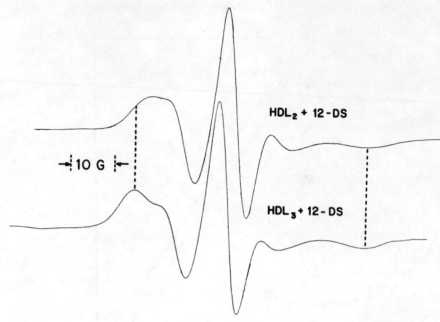

FIGURE 3. 9.1 GHz spectra (24°) of 12-doxylstearate incorporated into HDL₂ and HDL₃ at 23° C.

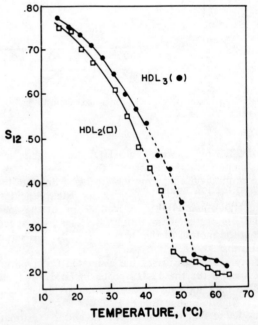

FIGURE 4. Estimated order parameters for 12-doxylstearate in HDL₂ and HDL₃ over the temperature range 15°–65° C.

motions that are intermediate on the ESR time scale (10^{-7}–10^{-9} sec) order parameters estimated directly from spectra may be greater than those determined with better estimates of $T_\perp$[18] or by rigorous treatment using computer simulated spectra.[14] However, the conclusions drawn from the calculated order parameters in the following discussion are based primarily upon comparisons of the same probe in very similar systems. Consequently, nonrigorous calculation of the order parameters is not expected to affect the inferences based on these comparisons. Moreover, the criteria [10, 11, 14] for rigorous application of the simple order parameter formalism are met over a substantial portion of the temperature range ($\sim$29–60° C for 5-DS and 30–40° C for 12-DS) and the order parameters estimated directly from the EPR spectra are expected to deviate very little from those determined by computer simulation.

The order parameters for nitroxides are related both to the orientation of the nitroxide ring system with respect to the major axis of probe reorientation and to the fluctuations in that orientation. For the doxyl-labeled fatty acids, the $2p\pi$ orbital containing the unpaired electron lies almost parallel to the long axis of the probe when the fatty acyl chain is in the all *trans* conformation. Consequently the order parameter is primarily related to the average amplitude of the rapid fluctuations in the doxyl ring orientation due to segmental motion of the fatty acyl chain.[13, 16] The data on 12-DS and 5-DS probes incorporated into lipoproteins indicate that both probes are slightly more ordered in HDL_3 than in HDL_2.

The best structural model for the plasma lipoproteins assumes that these particles consist of an inner core of neutral lipid surrounded by a monolayer of phospholipid, protein, and perhaps cholesterol.[19, 20] The amphipathic nature of the doxyl fatty acids makes it likely that when incorporated into lipoproteins, they are located primarily within the surface monolayer where their motions are affected by the motions of the surrounding intrinsic lipid constituents.‡ The results described above suggest that the surface monolayer of HDL_3 is slightly more ordered than in HDL_2.

In terms of a physical description of the motion of the doxyl ring within the surface monolayer, one may adopt two crude models.[13] In the first, the movement of the doxyl ring is characterized by rapid (on the ESR time scale, $\tau_c < 10^{-9}$ sec) motion about the monolayer normal with the π orbital (containing the unpaired electron) included at an angle θ to the monolayer normal. For this type of motion, the order parameter is given by

$$S_{NO} = \tfrac{1}{2}[3(\cos^2\theta) - 1]. \tag{2}$$

Another crude but more realistic model is one in which the doxyl ring undergoes rapid random motion within a cone of angle 2γ. In this case, the order parameter is given by [23]

$$S_{NO} = \tfrac{1}{2}(\cos\gamma + \cos^2\gamma). \tag{3}$$

The angles γ and θ calculated for some representative order parameters estimated for the doxyl-labeled fatty acid probes in HDL_2 and HDL_3 are shown in TABLE 2. Significantly, the small differences in order parameter are reflected

---

‡ A surface location for fatty acid analog probes in lipoproteins has been suggested by energy transfer experiments with fluorescent fatty acids [21] and by reduction of doxyl fatty acids with ascorbate.[22]

TABLE 2

ESTIMATED PARAMETERS FOR PHYSICAL MODELS OF DOXYL RING
MOTION IN HDL₂ AND HDL₃

Probe	Tempera-ture, °C	HDL$_2$			HDL$_3$		
		S_{NO}	θ *	γ †	S_{NO}	θ *	γ †
5-DS	20	0.710 ‡	26.1	37.6	0.734 ‡	24.9	35.8
	37	0.611	30.6	44.5	0.634	29.6	42.9
	60	0.476	36.2	53.4	0.500	35.3	57.8
12-DS	20	0.712 ‡	25.5	36.8	0.742 ‡	24.5	35.2
	37	0.520	34.5	50.5	0.568	32.5	47.4

* θ, estimated angle for static orientation of T_{zz} tensor with respect to long axis of fatty acid $\theta = \cos^{-1}[(2S_{NO}+1)/3]^{1/2}$ (see text).

† γ, estimated angle for limits of cone within which the T_{zz} tensor may undergo random motion $\gamma = \cos^{-1}\{[1 + (1 + 8S_{NO})^{1/2}]/2\}$ (see text).

‡ Parameters over-estimated due to presence of slow motions.

in rather small changes in the physical parameters characterizing these motional models. The estimated order parameters for the doxyl acid probes incorporated into HDL₂ and HDL₃ are considerably higher than for the same probes incorporated into phospholipid bilayer model systems (TABLE 3). However, they appear to be about the same magnitude as for doxyl fatty acids incorporated into biological membranes.

Several investigators have suggested that protein restricts the motions of lipids in mixed lipid–protein systems.[10, 11] It is likely that the presence of protein in the surface monolayer of HDL₂ and HDL₃ restricts the motion of fatty acyl chains in the surface region. This restriction in turn may be reflected in the increased order parameters for the probes in lipoproteins relative to the pure phospholipid bilayer model systems. The difference between the order parameters for the doxyl-labeled fatty acids in HDL and phospholipid bilayers could also be related to polarity differences between the interior of a phospholipid bilayer and the surface monolayer of a lipoprotein. These polarity differences may be associated with water penetration into the highly curved monolayer or to the presence of protein. However, it seems unlikely that polarity differences could make such a large difference in the derived order parameters since the difference in the isotropic hyperfine interaction for 8-DS in water and n-decane is only 12%.[8]

The differences in the order of acyl chains within the surface monolayer of HDL₂ and HDL₃ suggest that there might be similar differences within the hydrophobic core of these particles. This possibility has been investigated using the cholesteryl ester of 12-DS incorporated into HDL₂ and HDL₃.

While the motional characteristics of this probe are not as well established as those of the doxyl fatty acids, experiments in our laboratory have indicated that this probe faithfully reports the dynamics of a variety of neutral lipid systems such as triglycerides, cholesteryl esters and mixtures of these lipids. In addition, energy transfer experiments with fluorophore-labeled cholesteryl esters [21] and chemical reduction of spin-labeled cholesteryl esters [22] incorporated

TABLE 3

COMPARISON OF ORDER PARAMETERS FOR 5-DS AND 12-DS IN HDL₂ AND HDL₃ WITH ORDER PARAMETERS FROM PHOSPHOLIPID BILAYERS AND MEMBRANES

System	Temperature, °C	S_{NO} (5-DS)	S_{NO} (12-DS)
HDL₂	21–22	0.707	0.702
HDL₃	22–24	0.725	0.735
EYPC * multilayers [23]	23	0.47	0.20
EYPC multilayers [25]	20–23	0.35	0.15
EYPC-CH ‡ multilayers [13]	20–23	0.52	0.46
EYPC-CH multilayers (PL § probe) [7]		0.695	0.46
DPPC † multilayers (gel) (PL probe) [7]	35	0.6	0.4
DPPC multilayers (liquid crystal) (PL probe) [7]	40	0.5	0.2
EYPC liposomes [9]		0.56	
EYPC-CH liposomes [9]		0.59	
EYPC vesicles [9]		0.53	
EYPC-CH vesicles [9]		0.54	
Acholeplasma laidlawii membranes (oleic acid enriched) [10]	25	0.78	
Dispersed lipids		0.71	
Acholeplasma laidlawii membranes (palmitate and CH enriched) [10]	25		0.95
Dispersed lipids			0.61
Hamster adipose tissue mitochondria membranes [11]		0.86	
Dispersed lipids		0.78	

* EYPC, egg yolk phosphatidylcholine.
† DPPC, dipalmitoyl phosphatidylcholine.
‡ CH, cholesterol.
§ PL, phospholipid.

into lipoproteins have suggested that these probes are localized within the hydrophobic core of these particles. Furthermore, the presence of any cholesteryl doxylstearate in the form of microdispersions remaining in the aqueous phase, or in the HDL particles such that the spin-labeled esters are in close proximity (less than ~9Å separating the doxyl groups) is easily detectable by the observation of spin exchange between these moieties. The EPR spectrum of a mixture of HDL₃ and 12-doxylstearyl cholesteryl ester (12-DS-CE) containing an excess of probe is shown in FIGURE 5. The spin exchange phenomenon is characterized by the presence of a single broad line which may be eliminated by sufficiently increasing the center-to-center distance between the doxyl groups. In a homogeneous solution, this is easily achieved simply

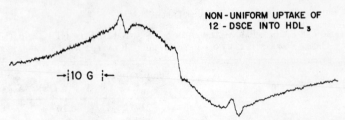

FIGURE 5. 9.1 GHz EPR spectrum (24° C) of 12-doxylstearate cholesteryl ester in HDL₃. The aqueous dispersion of spin-labeled lipid was added rapidly at 25° C, and the mixture stirred 10 min before recording the spectrum. Final concentrations: 86 mg HDL₃/ml, 0.3 mM spin label.

by dilution. In nonhomogeneous solutions which contain local concentrations of organized lipid arrays, it is important not only that a critical concentration of spin label not be exceeded, but also that the lipid probe be introduced in a manner which minimizes its clustering and maximizes its dispersal in the lipid domain. In FIGURE 5, the presence of a second population of 12-DS-CE not undergoing spin exchange is indicated by the three rather weak, narrow lines superimposed on the broader spin exchanged lines. At present, we have not determined whether the cholesteryl ester undergoing spin exchange is present within the lipoprotein or still within the bulk aqueous phase. FIGURE 6 com-

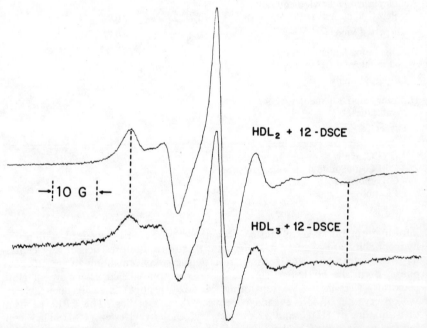

FIGURE 6. 9.1 GHz EPR spectra (37°) of 12-doxylstearate cholesteryl ester incorporated into HDL₂ and HDL₃. The aqueous dispersion of lipid was added slowly to a stirred solution of HDL at 45°–50° C. Final concentrations: 86 mg HDL₃/ml, 89 mg HDL₂/ml, 0.3 mM spin label.

pares the EPR spectra of 12-DS-CE (not exchange-broadened) incorporated into HDL_2 and HDL_3. The order parameters for these systems are compared over the temperature range 20°–60° C in FIGURE 7. In contrast to the behavior observed for the doxyl-labeled fatty acids, 12-doxylstearoyl cholesteryl ester exhibited order parameters in HDL_2 and HDL_3 which were indistinguishable within experimental error. This observation suggests that the motion of the fatty acyl chains of cholesteryl esters is quite similar in HDL_2 and HDL_3.

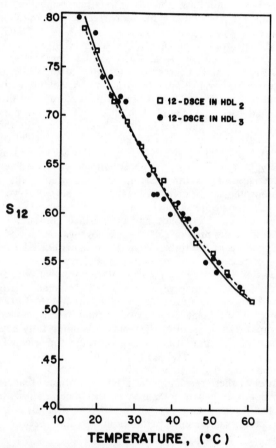

FIGURE 7. Estimated order parameters for 12-doxylstearate cholesteryl ester in HDL_2 and HDL_3 over the temperature range 15°–65° C.

^{13}C-NMR STUDIES OF HDL SUBFRACTIONS

Although spin-labeled lipids afford the advantages of high sensitivity and selectivity, the interpretation of results obtained with them necessarily involves the assumption that they faithfully reflect the properties of endogenous constituents, a situation that does not always prevail. ^{13}C-NMR, on the other hand, has relatively low sensitivity and in some cases poor selectivity, but it has the distinct advantage that it monitors the properties of molecules native to the system studied. While the formalism for the quantitative treatment of anisotropic motion, in terms of the measured NMR relaxation parameters, is not as well established as the formalism for the EPR measurements, several investigations have demonstrated the sensitivity of ^{13}C spin-lattice relaxation times and the observed linewidths of ^{13}C resonances to the dynamics within lipid systems.[24-26] Although a number of factors can affect the observed relaxation times, under certain conditions, shorter spin-lattice relaxation times and increased linewidths are associated with more restricted modes and/or slower rates of motion.

The ^{13}C-NMR spectra at 63.4 kG and 37° C for HDL_2 and HDL_3 are shown in FIGURE 8. Although the spectra are very similar, the greater proportion of protein in HDL_3 is reflected in the greater intensity of the broad protein amide resonance at approximately 178 ppm, the arginine ζ-guanidino carbon resonance at 157 ppm, and the resonance at 116 ppm which is presently unassigned to a specific amino acid carbon nucleus. Although both of these particles contain about 50% protein by weight, the narrow resonances within the spectra are those from lipid carbon nuclei. At 63.4 kG, the carbon nuclei of phosphorylcholine moiety (CH_2N, CH_2O, and $N(CH_3)_3$ in FIGURE 8) and of the glyceryl backbone moiety ($C\alpha$, $C\beta$, $C\gamma$) § of phospholipids yield resolved resonances, providing a selective probe of the dynamics of this region of the phospholipids within these lipoproteins. Resolved resonances are also observed for the C5, C6, C3, and C9 (among others) nuclei of the cholesteryl ring system. In addition, the C6 resonances of esterified and unesterified cholesterol are resolved. These resolved resonances provide selective probes for the motions and organization of at least portions of the three classes of lipids within HDL. On the other hand, a number of resonances have contributions from carbon nuclei in several different lipid classes, consequently their usefulness as selective probes is limited. Into this category fall the envelopes containing the resonances from the methylene and unsaturated carbons of the fatty acyl chains and the fatty acyl terminal methyl resonance. The relaxation behavior of these resonances may reflect the dynamics and organization of all of the lipids containing fatty acyl chains.

A comparison of the spin-lattice relaxation times for selected carbon resonances of HDL_2 and HDL_3 at 63.4 kG are shown in TABLE 4. Relaxation times for selected resonances at 23.2 kG are given in TABLE 5. Although the mean T_1 values for most of these resonances in HDL_2 are greater than for HDL_3, the differences are not large when compared to the uncertainties associated with the measurements. Consequently, within the uncertainties of our measurements, there appear to be no significant differences in T_1 values between the two particle populations.

Linewidths at 63.4 kG for selected single carbon resonances for HDL_2 and HDL_3 are compared in TABLE 6. The uncertainties associated with these values are the estimated upper limits on variations due to low signal/noise ratios, spectrometer H_0 drift, and variations in H_0 homogeneities derived from multiple measurements. Although for most resonances of HDL_2 and HDL_3 the differences in linewidths are small, for some resonances the differences are greater than can be accounted for by variations in instrumental contributions. In

---

§ Carbon nuclei of the glycerol backbone are identified by $C\alpha$, CH_2OP; $C\beta$, CHO; and $C\gamma$, CH_2O.

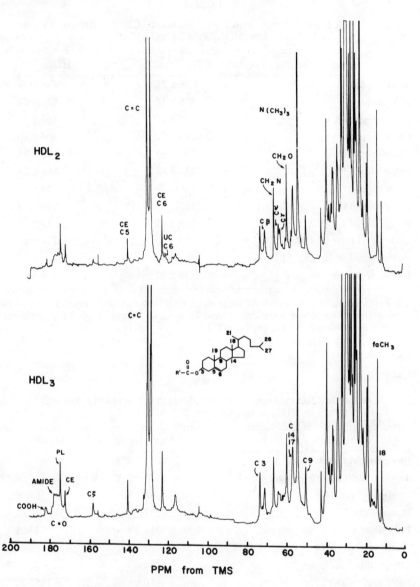

FIGURE 8. Proton decoupled natural abundance ^{13}C NMR spectra at 63.4 kG and 37° C of HDL$_2$ and HDL$_3$. HDL$_2$: 143 mg/ml, 16384 accumulations. HDL$_3$: 139 mg/ml, 32768 accumulations. Both spectra were recorded with a 0.714-sec pulse interval and were processed with 2.0 Hz exponential filtering.

TABLE 4

SPIN-LATTICE RELAXATION TIMES FOR SELECTED CARBON RESONANCES OF
HDL$_2$ AND HDL$_3$ AT 63.4 KG, 37° C *

Resonance	HDL$_2$ (msec)	HDL$_3$ (msec)
Mono olefin	526±21	433±29
Poly olefin	598±55	533±22
Cholesteryl ester C6	133±12	165±7
Cholesteryl ester C3	210±8	204±20
Phospholipid Cβ	195±15	192±23
Phospholipid POCH$_2$	381±18	361±21
Phospholipid Cα	128±13	123±11
Phospholipid Cγ	128±9	146±16
Phospholipid CH$_2$N	349±22	335±17
Cholesteryl ester C14,17	228±10	228±8
Phospholipid (CH$_3$)$_3$N	522±54	501±35
Cholesteryl ester C9	230±22	198±15

* Reported values are weighted means and weighted standard deviations from two experiments. The values were determined by a least squares fit of the experimental data to the equation $I = A + B \exp(-\tau/T_1)$.

TABLE 5

SPIN-LATTICE RELAXATION TIMES FOR SELECTED CARBON RESONANCES OF
HDL$_2$ AND HDL$_3$ AT 23.2 KG, 37° C *

Resonance	HDL$_2$ (msec)	HDL$_3$ (msec)
Phospholipid C=O	1830±278	1870±169
Triglyceride/Cholesteryl ester C=O	1150±238	1370±282
Cholesteryl ester C5	896±100	896±110
Mono olefin	277±4	287±6
Poly olefin	318±4	330±5
Cholesteryl ester C6	51±13	50±13
Phospholipid (CH$_3$)$_3$N	438±9	416±7
Fatty acyl t-CH$_3$	1860±167	1550±84
Cholesteryl ester C18	328±24	269±55

* Reported values are weighted means and weighted standard deviations from four (HDL$_2$) and five (HDL$_3$) measurements. Values were determined by a least squares fit of the experimental data to the equation $I = A + B \exp(-\tau/T_1)$.

particular, resonances from the cholesteryl ester C6 and the phospholipid $C\alpha$ are broader in HDL_3 than in HDL_2. Linewidths for selected carbon resonances at 23.2 kG are shown in TABLE 7. Spectra at lower field show significantly broader resonances for cholesteryl ester C6 and the fatty acyl terminal methyl resonances of HDL_3. While almost all of the other resonances at 63.4 and 23.2 kG show slightly greater linewidths in HDL_3 than in HDL_2, these differences may not be outside the possible instrumental contributions and hence are presently regarded as more suggestive than definitive.

TABLE 6

LINEWIDTHS FOR SELECTED CARBON RESONANCES OF HDL_2 AND HDL_3 AT 63.4 KG, 37° C *

Resonance	HDL_2 (Hz)	HDL_3 (Hz)
Triglyceride, Cholesteryl ester C=O	9.2 ± 2	12.8 ± 3
Cholesteryl ester C5	8.7 ± 2	12.1 ± 2
Cholesteryl ester C6	12.6 ± 2	18.2 ± 2
Cholesteryl ester C3	20.1 ± 4	23.7 ± 4
Phospholipid $C\beta$	36.8 ± 5	37.4 ± 6
Phospholipid CH_2N	17.2 ± 2	18.6 ± 2
Phospholipid $C\alpha$	18.0 ± 3	32.5 ± 4
Phospholipid $C\gamma$	34.0 ± 5	45.0 ± 7
Phospholipid $POCH_2$	11.4 ± 2	12.0 ± 2
Phospholipid $(CH_3)_3N$	9.4 ± 2	13.3 ± 2
Cholesteryl ester C9	20.6 ± 4	23.5 ± 4
Fatty acyl t-CH_3	7.6 ± 2	10.4 ± 2
Cholesteryl ester C18	8.9 ± 2	10.3 ± 2

* The reported values were determined by least squares fit of well-resolved resonances to a Lorenzian line shape using the Nicolet NTCFT software. For partially resolved resonances, the data were plotted out on an expanded scale and the overlapping portions of the resonances reconstructed assuming symmetrical peak shapes. The errors were estimated from the standard deviations from the NTCFT program plus an estimate of the instrumental contribution. Reported values include 2.0 Hz exponential line broadening applied during processing.

The ^{13}C-NMR relaxation data suggest that there are subtle differences in the dynamics of the lipids within HDL_2 and HDL_3. Increased linewidths for selected single carbon resonances suggest that the motions contributing to spin-spin relaxation for the cholesteryl ester C6, phospholipid $C\alpha$ and $C\gamma$, and the fatty acyl methyl carbon are more restricted and/or slower in HDL_3 than in HDL_2. In contrast, the motions contributing to spin-lattice relaxation for these carbons, as well as several other carbons with resolved resonances, are very similar for the two particle populations.

In systems where the motion may be characterized as anisotropic, spin-spin and spin-lattice relaxation are sensitive to different types of motion. Spin-spin relaxation and the related natural linewidth are more sensitive to motions with frequencies below the Larmor frequency, whereas spin-lattice relaxation is more sensitive to motions at or above this frequency.[24, 27, 28] Consequently, the ^{13}C-NMR data suggest that the largest dynamic differences between HDL_2 and HDL_3 reside primarily in those motions with correlation times longer than 10^{-6} sec. For fatty acyl chains in liquid crystalline phases, it has been suggested that motions in this time frame are mostly uncoupled *trans-gauche* rotations,[24] or rigid body reorientations of the fatty acyl chains.[28] These types of motions in doxyl fatty acid probes would result in changes in the average orientation of the doxyl ring with respect to its major axis of rapid rotation. Consequently,

TABLE 7

LINEWIDTHS OF SELECTED RESONANCES OF HUMAN HDL_2 AND HDL_3 AT 23.2 KG, 37° C *

Resonance	HDL_2 (Hz) †	HDL_3 (Hz) ‡
Phospholipid C=O	4.29±0.54	5.04±0.91
Triglyceride C=O	3.3 ±0.89	5.32±0.88
Cholesteryl ester C5	4.19±0.80	5.65±0.81
Fatty acyl C=C (down field)	6.86±0.60	7.84±0.78
Fatty acyl C=C (up field)	6.80±0.54	8.82±0.87
Cholesteryl ester C6	9.85±0.66	17.1 ±1.70
Phospholipid $(CH_3)_3N$	5.65±0.61	6.71±0.74
Fatty acyl CH_3	2.80±0.70	5.68±0.74
C18	6.01±1.00	—

* Reported values were determined by a least squares fit of resolved resonances to a Lorenzian line shape using the Nicolet NTCFT software. Fits were performed on spectra processed *without exponential line broadening*. Reported errors were estimated from the standard deviations given by the NTCFT program plus an estimate of the instrumental contribution.

† Weighted means±weighted uncertainties for two separate measurements on each of two different preparations.

‡ Weighted means±weighted uncertainties from two separate measurements on a single preparation.

the trends in linewidths of the phospholipid Cα and fatty acyl methyl carbon resonances, and in the order parameters for the 5-DS and 12-DS probes both suggest that motion of the phospholipids with correlation times greater than 10^{-6} sec are more restricted within HDL_3 than within HDL_2.

ACKNOWLEDGMENTS

The authors are indebted to Ms. Debbie Mason and Ms. Kaye Shewmaker for their assistance in preparation of the manuscript, and to A. O. Clouse, R. Addleman, D. Wenkert, and R. K. Stockton for technical support. TTGA.

REFERENCES

1. EISENBERG, S. & D. RACHMILEWITZ. 1975. J. Lipid Res. **16**:341–351.
2. REDGRAVE, T. G. & D. M. SMALL. 1979. J. Clin. Invest. **64**:162–171.
3. PATSCH, J. R., A. M. GOTTO, JR., T. OLIVECRONA & S. EISENBERG. 1978. Proc. Natl. Acad. Sci. USA **75**:4519–4523.
4. FOURCANS, B. & M. K. JAIN. 1974. Adv. Lipid Res. **12**:147–226.
5. PAPAHADJOPOULOS, D., K. JACOBSEN, S. NIR & T. ISAC. 1973. Biochim. Biophys. Acta **311**:330–348.
6. PATSCH, J. R., S. SAILER, G. KOSTNER, F. SANDHOFER, A. HOLASEK & H. BRAUN-STEINER. 1974. J. Lipid Res. **15**:356–366.
7. HUBBELL, W. F. & H. M. MCCONNELL. 1971. J. Amer. Chem. Soc. **93**:314–326.
8. SEELIG, J. 1970. J. Am. Chem. Soc. **92**:3881–3887.
9. MARSH, D., A. D. PHILLIPS, A. WATTS & D. F. KNOWLES. 1972. Biochim. Biophys. Acta **49**:641–648.
10. BUTLER, K. W., K. G. JOHNSON & I. C. P. SMITH. 1978. Arch. Biochem. Biophys. **191**:289–297.
11. CANNON, B., C. F. POLNASEK, K. W. BUTLER, L. E. GÖRAN ERIKSSON & I. C. P. SMITH. 1975. Arch. Biochem. Biophys. **167**:505–581.
12. JOST, P., O. H. GRIFFITH, R. A. CAPALDI & G. VANDERKOOI. 1973. Proc. Natl. Acad. Sci. USA **70**:480–484.
13. SCHREIER-MUCCILLO, S., D. MARSH, H. DUGAS, H. SCHNEIDER & I. C. P. SMITH. 1973. Chem. Phys. Lipids **10**:11–27.
14. SCHREIER, S., C. F. POLNASZEK & I. C. P. SMITH. 1978. Biochim. Biophys. Acta **515**:375–436.
15. SEELIG, J. 1976. *In* Spin Labeling Theory and Applications. L. J. Berliner, Ed., Chap. 10: 373–410. Academic Press, New York, N.Y.
16. SMITH, I. C. P. & K. W. BUTLER. 1976. *Ibid.* Chap. 11: 411–453.
17. GRIFFITH, O. H. & P. C. JOST. 1976. *Ibid.* Chap. 12: 454–524.
18. GAFFNEY, B. J. 1976. *Ibid.* Appendix 4: 567–571. Academic Press, New York, N.Y.
19. CHEN, B., A. M. SCANU & F. D. KÉZDY. 1977. Proc. Natl. Acad. Sci. USA **74**: 837–841.
20. JACKSON, R. L., J. D. MORRISETT & A. M. GOTTO, JR. 1976. Physiol. Rev. **56**: 259–316.
21. SKLAR, L., M. DOODY, A. M. GOTTO & H. J. POWNALL. Biochemistry. In press.
22. KEITH, A. D., R. J. MEHLHORN, N. K. FREEMAN & A. V. NICHOLS. 1973. Chem. Phys. Lipids **10**:223–236.
23. JOST, P., L. J. LIBERTINI, V. C. HERBERT & O. H. GRIFFITH. 1971. J. Mol. Biol. **59**:77–98.
24. GENT, M. P. N. & J. H. PRESTEGARD. 1977. J. Magn. Reson. **25**:243–262.
25. GODICI, P. E. & F. R. LANDSBERGER. 1975. Biochemistry **14**:3927–3933.
26. HAMILTON, J. A., C. TALKOWSKI, R. F. CHILDERS, E. WILLIAMS, A. ALLERHAND & E. H. CORDES. 1974. J. Biol. Chem. **249**:4872–4878.
27. SEITER, C. H. A. & S. I. CHAN. 1973. J. Am. Chem. Soc. **95**:7541–7553.
28. PETERSON, N. O. & S. I. CHAN. 1977. Biochemistry **16**:2657–2667.

DISCUSSION OF THE PAPER

DR. P. C. JOST: I am a little bit concerned about the use by several speakers today of the outside splitting (2 $T_\parallel$) in a heterogeneous system as being indicative of fluidity. The reason I say this is because when we have looked at acyl chain motion between carbons 5 and 12, we can demonstrate the same effect that I spoke of earlier at carbon 16. One can take two different systems, for instance, even HDL_2 and HDL_3, put them in separate capillaries in the same cavity at different proportions or take albumin plus phospholipid bilayer and vary their proportions and you will discover that as the protein associates with the lipids, the net effect is the alteration of the outside lines without apparent changes in line shape. Before one could evaluate from the ESR data that there was more or less fluidity in the presence of proteins, I think model experiments must be carried out because the splitting may in fact reflect hydrophobic protein in contact with the phospholipid bilayer.

DR. J. D. MORRISETT: Several years ago we did a set of experiments with dimyristoylphosphatidylcholine to which increasing amounts of apoC-III were added. In this system, the physical form of the lipid actually changed, i.e., from a single bilayer vesicle to a micellar structure. It seems to me that to do correctly the experiment which you just described you need to insure that the physical form of the lipid structure is *not* changing.

DR. JOST: That is the reason that I was suggesting that two separate capillaries be used in the cavity at the same time over a range of lipid–protein ratios to see how the outside splittings differ as you change the ratios in the two separate capillaries.

DR. MORRISETT: We have not done the experiment you describe. If I correctly perceive the point of your comment, it is that we cannot simply say the bulk surface phospholipids of HDL_3 are less fluid than those of HDL_2; the spectral results we obtain may also be attributable to greater motional restriction in the phospholipids of HDL_3 due to their greater interaction with the larger proportion of apoprotein present; i.e., the data may be a combination of bulk and boundary lipid motion. If this is your point, I totally agree.

DR. JOST: Do you see differences between HDL_2 and HDL_3 in the motion of the phospholipid hydrocarbon chains? If I remember correctly, you see little difference in the motion of the cholesterol part of cholesteryl esters in HDL_2 and HDL_3, but you see significant difference in the cholesteryl ester fatty acyl chain motions. Would that not indicate something?

DR. MORRISETT: It is just the reverse. There are no observable differences in the motions of the fatty acyl chains in the cholesterol esters of HDL_2 and HDL_3, but the steroid ring motion does seem to be slower in HDL_3 as judged by ^{13}C-NMR linewidths.

COMMENT: Then, one would think that these differences arise from the fact that the cholesterol moiety of the cholesteryl esters would be closer to the surface monolayer.

DR. MORRISETT: Well, that is one possibility. There is another one too. Recall a paper by Verdery and Nichols several years ago on HDL models. Their model proposed different conformations for the cholesteryl esters in HDL_2 and HDL_3. The HDL_3 with its smaller radius would require that a large portion of the cholesteryl esters be folded with the acyl chain bent back over the steroid nucleus. This would not be obligatory in HDL_2.

Along the same line, we have other data that are interesting in this context. If you look at the motion of cholesteryl esters in a larger particle which by other criteria is shown to have higher microscopic viscosity (for example, the cholesteryl ester in the VLDL of cholesterol-fed rabbits) the rate and/or amplitude of acyl chain motion is large as reflected in the ESR spectra; but the steroid motion is restricted in the very broad ^{13}C C5 and C6 linewidths as you lower the temperature. At 37°, the cholesterol carbons are so broad that you can hardly see them. So, here are two contrasting situations which may be partly explainable in terms of the particle size.

DR. P. LAGGNER: I just want to add that the necessity of the acyl chain folding back in Nichols' model arose from the very small diameters that he obtained from negative stain electron microscopy; I think the x-ray studies would indicate the acyl chain fold-back is not necessary.

DR. MORRISETT: In HDL_3?

DR. LAGGNER: In HDL_3 and HDL_2.

DR. D. M. SMALL: I have three questions. First, the spin-labeled cholesteryl esters that you used—what transition temperature did they have?

DR. MORRISETT: The DSC thermogram of 12-doxylstearate cholesteryl ester shows an endotherm at 26.2° and an exotherm at 20.8°.

DR. SMALL: Have you put this spin label into LDL and been able to see a transition?

DR. MORRISETT: Not LDL, but we have examined rabbit VLDL enriched with cholesteryl oleate and found a transition temperature higher than 48°, which surprised us.

DR. SMALL: You mean it is higher than it would be by differential scanning calorimetry?

DR. MORRISETT: Yes.

DR. SMALL: Finally, another question on methodology. When you look at the fatty acyl chains and calculate the T_1 of carbons near double bonds, these T_1 values arise from acyl chains in both cholesteryl esters and phospholipids in the particle. Then the T_1 is really a combination of the two?

DR. MORRISETT: Yes. About 60% of the fatty acyl chains in HDL belong to the surface monolayer phospholipids and about one-third belong to acyl chains of the cholesteryl esters and triglycerides. This is an unfortunate limitation of natural abundance ^{13}C-NMR.

DR. SMALL: The question is, can you see the difference in the chemical shift between them?

DR. MORRISETT: No, they are not resolvable. The most direct way of distinguishing between fatty acyl carbons of triglycerides, cholesteryl esters, and phospholipids is to dope the system with a single lipid type containing fatty acyl chains enriched at one or more specific carbons with ^{13}C.

VIEW FROM FLUORESCENCE ANALYSES: INTERACTION OF APOLIPOPROTEIN A-I WITH L-α-DIMYRISTOYLPHOSPHATIDYLCHOLINE VESICLES *

Ana Jonas,† Susan M. Drengler, and Bruce W. Patterson

Department of Biochemistry
School of Basic Medical Sciences
University of Illinois
Urbana, Illinois 61801

INTRODUCTION

Apolipoprotein A-I (apoA-I) interactions with phospholipids are intimately involved in the biogenesis of high-density serum lipoproteins (HDL) and in their transformations while in circulation. We investigated some aspects of these problems by studying the binding of apoA-I with phospholipid bilayer surfaces, the stoichiometric conditions required for the breakdown of the bilayers into small complexes of the general size of HDL, and the kinetics of both of these processes. In this work, we used the model system of human apoA-I with sonicated dimyristoylphosphatidylcholine (DMPC) vesicles. Fluorescent labeled apoA-I (dansyl apoA-I) was added to DMPC preparations covering DMPC:apoA-I molar ratios from 4000:1 to 50:1, and the reactions were followed by means of fluorescence polarization. At equilibrium, rotational relaxation times were determined, and the mixtures were fractionated by gel filtration on a Sepharose CL-4B column.

The equilibrium results indicate the existence of only two types of complexes: vesicles with 3–4 or less apoA-I molecules bound to them and micellar complexes with a DMPC to apoA-I molar ratio of 95:1 and 3 protein monomers per particle. Kinetic data were obtained from fluorescence measurements on 4000:1 and 100:1 DMPC:apoA-I (mol/mol) reaction mixtures, representing apoA-I binding to vesicles and interactions leading to the formation of micellar complexes, respectively. The binding of apoA-I to vesicles occurs rapidly (within minutes) and is accompanied by major changes in protein structure, without significant effects on the lipid phase. The breakdown of vesicles into micellar complexes is a much slower, first-order process with a $t_{1/2} = 3$ hr 9 min, which causes major changes in the lipid phase but does not affect noticeably the spectral properties of the apoA-I already bound to lipid.

Apolipoprotein A-I (apoA-I) is the major protein component of all high-density serum lipoproteins (HDL) investigated so far.[1, 2] As the major informational molecule of HDL, it probably plays a fundamental role in defining the structure and function of this lipoprotein class. Studies of apoA-I inter-

* This work was carried out under the support of grants: HL-16059 from the National Institutes of Health, C-5-1979 from the Illinois Heart Association, and the Eagles Max Baer Heart Research Award to A. Jonas.
† Established Investigator of the American Heart Association.

actions with synthetic lecithins, in particular dimyristoylphosphatidylcholine (DMPC), have shown that apoA-I can form well-defined micellar complexes, of the general size of HDL, starting from particulate DMPC dispersions.[3-7] The interaction of apoA-I with phospholipid bilayer membranes and its surfactant-like action on them are probably important processes in the biogenesis of HDL precursor particles in intestinal and liver cells or from excess surface components of triglyceride-rich lipoproteins undergoing lipolysis.[8-10] As in the model systems, the type and extent of interaction between apoA-I and naturally occurring phospholipid bilayers may depend on the local proportions of lipid to apoA-I, on the chemical composition of the bilayer (in particular its cholesterol content),[11-13] on the physical state of the bilayer,[4, 12] and on the kinetics of the interaction.[7] Pownall *et al.*[7, 12] have shown that the interaction of apoA-I with DMPC liposomes, with or without cholesterol, is kinetically determined; the maximum rate of micellar complex formation occurs at the transition temperature of the lipid, and decreases markedly as the temperature is lowered or increased.

In this paper, we examine in some detail the interaction of human apoA-I with excess DMPC vesicles in attempts to elucidate the mode of interaction of apoA-I with phospholipid bilayer structures, the stoichiometric conditions required for the formation of the micellar complexes, and the kinetics of these processes.

MATERIALS AND METHODS

Preparation of apoA-I. The procedures used in the isolation and purification of human apoA-I have been described previously [14, 15] except that 3 M guanidine hydrochloride and two (2.0 × 90 cm) Sephacryl-200 columns in series (Pharmacia Fine Chemicals) were employed in the apolipoprotein fractionations. After desalting, lyophilization, and solution in 3 M guanidine hydrochloride, the apolipoprotein was rechromatographed on the Sephacryl-200 columns in order to remove any traces of apoA-II. By polyacrylamide gel electrophoresis in 0.01% sodium dodecyl sulfate, 7.5% acrylamide, apoA-I showed a single band up to 100 μg protein loading on the gels. ApoA-I preparations were stored at $-20°$ C in lyophilized form. Before use, the solid protein was dissolved in 3 M guanidine hydrochloride and was dialyzed extensively against buffer. All the experiments described in this work were performed in 0.1 M Tris-HCl, pH 8.0, 0.001% EDTA, and 10^{-3} M NaN$_3$ buffer. Covalent labeling of the apolipoprotein with dansyl chloride (Dns-Cl) (Eastman Kodak Co.) to an extent of 1.5–3 Dns groups per apoA-I monomer, was performed as described previously.[16, 17] Extensive dialysis against buffer and against two changes of Dowex-2X resin in hydroxyl form ensured the complete removal of free Dns label from the covalent conjugates with the apolipoprotein. Absence of free Dns was confirmed by chromatography on TLC silica gel plates (Eastman Kodak Co.), with a solvent system of (60:40, vol/vol) 0.2 M sodium acetate:ethanol, and by observation of fluorescence under a UV lamp. In previous work, we showed that Dns labeling of apoA-I proteins does not affect their secondary structure, nor the shape of the monomers in solution, even though it weakens the self-association of the human apoA-I.[18] In terms of the complexes formed with DMPC, we demonstrated that labeled and unlabeled apoA-I proteins form identical structures at equilibrium.[4] Therefore, we feel confident that the results obtained in this work with Dns-labeled apoA-I also apply to the unlabeled protein. Dimyristoylphosphatidylcholine (DMPC) was purchased from Sigma Chemical Co., St. Louis. The purity of this commercial preparation was checked by TLC chromatography on silica gel plates developed in a chloroform:methanol:H_2O (65:25:5, vol/vol) solvent and detected by acid spray and charring. ^{14}C-labeled DMPC was obtained from P. J. Cobert Associates, St. Louis, and was found to be >97% pure in the TLC system described above. The spots were detected by autoradiography. At the end of several experiments, DMPC was extracted from complexes using a chloroform: methanol (2:1, vol/vol) solvent and was chromatographed again. In all cases, there was no major degradation of the phospholipid during the sonication, incubation, and analytical steps that were carried out at 25° C for a maximum period of 3 days.

Vesicles of DMPC were prepared by mixing DMPC and [^{14}C]DMPC (about 1.5×10^6 cpm) in redistilled chloroform and evaporating the solvent under N_2. Dispersions of DMPC in buffer (10 mg DMPC/ml) were then sonicated with a Heat Systems–Ultrasonics, Inc. sonifier, Model W185, using a power setting of 4–5. Temperature was controlled between 25° and 40° C with a water bath during the 30 min sonication in 3–4 min bursts. Sonication was followed by centrifugation at 30° C, 16,000 rpm for 40 min. The specific activity of the vesicle preparations was determined from the weight of DMPC and the [^{14}C] cpm measured in a Beckman LS-100 scintillation counter on known volumes of the unsonicated dispersion. Quenching by different amounts of buffer was taken into account. This specific activity, in the range of 20,000 cpm/mg DMPC, was employed in the quantitation of DMPC in all other experiments. In a few cases, we confirmed the accuracy of this determination by using the method of Chen et al.[19] for the analysis of organic phosphorus. Both methods agreed within ±5%.

The DMPC vesicles prepared in this manner gave only one peak upon chromatography on a Sepharose CL-4B (Pharmacia Fine Chemicals) column (2.3 × 40 cm) and were shown to contain fairly uniform single-bilayer Huang-type vesicles[20] by electron microscopy using negative staining with phospho-tungstic acid.[21] Unfractionated, centrifuged DMPC vesicle preparations were used immediately for all experiments, but storage for 2 days at 25° C resulted only in a 10%–20% conversion into multilamellar liposomes as judged by gel filtration on the Sepharose CL-4B column.

Mixtures of DMPC vesicles with apoA-I were prepared at 25° C by adding a concentrated stock protein solution (1.25×10^{-4} M), gradually (over 10 min) with intermittent vortexing, to a DMPC vesicle dilution to give a final 2.0 ml sample of 1.5×10^{-6} M protein with a 4000- to 50-fold molar excess of DMPC monomers. The reaction mixtures were incubated in a shaking water bath for 5–20 hr at 25° C for the equilibrium experiments. In the kinetic experiments, apoA-I was added to a fluorescence cuvette containing the appropriate DMPC preparation in order to start the reaction.

Gel Filtration. Reaction mixtures containing DMPC to apoA-I molar ratios from 4000:1 down to 50:1 in 2.0 ml of solution were applied to a Sepharose CL-4B column (1.8 × 35 cm) pre-equilibrated with the equivalent of the 4000:1 preparation of vesicles alone. The elution time was approximately 3 hr at 25° C for 50–60 fractions, each containing 1.7 ml. The column fractions were assayed by obtaining ^{14}C cpm on 0.5 ml or 1.0 ml aliquots (Beckman LS-100 scintillation counter) and by measuring the fluorescence intensity of the Dns-labeled proteins in a Perkin Elmer MPF-3 spectrofluorometer. Exciting light was 340 nm and fluorescence was observed at 500 nm. Under the conditions of our experiments, the light-scattering contributions from the most concentrated DMPC samples did not amount to more than 10% of the maximum fluorescence signal. Protein elution was quantitated by measuring the fluorescence of the fractions against a standard of human apoA-I-Dns solution of known concentration. Corrections were applied for a 25% or 15% increase in the Dns fluorescence in micellar or vesicular complexes of apoA-I-Dns, respectively. Stock protein concentrations were determined from known extinction coefficients [22] or from the Lowry *et al.* assay.[23] The protein and DMPC yields from this column were >85% and the reproducibility of results for a series of 10 column runs was ±10% for both components.

Fluorescence Methods. Fluorescence intensities and uncorrected intrinsic protein fluorescence spectra were recorded on a Perkin Elmer MPF-3 spectrofluorometer at 25° C. At high molar ratios of DMPC:apoA-I, the appropriate DMPC controls were used in order to subtract the contribution of vesicle light scattering to the fluorescence signal.

Fluorescence polarization of apoA-I-Dns, free in solution or in complexes with DMPC, was measured at 25° C in the SLM Series 400 polarization spectrofluorometer. Exciting light of 340 nm, Corning glass 3–72 filters, and 8 nm slits were used for these measurements. Corrections for vesicle light scattering were not necessary in most cases. Fluorescence polarization of 1,6-diphenyl-1,3,5-hexatriene (DPH) (Aldrich Chemical Co.) dissolved in DMPC vesicles and in unlabeled apoA-I complexes with DMPC was measured using 366 nm exciting light, Corning glass 3–74 filters, and 4 nm slits. Temperature was regulated to ±0.1° C with a Forma Scientific circulating water bath. Fluorescence lifetimes were measured in Professor G. Weber's laboratory using his cross-correlation phase fluorometer.[24]

Rotational relaxation times of apoA-I-Dns and of DMPC:apoA-I-Dns complexes were calculated from Perrin's equation,[25] as adapted by Weber [26] to macromolecules approaching the shape of simple ellipsoids of revolution:

$$(1/p - 1/3) = (1/p_0 - 1/3) (1 + 3 \ \tau/\rho_h)$$

ρ_h, the harmonic mean of the rotational relaxation times about the major axes, can be approximated by the expression: $\rho_h = 3 \ V\eta/RT$, for a sphere.

In the above equations, p, fluorescence polarization equals: $(I_\| - I_\perp)/ (I_\| + I_\perp)$, where $I_\|$ and $I_\perp$ are the fluorescence intensities parallel and perpendicular to the plane of polarization of the exciting light; p_0 is the intrinsic polarization in the absence of Brownian rotations: τ is the fluorescent lifetime of the probe; V is the molar volume of the fluorescent particles; η is the viscosity of the medium; R is the gas constant; and T is absolute temperature. In practice, ρ_h values are calculated from fluorescence lifetime data and from $1/p$ versus T/η plots (Perrin plots); the latter can be obtained by varying temperature or by changing viscosity isothermally. Viscosity is changed by adding appropriate amounts of sucrose to the sample. For relatively small particles where the labels are tightly bound, the isothermal data and the results obtained by varying temperature are identical. However, for some large proteins [27, 28] and for lipoproteins,[22] this is not the case. Whereas isothermal experiments yield ρ_h values that correspond to the rotational motion of the whole particle, temperature variation data give considerably lower ρ_h values that can be attributed to temperature-induced rotations of flexible segments of the macromolecule, adjacent to the probe.[27] In short, in this work we use

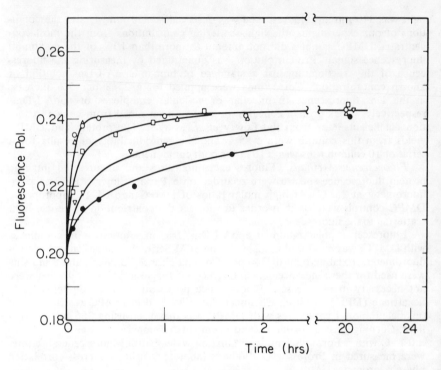

FIGURE 1. Changes in dansyl-labeled apolipoprotein A-I (apoA-I-Dns) fluorescence polarization, at 25° C, with time for various molar ratios of DMPC:apo A-I-Dns: 4000:1 (◯), 1000:1 (△), 500:1 (□), 200:1 (▽), 100:1 (●). The protein concentration was held constant at 4×10^{-6} M for all the samples. The initial polarization was obtained on an equivalent apoA-I-Dns solution.

isothermal ρ_h values to report on overall volume and shape changes of apoA-I and their complexes, and temperature variation ρ_h data to provide information on flexibility and local motions within the particles.

The phase transitions of DMPC vesicles, liposomes, and DMPC:apoA-I mixtures were observed by measuring fluorescence polarization changes of the lipophilic probe DPH dissolved in the samples, as a function of temperature.[29] DPH was prepared as a 10^{-3} M solution in tetrahydrofuran; 5 μl of this solution were added with stirring to 2 ml of the samples containing from 5×10^{-5} to 8×10^{-3} M DMPC. After a ½ hr incubation at 25° C, tetrahydrofuran was removed by blowing N_2 through the samples. For the equilibrium experiments, the samples were incubated at 25° C for 6 hr, prior to fluorescence polarization measurements between 45° and 5° C. In the kinetic experiments, the reactions were initiated by adding apoA-I to DMPC samples, and were observed by means of fluorescence polarization at 25° C for 20 hr.

RESULTS

FIGURE 1 demonstrates the interaction of apoA-I-Dns at constant concentration (4×10^{-6} M), with increasing amounts of DMPC vesicles: from

100:1 to 4000:1, DMPC:apoA-I-Dns molar ratios. For each sample, the reaction was initiated by adding concentrated apoA-I-Dns to the appropriate DMPC preparation in a fluorescence cuvette equilibrated to 25° C in the fluorescence polarization instrument. Changes in fluorescence polarization of the Dns probe were then followed at timed intervals for 20 hr. Clearly at lower DMPC:apoA-I ratios the interaction is slower, but all the complexes at equilibrium have very similar polarization values (0.243).

In order to characterize the equilibrium complexes, we proceeded to determine their rotational relaxation times from 1/fluorescence polarization versus T/η plots (i.e., Perrin plots) (FIGURE 2). In these experiments, we varied T/η

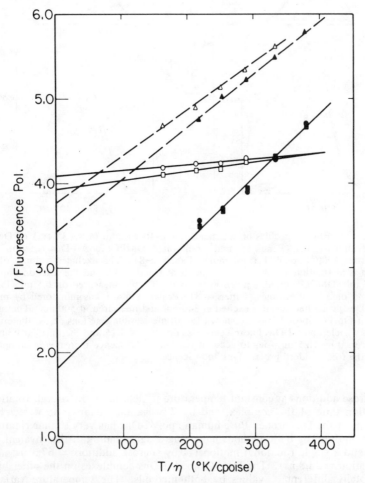

FIGURE 2. Perrin plots 1/(fluorescence polarization) versus T/η for human apoA-I-Dns ($\triangle$, $\blacktriangle$); DMPC:apoA-I-Dns, mol/mol, 2000:1 ($\bigcirc$, $\bullet$); and DMPC:apoA-I-Dns, mol/mol, 100:1 ($\square$, $\blacksquare$). The open symbols represent measurements carried out at 25° C, varying η by sucrose additions. The closed symbols correspond to measurements where T was varied. Rotational relaxation times at 25° C were obtained from: $\rho_h = (1/p_o - 0.333)\ \tau/(\text{slope} \times 1.11)$.

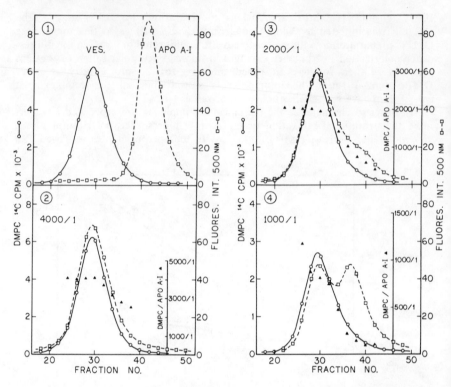

FIGURE 3. Elution profiles on a Sepharose CL-4B column (1.8×35 cm) of DMPC vesicles, apoA-I-Dns (Panel 1), and equilibrated DMPC:apoA-I-Dns reaction mixtures from 4000:1 to 50:1 (mol/mol) (Panels 2–8). The excluded volume of the column is at fraction 16, the total volume is at fraction 49, and the fraction volumes are 1.7 ml. DMPC elution is given in terms of ^{14}C cpm measured on 0.5 ml (Panels 1–3) and on 1.0 ml samples (Panels 4–8). Protein elution was monitored by means of the Dns probe fluorescence excited at 340 nm and measured at 500 nm. The molar ratios of DMPC:apoA-I-Dns are shown for all measurable fractions across the elution peaks. Vesicle:apoA-I-Dns fluorescence was divided by 1.15 and the micellar complex fluorescence by 1.25 in order to account for Dns fluorescence increases in complexes versus the free standard protein-Dns fluorescence.

by sucrose additions at constant temperature to determine the overall rotational relaxation time of the complex, and by T variations in order to detect local rotations of the Dns probe. Pure human apoA-I-Dns has very similar rotational relaxation times by both methods indicating a tight binding of the covalent Dns probe and a single rotational motion (ρ_h by sucrose additions = 67.3 ns; ρ_h by T variation = 58.8 ns). The DMPC–apoA-I-Dns complexes on the other hand, give totally different ρ_h values by both methods. The temperature variation method yields a ρ_h near 21 ns for all the molar ratios of DMPC:apoA-I-Dns, indicating that the Dns probe and its adjacent polypeptide chains become much more free to move in the DMPC complexes compared to the pure protein. From this observation, the protein can be inferred to change its structure

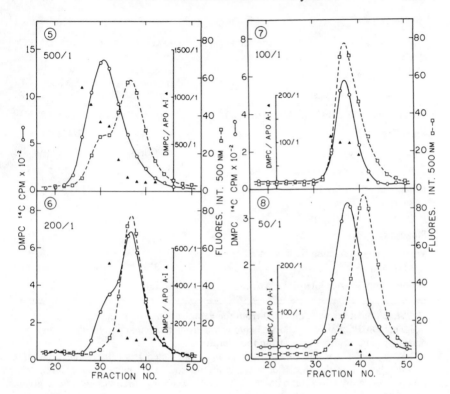

FIGURE 3 (*continued*).

drastically in going from the free to the lipid-bound state. The rotational relaxation times of the complexes determined from sucrose additions ranged from 270 ± 30 nsec for the 100:1 sample to >1000 nsec for the 4000:1 sample. Thus at the different molar ratios, the complexes have different average sizes (from a Stokes radius of 47 Å to a Stokes radius >73 Å). A summary of these results is presented in TABLE 1, together with other properties of DMPC complexes with apoA-I. Since the rotational relaxation times strongly suggested the presence of different complexes of DMPC:apoA-I-Dns at different molar ratios, we turned to gel filtration chromatography in order to fractionate various reaction mixtures of DMPC with apoA-I-Dns.

Gel Filtration. FIGURE 3, Panels 1–8, show the elution profiles of DMPC–apoA-I mixtures at equilibrium, on a Sepharose CL-4B column. The first panel illustrates the elution positions and the extent of separation of DMPC vesicles and apoA-I-Dns passed individually through this column. The remaining panels (2–8) show the elution profiles of reaction mixtures ranging from 4000:1 down to 50:1 DMPC:apoA-I-Dns (mol/mol). At the highest molar ratios, most of the protein elutes with the DMPC at the position corresponding to DMPC vesicles (fraction 29). These complexes have DMPC:apoA-I-Dns molar ratios

TABLE 1

PROPERTIES OF VESICULAR AND MICELLAR COMPLEXES OF APOA-I AND DMPC

Property	Vesicular DMPC–apoA-I Complexes	Micellar DMPC–apoA-I Complexes
Stoichiometry (DMPC:apoA-I, mol/mol) *	$\geq 900 \pm 200$	95 ± 15
DMPC:particle	2850 ± 140 [30]	280 ± 40 †
ApoA-I:particle	≤ 3 or 4	3
Fluorescence lifetime (Dns, nsec) ‡	9.07	9.52
Rotational relaxation time (nsec) ‡ Sucrose additions	>1000	270 ± 30
Temperature variation	21.2	20.8
Stokes radius (Å) §	>73	47
Wavelength—maximum fluorescence (Trp, nm) ¶	329	329
Relative fluorescence intensity (Trp) **	156	152

* Stoichiometries were obtained from the gel filtration experiments.

† This DMPC:particle ratio was calculated from molecular weight data [4] and from partial-specific volumes taken from the literature.

‡ Rotational relaxation times at 25° C were calculated from fluorescence polarization data and from the phase fluorescence lifetimes given in the table (the fluorescence lifetime for apoA-I in solution was 10.2 nsec). For these lifetimes, ρ_h values greater than 500 nsec cannot be calculated accurately.

§ Stokes radii were calculated from the "sucrose addition" rotational relaxation times.

¶ Human apoA-I in solution has an intrinsic fluorescence maximum at 333 nm.

** Fluorescence intensities are relative to the free protein taken as 100.

similar to those of the starting reaction mixtures. At molar ratios from 1000:1 to 100:1, progressively larger proportions of the protein elute in a peak with a maximum at fraction 37, intermediate between the vesicle elution and free protein elution. This complex has a stoichiometry of 95 ($\pm$15) DMPC:apoA-I-Dns (mol/mol) and corresponds to the complex we described previously.[4] In this series of column elutions (Panels 4–6) the remainder of the protein still elutes with the bulk of DMPC lipid at the position of vesicles. The molar ratios found in the latter complexes range from 1000 to 700 DMPC:apoA-I-Dns. This appears to be the lower limit for the stoichiometry of this type of complex. The last panel (Panel 8) shows the elution profile for a sample of 50:1, DMPC: apoA-I-Dns (mol/mol). Here, essentially all of the DMPC elutes with a maximum at fraction 37, but the protein peak is displaced toward the position of free protein elution (fraction 41).

It is noteworthy that the positions of maximum DMPC elution were, in all cases, at fraction 29 and fraction 37, and for protein at fraction 29, fraction 37, and fraction 41, without any intermediate species. Thus, the gel filtration results point toward the existence of two distinct complexes of DMPC and apoA-I. Also, it is evident that in the presence of large amounts of DMPC, all of the protein is associated with lipid. On the other hand, below 100:1 molar ratios free protein is recovered.

Phase Transition Behavior. The fluorescence polarization of DPH as a function of temperature is given in FIGURE 4 for vesicles and liposomes of DMPC and various molar ratios of DMPC:apoA-I. Pure vesicles have a fairly broad phase transition with a midpoint at 22° C, the 100:1 complexes have an increased polarization at all temperatures and a broadened phase transition with midpoint at 25° C. All the higher molar ratios of DMPC to apoA-I have polarizations intermediate between these two extremes, with the 4000:1 and 2000:1 ratios most closely approaching the behavior of pure vesicles. Interestingly, mixtures behave at high temperatures more like vesicles but, at low temperatures, resemble more the micellar complexes.

Hydrodynamic and Spectroscopic Results. TABLE 1 summarizes hydrodynamic and spectroscopic data on the vesicle:apoA-I complexes and on the micellar complexes of apoA-I and DMPC. The stoichiometries of the com-

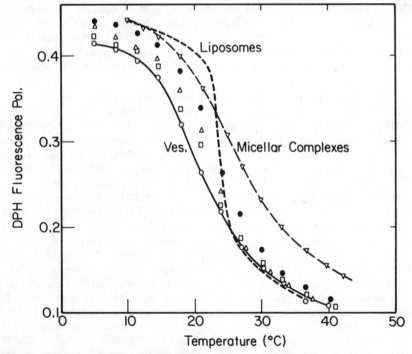

FIGURE 4. DPH fluorescence polarization as a function of temperature for DMPC vesicles (○), and DMPC:apoA-I reaction mixtures of molar ratios 4000:1 (□), 2000:1 (△), 500:1 (●), and 100:1 (▽). The dotted line represents the phase transition behavior of multilamellar DMPC liposomes.

plexes from the gel filtration experiments are 900:1 or greater (DMPC:apoA-I, mol/mol) for the vesicle–apoA-I complexes and 95($\pm$15):1 for the micellar complexes. The number of DMPC molecules per particle was taken from the literature in the case of DMPC vesicles,[30] and was calculated from the molecular weight of micellar complexes (270,000) determined from ultracentrifugal data [4] and the partial specific volume of DMPC vesicles at 18° C.[30] In the vesicles, a maximum of 3 or 4 molecules of apoA-I can be found; the micellar complexes contain 3 apoA-I monomers per particle. The rotational relaxation times (ρ_h) at 25° C, calculated from fluorescence polarization data as a function of T/η (sucrose additions) and fluorescence lifetimes, are consistent with very large particles for the vesicle–apoA-I complexes ($\rho_h > 1000$ nsec) and with particles of the size of HDL ($\rho_h = 270 \pm 30$ nsec) for the micellar complexes. The ρ_h determined from temperature variation experiments was 21 nsec for both types of complexes. From the latter ρ_h values and the spectral properties, it is evident that interaction with DMPC, whether in vesicle form or in micellar complexes, alters the structure of apoA-I to a similar extent. Fluorescence wavelength maxima of apoA-I tryptophanyl residues shifts toward the blue upon interaction with DMPC (a 4 nm shift) and the fluorescence intensity increases at the maxima by about 50%.

Fluorescence–Kinetic Experiments. Since a 4000:1 reaction mixture of DMPC:apoA-I-Dns (mol/mol) was shown to give, at equilibrium, over 98% of vesicular complexes of apoA-I with DMPC (FIGURE 3) we selected it for the kinetic experiments as being representative of DMPC–apoA-I interactions which do not lead to breakdown of the bilayer. On the other hand, the 100:1 ratio was selected as the stoichiometric mixture for the formation of micellar complexes at equilibrium.

FIGURE 5 (FIGURE 1) shows the fluorescence polarization changes (from 0.197 to 0.243) of apoA-I-Dns as it interacts with DMPC vesicles in a 4000:1 DMPC:apoA-I-Dns (mol/mol) reaction mixture. Evidently the reaction is complete within 5 min, even though measurements were continued for 20 hr. Dilution of the samples by about five-fold did not decrease the rate of interaction significantly; therefore, the measurement of apoA-I interaction kinetics with DMPC vesicles would require faster detection methods than those employed by us. Intrinsic fluorescence changes (from 23 to 35 fluorescence units) at 335 nm are also complete after 5 min and parallel very closely the fluorescent polarization changes with time. These results indicate that the environment of the tryptophanyl residues of apoA-I changes simultaneously with the formation of the vesicular complexes. Fluorescence polarization changes in a 100:1 DMPC:apoA-I-Dns (mol/mol) sample with time, are also shown in FIGURE 5. In this experiment, the product of the apoA-I-Dns and DMPC concentrations was identical to their product in the 4000:1 sample, to allow comparison between the two samples in the absence of concentration effects (assuming second order kinetics). Clearly the rate of change of fluorescence polarization for the 100:1 sample is considerably slower than that for the 4000:1 sample. Also the 100:1 curve appears biphasic, with a fast and a slow component. Since the final micellar complexes have the same fluorescence polarization value (0.243) as the vesicular complexes, it appears that not all of the apoA-I can bind to vesicles prior to the breakdown step. Rather, the observed fluorescence polarization for the 100:1 sample must represent the composite of vesicle–apoA-I-Dns precursor, micellar complex, and free apoA-I-Dns fluorescence polarizations.

FIGURE 6 shows the time course of DPH fluorescence polarization in three samples of 100:1 DMPC:apoA-I molar ratios. ApoA-I concentrations varied from 4×10^{-6} M to 5×10^{-7} M. A 4000:1 DMPC:apoA-I (mol/mol) sample was used as a control. The initial small change in fluorescence polarization in the 4000:1 sample corresponds to the binding of apoA-I to DMPC vesicles as shown in FIGURE 4, the subsequent slow change can be attributed to the transformation of DMPC vesicles into liposomes over a period of days. Since apoA-I binding to DMPC vesicles causes only minor changes in DPH polariza-

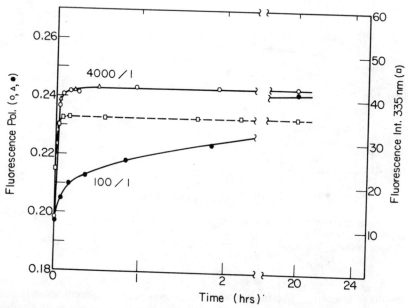

FIGURE 5. Fluorescence polarization changes (full lines) and fluorescence intensity changes (broken line) of apoA-I-Dns with time in the presence of a 4000:1 molar excess of DMPC (open symbols), or a 100:1 molar excess of DMPC (●). The 4000:1 samples represent the formation of vesicle:apoA-I-Dns complexes, for apoA-I-Dns concentrations from 2×10^{-6} M (○) to 5×10^{-7} M (△).

tion, the polarization changes observed with the 100:1 samples are mostly due to the formation of micellar complexes. After subtracting the polarization of the 4000:1 sample from the observed polarizations for the 100:1 samples, we analyzed the kinetic data by plotting ln(DPH polarization) versus time and 1/(DPH polarization) versus time, assuming that the DPH fluorescence polarization changes are proportional to the concentration of micellar complexes. The resulting plots of ln(fluorescence polarization) versus time (FIGURE 7) are linear for the two lower protein concentrations between ½ and 4½ hr; the deviations below ½ hr are probably due to the rapid changes in the polarization when apoA-I binds to vesicles, which are not completely accounted for by

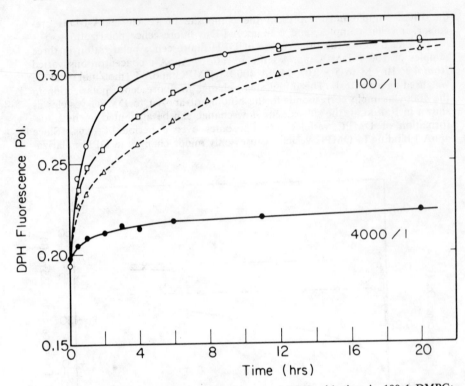

FIGURE 6. Fluorescence polarization changes of DPH with time in 100:1 DMPC: apoA-I (mol/mol) reaction mixtures (open symbols) and in a 4000:1 reaction mixture (●). The apoA-I concentrations in the 100:1 reaction mixtures were 4×10^{-6} M (○), 10^{-6} M (□), and 5×10^{-7} M (△).

the 4000:1 control. The sample with the highest protein concentration is linear between 1 and 3 hr. At longer times, approach to equilibrium precludes a meaningful analysis of the data. The slopes of all three ln(fluorescence polarization) versus time plots are very similar and average out to a first order rate constant $k = 0.22 \ h^{-1}$. The 1/(fluorescence polarization) versus time plots (not shown) were not at all linear indicating that our system does not follow second order kinetics for stoichiometric amounts of apoA-I and vesicles.[31]

CONCLUSIONS

1. Human apoA-I interaction with DMPC vesicles yields two types of stable complexes at equilibrium: Vesicle:apoA-I complexes and apoA-I micellar complexes with DMPC.

2. The vesicle:apoA-I complexes contain less than 3 or 4 protein monomers per complex.

3. Micellar complexes of apoA-I and DMPC have a stoichiometry of 95 (±15) DMPC:apoA-I (mol/mol) and three protein monomers per particle.

4. ApoA-I changes its structure drastically in going from solution to the DMPC-bound state, but the structural changes are very similar for the vesicle-bound apoA-I and the apoA-I in micellar complexes.

5. The binding of apoA-I to DMPC vesicles is a rapid process which is complete in several minutes.

6. Breakdown of vesicles to give micellar complexes is a much slower process, following first order kinetics.

7. The first order rate constant for micellar complex formation is $k = 0.22$ h^{-1} and the half life is $t_{1/2} = 3$ hr 9 min.

8. It may be significant for apoA-I distribution in circulation, that apoA-I can bind rapidly to phospholipid bilayers. On the other hand, slow formation of micellar complexes may help regulate the levels of HDL precursor particles.

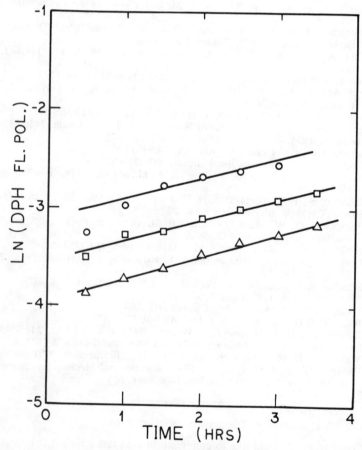

FIGURE 7. Plot of ln(DPH fluorescence polarization) versus time of the kinetic data shown in FIGURE 6 for the 100:1 DMPC:apoA-I (mol/mol) reaction mixtures. The apoA-I concentrations were 4×10^{-6} M (○), 10^{-6} M (□), and 5×10^{-7} M (△).

REFERENCES

1. SCANU, A. M., C. EDELSTEIN & P. KEIM. 1975. *In* The Plasma Proteins. F. W. Putnam, Ed. Vol. 1: 317–389. Academic Press, New York.
2. JACKSON, R. L., J. D. MORRISETT & A. M. GOTTO, JR. 1976. Physiol. Rev. **56:** 259–316.
3. ATKINSON, D., H. M. SMITH, J. DICKSON & J. P. AUSTIN. 1976. Eur. J. Biochem. **64:**541–547.
4. JONAS, A., D. J. KRAJNOVICH & B. W. PATTERSON. 1977. J. Biol. Chem. **252:** 2200–2205.
5. TALL, A. R., D. M. SMALL, R. J. DECKELBAUM & G. G. SHIPLEY. 1977. J. Biol. Chem. **252:**4701–4711.
6. REYNOLDS, J. A., C. TANFORD & W. L. STONE. 1977. Proc. Natl. Acad. Sci. USA **74:**3796–3799.
7. POWNALL, H. J., J. B. MASSEY, S. K. KUSSEROW & A. M. GOTTO, JR. 1978. Biochemistry **17:**1183–1188.
8. GREEN, P. H. R., A. R. TALL & R. M. GLICKMAN. 1978. J. Clin. Invest. **61:** 528–534.
9. HAMILTON, R. L. & H. J. KYDEN. 1974. *In* Biochemistry of Disease. F. F. Becker, Ed. pp. 531–572. Dekker, New York.
10. TALL, A. R., P. H. R. GREEN, R. M. GLICKMAN & J. W. RILEY. 1979. J. Clin. Invest. In press.
11. JONAS, A. & D. J. KRAJNOVICH. 1978. J. Biol. Chem. **253:**5758–5763.
12. POWNALL, H. J., J. B. MASSEY, S. K. KUSSEROW & A. M. GOTTO, JR. 1979. Biochemistry **18:**574–579.
13. TALL, A. R. & Y. LANGE. 1978. Biochim. Biophys. Acta **513:**185–197.
14. EDELSTEIN, C., C. T. LIM & A. M. SCANU. 1972. J. Biol. Chem. **247:**5842–5849.
15. JONAS, A. 1975. Biochim. Biophys. Acta **393:**460–470.
16. WEBER, G. 1953. Discuss. Faraday Soc. **14:**33–39.
17. JONAS, A. 1975. Biochim. Biophys. Acta **393:**471–482.
18. BARBEAU, D. L., A. JONAS, T. TENG & A. M. SCANU. 1978. Biochemistry **18:** 362–369.
19. CHEN, P. S., T. Y. TORIBARA & H. WARNER. 1965. Anal. Chem. **28:**1756–1758.
20. HUANG, C. 1969. Biochemistry **8:**344–352.
21. ANDERSON, D. W., A. V. NICHOLS, T. M. FORTE & F. T. LINDGREN. 1977. Biochim. Biophys. Acta **493:**55–68.
22. JONAS, A. & D. J. KRAJNOVICH. 1977. J. Biol. Chem. **252:**2194–2199.
23. LOWRY, O. H., N. J. ROSEBROUGH, A. L. FARR & R. J. RANDALL. 1951. J. Biol. Chem. **193:**265–275.
24. SPENCER, R. D. & G. WEBER. 1969. Ann. N.Y. Acad. Sci. **158:**361–376.
25. PERRIN, F. 1926. J. Physique **7:**390–401.
26. WEBER, G. 1953. Adv. Protein Chem. **8:**415–459.
27. WAHL, P. & G. WEBER. 1967. J. Mol. Biol. **30:**371–382.
28. RAWITCH, A. B., E. HUDSON & G. WEBER. 1969. J. Biol. Chem. **244:**6543–6547.
29. SHINITZKY, M. & Y. BARENHOLZ. 1974. J. Biol. Chem. **249:**2652–2657.
30. WATTS, A., D. MARSH & P. F. KNOWLES. 1978. Biochemistry **17:**1792–1801.
31. FROST, A. A. & R. G. PEARSON. 1961. Kinetics and Mechanism. 2nd edit. pp. 10–19. John Wiley and Sons, Inc., New York, N.Y.

◆

DISCUSSION OF THE PAPER

COMMENT: I would like to comment on that last slide. It is interesting to note that we performed similar experiments with apoC-III and DMPC and showed the same effect. What I want to say is that when you took egg yolk lecithin to start with instead of DMPC the last step did not occur.

DR. A. JONAS: That is very likely. I think it depends very much on the stability of the vesicles that you start out with, and I think some of the controversy we had previously as to whether some apoprotein would bind to vesicles and whether it would or would not clarify a lipid system depends very much on the type of lipid that we are dealing with.

As you probably gathered, so many of us chose the DMPC system because it readily forms micellar complexes, and we are currently working on other phospholipids trying to solve the problem of exactly how these processes are controlled.

COMMENT: We did exactly the same type of experiment with DMPC and compared the binding of apoA-I and apoA-II; we found that at any temperature apoA-II associates faster by a factor of about ten compared to apoA-I. We also looked at the effect of cholesterol in that system and it seems that in the presence of cholesterol the rate of association of apoA-I increases by a factor of ten. Instead, the association of apoA-II was not so sensitive to the presence of cholesterol. So, I think that cholesterol is very important in the association of apoA-I to vesicles.

DR. JONAS: Thank you. I appreciate the comment, but I cannot add anything to it at this point.

DR. G. G. SHIPLEY: It was rather interesting that the binding of apoA-I to the vesicles did not in fact restrict the access of lanthanide to the phosphate. How do you account for that?

DR. JONAS: I did not show that in my data. I have a table which is going to appear in a full manuscript and which shows the degree of chemical shift between the initial peak and the shifted peak, that is to say, the difference between the two as a function of the amount of apolipoprotein on the vesicle surface. It decreases the more protein you have. What it means exactly in terms of the access of the lanthanide, I do not know. Maybe, somebody can comment on that.

DR. A. R. TALL: These are very nice studies and I think they help to clarify some of the confusion there has been about whether lipoprotein complexes are primarily vesicular in nature or primarily micellar or discoidal and I think you have very nicely shown that it depends very heavily on the incubation conditions, particularly the lipid–protein ratio.

I was surprised by your comment afterwards when you said that with egg yolk lecithin vesicles you showed binding of apoA-I to the vesicles, but that they did not break down any further. I may be wrong about this, but I seem to recall that you published with Dr. Scanu in *BBRC* about two years ago a paper which demonstrated that if you incubated egg yolk lecithin vesicles with apoA-I, you formed HDL-size particles which eluted in a different region of the column profile.

DR. JONAS: Those data were preliminary. The change in fluorescence polarization and rotational relaxation time would have gone with the size of a small particle. I believe that it is a question of interpretation and we are looking at this problem.

DR. TALL: I would like to ask Dr. Scanu what is his opinion about this point.

DR. SCANU: I would like to confine my comment to what we have been doing recently. I would say that in studies of this kind it appears obvious that the nature of the lipid plays a very important role. There is a difference whether you use DMPC or egg yolk lecithin and moreover whether cholesterol is in the system. It is also important that one uses the appropriate technology to distinguish a vesicle from a disc.

When you add apoA-I much will depend upon its physical state in solution and how gradual its addition to the system is. So, in the future I am sure our experimental conditions have to be defined very precisely.

DR. SMALL: Dr. Jonas, I think there is a fundamental difference in what Drs. Tall and Shipley and I found with DMPC and apoA-I and what you have reported. The difference is that you are saying that there is a vesicle complex when you approach a phospholipid:protein ratio of 900 to 1 and only a disc at a ratio of about 100 to 1.

What Dr. Tall found was that there are a series of differently sized discs which depend upon the lipid to protein initial ratio, and I think that the data are sound in both cases. The difference may lie in the incubation temperature or something like that, but it could well lie in the fact that you are using vesicles to start with where we were using myelinic figures. In vesicles you have to put energy into that system to begin with and, therefore, you have raised the general energy of the system that you are starting with and the end product that you get may be rather different. I think that it is a point that should be taken into consideration.

DR. JONAS: During this Conference I have been talking to several people who are working on similar problems starting with liposomes and we noted some discrepancies. So, I would like to indicate that there may be indeed a difference depending on the starting material.

DR. J. C. OSBORNE: First of all, I would like to compliment you on your studies. At NIH, using a different technique, and DPPC vesicles, we found similar types of structures as you found also at very high lipid-to-protein ratios. We actually viewed them first under the electron microscope and they looked like very large discs, but I think your evidence that they are really vesicles is very nice and now one really has to conceptionally think why the number of three or four gives an upper limit to how much lipid this vesicle can contain.

DR. J. A. HUNTER: We have recently done some experiments incubating human lecithin vesicles with HDL subclasses, HDL_2 and HDL_3. After incubation we have fractionated the products by an equilibrium gradient ultracentrifugation. With HDL_2 we also see some transfer of protein into the vesicle density region and also see the formation of discoidal complexes as seen under the negative stain of electron microscopy. The size of these discs is very large. They seem to be about 250 Å in diameter. We also noted discs of that size with HDL_3. If you increase the lecithin loading, there is ultimately a shift in the vesicle position; that is, there is a sort of sudden shift in density. Preliminary studies indicate that there is definitely a decrease in apoA-I concentration in the HDL fraction isolated from gradient ultracentrifugation, but not a significant change and not a significant transfer, apparently, of apoCs.

DR. JONAS: I think the best person for you to talk to is Alan Tall who has done some of those experiments in Dr. Small's laboratory. He sees, and I believe that I am quoting him correctly, that apoA-I comes off the HDL and appears in disc-like complexes.

STRUCTURE OF PLASMA LIPOPROTEINS:
VIEW FROM CALORIMETRIC STUDIES *

Alan R. Tall

Gastroenterology Division
Department of Medicine
Columbia University College of Physicians & Surgeons
New York, New York 10032

X-ray scattering and electron microscopic studies have shown that plasma lipoproteins are quasi-spherical particles in which a core of apolar lipids is surrounded by a more polar surface of lipids and proteins.[1-3] A more detailed description of the structure of the apolar lipid core of the lipoproteins became available with the advent of studies employing differential scanning calorimetry (DSC). These investigations were motivated by the observations of Small [4] that the physiological cholesterol esters, cholesterol oleate and linoleate, displayed liquid crystalline transitions in the vicinity of body temperature. Plasma low-density lipoproteins (LDL), the major cholesterol transporting lipoproteins of plasma, contain about 45 weight% of cholesterol ester, and Deckelbaum et al.[5] were able to show that liquid crystalline transitions of cholesterol ester could be observed in intact LDL. These and subsequent studies [6-8] established that human plasma LDL displayed order–disorder transitions of cholesterol esters between about 20° and 40° C. The problem then became to determine how the organization of the lipoprotein core lipids varied as a function of lipoprotein size and composition. The relation between lipoprotein size and structure of the core lipids will be reviewed here. In addition, the calorimetric studies of HDL,[9] its apoproteins,[10] and its recombinants [11, 12] led to an investigation of the interactions of intact HDL with phospholipids.[13, 14] The metabolic and structural consequences of the uptake by HDL of phospholipid from vesicles [15] or lipolyzed chylomicrons [16] will also be discussed.

The thermal behavior of the lipoprotein core lipids is greatly influenced by both the overall size of the lipoprotein particle and by the composition of the core lipids. In FIGURE 1 DSC curves of a variety of lipoproteins are shown, arranged in order of decreasing size. The particles have been heated from 0° to 100° C. All particles display an irreversible endotherm at high temperature, associated with lipoprotein denaturation.

At lower temperatures, some particles display reversible thermal transitions of cholesterol esters, as typified by human LDL (LDL_N). This transition, occurring between about 20° and 40° C, is probably due to a reversible change of the LDL cholesterol esters from a smectic-like (layered) state below the transition to a more disordered state above the transition. The evidence for this is that pure cholesterol esters display smectic-to-liquid transitions of similar temperature and enthalpy,[5, 6, 17] and that below the transition there is a maximum at $1/36$ $Å^{-1}$ in the x-ray scattering profile of LDL which seems to result

* A part of this work was supported by National Institutes of Health Grant HL-22682 and by a Grant-in-Aid from the American Heart Association (316–3070–2286, New York Affiliate).

from a layered arrangement of core cholesterol esters.[8, 18] The temperature of this transition is correlated with the cholesterol ester/triglyceride ratio and with the degree of saturation of the cholesterol ester fatty acids.[6, 17, 18] Human VLDL (not shown) displays no thermal transitions of its cholesterol esters because they are completely dissolved in the liquid triglyceride core.[19] The density 1.006 to 1.02 fraction (intermediate density lipoprotein) of hypercholesterolemic rabbits contains large cholesterol ester-rich particles which display reversible transitions of cholesterol ester (FIGURE 1, IDL$_c$). For these particles the transition enthalpy, ~1 cal/g, is similar to that of pure cholesterol ester. Hypercholesterolemic monkey LDL (LDL$_c$) and hypercholesterolemic swine LDL (not shown) display similar transition to human LDL.[17, 18] However, the temperature of the transitions is elevated in these hypercholesterolemic LDL due to a low content of triglyceride in the lipoprotein core and to a high content of more saturated cholesterol esters.[17, 18] These changes in core structure of hypercholesterolemic swine and monkey LDL mean that the LDL cholesterol esters circulate in a more ordered state than in normal animals or

TABLE 1

INFLUENCE OF LIPOPROTEIN SIZE ON THE ENTHALPY OF CHOLESTEROL ESTER (CE) LIQUID CRYSTALLINE TRANSITIONS

Lipoprotein	Diameter (Å)	ΔH (cal/g CE)
Hypercholesterolemic rabbit	>300	1.0
Hypercholesterolemic monkey	230–280	0.7
Human LDL	220	0.7
Swine HDL$_c$	150–190	0.7–0.8
Bovine HDL	90–150	0–0.6
Human HDL$_2$	110	0
Human HDL$_3$	90	0

humans, a factor which may contribute to atherosclerosis in these animal models.[17, 18] HDL$_c$, isolated from hypercholesterolemic swine, is intermediate in size between HDL and LDL but still displays cholesterol ester transitions like those of LDL (FIGURE 1).[17, 20] Lactating cows develop very high levels of plasma HDL, including larger HDL particles of diameters between 110 and 150 Å.[21] These larger HDL particles display cholesterol ester transitions (FIGURE 1, HDL$_1$) which have transitions with enthalpies less than LDL.[22] The smaller bovine HDL and human HDL$_2$ (FIGURE 1) and HDL$_3$ display no cholesterol ester transitions.[9]

To summarize, the cholesterol ester-rich lipoproteins show order–disorder transitions of their cholesterol esters over a wide range of sizes (TABLE 1, FIGURE 2). In the very largest particles, this transition has an enthalpy similar to the smectic-liquid melt of pure cholesterol esters (1.1 cal/g). However, in particles ranging in size from about 150 to 280 Å this transition has an enthalpy of 0.7 cal/g cholesterol ester (TABLE 1). The reduced enthalpy is probably due to some degree of persistent ordering of cholesterol esters above the transi-

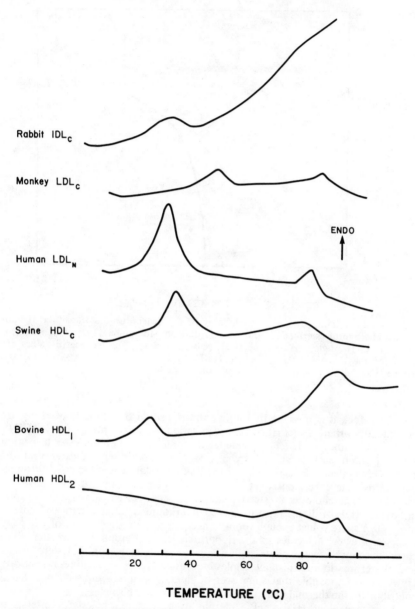

FIGURE 1. Differential scanning calorimetry heating curves of intermediate-density lipoprotein from hypercholesterolemic rabbits, low-density lipoproteins from hyperlipidemic monkeys, low-density lipoproteins from normal humans, HDL$_c$ from hyperlipidemic swine, HDL$_1$ (density ~1.06) from lactating cow and human HDL$_2$ (density 1.063 to 1.125). All lipoproteins were heated at 5° C/minute. ENDO indicates the direction of endothermic transitions.

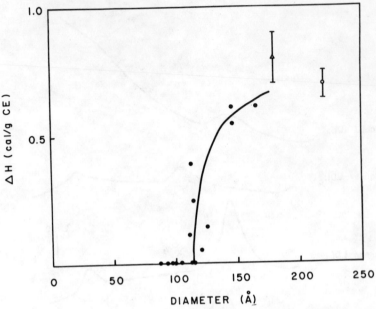

FIGURE 2. Relation between the enthalpy of the order–disorder transition of lipo-protein cholesterol esters (CE) and particle diameter for human LDL (open circle), swine HDL$_c$ (triangle), and bovine HDL (closed circles). The mean±SE values are given for the human LDL and swine HDL$_c$. Individual values are given for the bovine HDL between diameters 170 to 90 Å.

tion.[17] In fact, it is possible that above the transition the cholesterol esters are in a radially oriented, nematic-like organization,[17] as exemplified for an HDL$_c$ particle in FIGURE 3. The lack of dependence of the cholesterol ester transition enthalpy upon particle size between 150–280 Å diameter indicates that the constraining effects of the particle on the liquid crystal melt are exerted through-out the particle core, consistent with a radial nematic organization above the transition. The cholesterol ester transition decreases in enthalpy quite abruptly in bovine HDL of diameters 150 to 120 Å (FIGURE 2). At a critical diameter of ~140 Å there is just enough room to accommodate a single layer of extended cholesterol ester molecules in the lipoprotein core (FIGURE 3). Smaller HDL particles cannot accommodate such a layered arrangement of cholesterol esters and therefore do not display cholesterol ester liquid crystalline transitions. However, it is possible that some sort of lipid–lipid interactions do occur and contribute to the thermal denaturation of these smaller particles.

Although intact HDL lacks thermal transitions of cholesterol esters, its thermal denaturation is quite characteristic and has provided insights into lipid–protein interactions in HDL. The thermal denaturation of human HDL consists of a double-peaked endotherm (FIGURE 4).[19] The first component is broad and associated with release of apoA-I, while the second component is sharp and associated with a more generalized disruption of lipoprotein structure, including release of cholesterol esters from the lipoprotein particle.[19] Following lipo-

protein denaturation there is a reversible phase transition of liberated cholesterol esters as well as the reversible thermal denaturation of lipid-free apoA-I
(FIGURE 4). The evidence that the first broad component of the denaturation
of HDL is due to release of apoA-I is based on calorimetric and biochemical
studies. The thermal denaturation of apoA-I (of mid-point temperature 54° C)
was used to monitor the release of apoA-I from HDL. Heating HDL through
the first broad component resulted in liberation of most of the apoA-I as illustrated in FIGURE 5.[22] That apoA-I was released over this temperature range
was also verified by preparative ultracentrifugation of heated human HDL and
quantitation of free apoA-I in the density 1.21 bottom. Release of cholesterol
esters, as judged by the appearance of cholesterol ester liquid crystalline transitions at low temperature, only occurred when HDL was heated through the
second, sharp component of the denaturation endotherm (FIGURES 4 & 5). In
studies of human HDL the second high temperature peak was also associated
with release of apoA-II from HDL. However, calorimetric studies of the
thermal denaturation of bovine HDL (FIGURE 5) and swine HDL have shown
a similar double-peaked configuration of the denaturation endotherm, even
though the HDL apoproteins from these species consist almost entirely of an

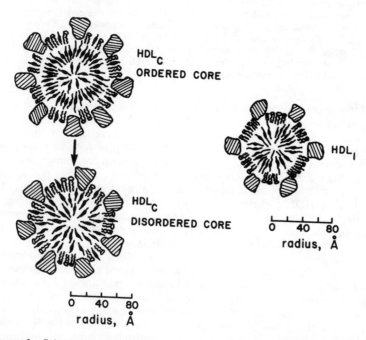

FIGURE 3. Schematic representation of the thermotropic order–disorder transition
of the core cholesterol esters of HDL$_c$. This transition may result from a change of
the cholesterol esters from a layered arrangement to a more disordered structure,
where there may still be some radial alignment of cholesterol ester molecules. As
particles become smaller than HDL$_c$, the core becomes too small to accommodate a
layered arrangement of cholesterol esters. The smallest particle that could accommodate a layered arrangement of extended cholesterol ester molecules would have a
diameter of about 140 Å, as illustrated for HDL$_1$.

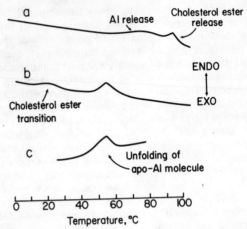

FIGURE 4. Differential scanning calorimetry heating curve for human HDL₂ (density 1.063–1.125). In (a) the curve for the intact lipoprotein demonstrating the characteristic double-peaked denaturation endotherm is shown. In (b) the sample has been previously denatured by heating to 100° C. In (c) the endotherm associated with reversible unfolding of a sample of pure, lipid-free apoA-I is shown. The first component of the denaturation endotherm of intact HDL is associated with release of apoA-I while the second component is associated with release of cholesterol esters and apoA-II. Following thermal denaturation of HDL, there are transitions due to released cholesterol esters and apoA-I.

apoA-I-like protein with no, or very little apoA-II-like protein.[17, 22] Thus, the sharp peak at high temperature may reflect the thermal disruption of stabilizing forces due to lipid–lipid interactions or due to interactions of lipid with a tightly bound subfraction of apoA-I. It is interesting to note that the entropy change associated with the high temperature endotherm for human and bovine HDL is about 0.0032 cal/g cholesterol ester per ° C, a value similar to the entropy change of the smectic-liquid transition of pure cholesterol esters. Thus, in the smaller HDL particles melting of an ordered structure involving core lipids may not be possible at lower temperatures because of size constraints. Melting of this ordered structure only becomes possible when most of the apoA-I has been removed and the particle is disrupted.

The fact that part of the apoA-I could be released from HDL, leaving a relatively stable lipoprotein particle, prompted an investigation of the interaction of HDL with phospholipids.[13, 14] Incubation of multilamellar liposomes of dimyristoyllecithin with HDL resulted in the solubilization of the lecithin because of the formation of dimyristoyllecithin–apoA-I discoidal lipoproteins.[13, 14] In these studies there was a concomitant decrease in hydrated density and an increase in size of HDL₃, interpreted to be due to fusion of apoA-I depleted HDL, or to insertion of phospholipid into the surface of apoA-I-depleted HDL₃.[14] Nichols and co-workers have presented similar results for the interaction of unilamellar vesicles of dimyristoyl lecithin with HDL₂ᵦ (density 1.063 to 1.10).[23] However, their detailed studies suggest that dimyristoyl lecithin initially inserts into the surface of HDL₂ᵦ and displaces apoA-I, which then becomes available for formation of discoidal complexes.[23] Incubation of egg yolk lecithin unilamellar vesicles in plasma also results in uptake of phospholipid by the HDL fraction; this interaction depends on the presence of pre-existing HDL.[24] At higher ratios of egg lecithin vesicles to HDL, a small amount of the HDL protein became associated with the vesicles. However, in the presence of a relative excess of HDL (vesicle phospholipid/HDL protein <1.0) the major mechanism of phospholipid uptake appears to involve insertion of phospholipid into pre-existing HDL.

These studies demonstrating the ability of the plasma HDL fraction to dissolve phospholipid led to speculation that one of the biological roles of HDL

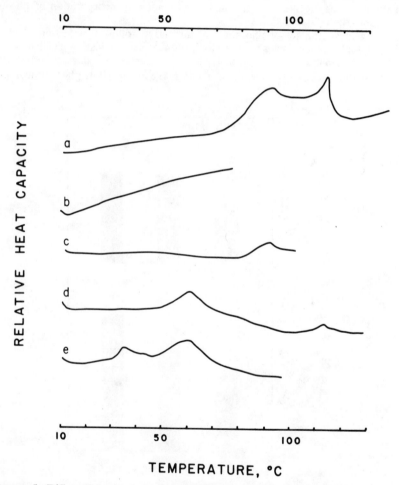

FIGURE 5. Differential scanning calorimetry heating curves of bovine HDL (density 1.12). In (a) the sample was heated from 0 to 130° C. In (b)–(e) a second, smaller sample was heated to 80° C, cooled, heated to 105°, cooled, heated to 130° C, cooled, and then heated to 100° C. The experiment shows that a major fraction of the apoA-I is released in association with the first broad component of the denaturation endotherm. Cholesterol esters are only released when the sample is heated through the higher temperature, sharp component of denaturation.

might be to remove phospholipids from other lipoproteins or cell membranes.[25] For example, during lipolysis, chylomicron phospholipids might be transferred into plasma HDL.[25] The latter hypothesis was also suggested by studies showing that HDL phospholipid rises following a fatty meal[26] and that during lipolysis phospholipids are removed from chylomicrons.[27] Subsequent investigations in the rat have, in fact, confirmed that during lipolysis of chylomicrons a major fraction of phospholipid is transferred into HDL.[16] Following injection of chylomicrons, a part of this phospholipid is initially released as a vesicle which is subsequently incorporated into the HDL fraction.[16] Similarly, injection of unilamellar egg lecithin vesicles in the rat results in incorporation of phospholipid into the HDL fraction.[15]

The mass transfer of phospholipid into HDL following injection of mesenteric lymph chylomicrons or vesicles produced by sonication is illustrated in FIGURE 6. Following injection of chylomicrons or unilamellar egg yolk lecithin vesicles there was an increment of about 1 mg in the HDL phospholipid mass,

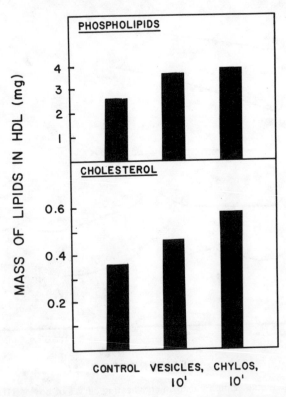

FIGURE 6. Changes in the mass of lipids in the high density lipoprotein (density 1.063–1.21) fraction of rat plasma, occurring 10 minutes after the injection of unilamellar egg lecithin vesicles or rat mesenteric lymph chylomicrons. The increment of HDL phospholipid approximates the mass of injected phospholipid in the vesicles or chylomicrons, indicating transfer of a major fraction of vesicle or chylomicron phospholipid into HDL. Simultaneously there is an increase in mass of unesterified cholesterol in HDL (bottom panel).

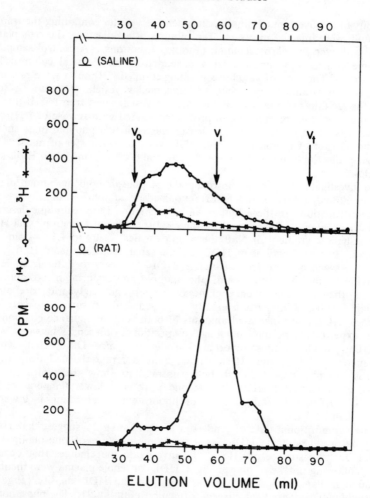

FIGURE 7. Agarose gel chromatography of unilamellar egg lecithin vesicles following injection into saline or into a rat. The vesicles of [14C]-phosphatidylcholine contained trapped [3H]inulin. Following injection into saline they were reisolated as vesicles containing trapped [3H]inulin. Following injection into the rat there is transfer of lecithin radioactivity into the HDL region of the column elution profile, associated with release of the trapped [3H]inulin. V_o and V_t represent the column void and total volumes. V_1 is the elution volume of control HDL.

representing most of the phospholipid injected with the chylomicrons or vesicles. Simultaneous with the increase in HDL phospholipid there was an increase in the mass of unesterified cholesterol (FIGURE 6) showing an influx of cholesterol into HDL following acquisition of phospholipid. During lipolysis, most of the mass of apoA-I of mesenteric lymph chylomicrons is also transferred into HDL.[16] The uptake of phospholipid from injected unilamellar egg yolk vesicle lecithin is further illustrated in FIGURE 7. In these experiments, the lecithin was sonicated in the presence of [3H]inulin, purified by Sepharose 4B chromatography to remove free [³H]inulin, and then the vesicles containing the trapped [³H]inulin were injected into rats. Ten minutes after injection, the rat's plasma was passed over an agarose column (FIGURE 7, bottom). A control sample of the same vesicles was simultaneously reisolated on an identical column (FIGURE 7, top). The control vesicles containing trapped [³H]inulin were reisolated at an elution volume appropriate for unilamellar vesicles (FIGURE 7, top), while the lecithin radioactivity of the injected vesicles was transferred into the HDL region of the column elution profile, associated with release of [³H]inulin radioactivity (FIGURE 7, bottom). Measurements of phospholipid mass showed that the transfer of radioactivity into HDL was due to transfer of mass. Thus, following injection the vesicles were disrupted and transformed into HDL-sized particles.

To investigate the mechanism of uptake of phospholipid by human plasma HDL in more detail, HDL was first fractionated by equilibrium density gradient ultracentrifugation. In these studies we have employed the technique described by Anderson et al.,[28, 29] who resolved three subfractions of human plasma HDL, using a shallow gradient of NaBr between densities ~1.09 to 1.15. Using this technique, two subfractions of HDL_2 can be separated, designated HDL_{2a} and HDL_{2b}. As can be seen from TABLE 2, HDL_{2a} appears to differ from HDL_3 by having an increased number of phospholipid and apoprotein molecules; by contrast, the core constituents, cholesterol ester and triglyceride are almost invariant. Thus, HDL_{2a} has a greatly increased ratio of surface to core constituents. HDL_{2b} has increased amounts of both core and surface components. In our experiments we have obtained compositional differences between HDL_3 and HDL_{2a} similar to those reported by Anderson et al.[28] Differential scanning calorimetry of HDL_3 and HDL_{2a} shows quite different thermal denaturation patterns (FIGURE 8). Although both subfractions show the typical double-peaked endotherm, for HDL_{2a} the second peak is at lower temperature than in HDL_3. Also, the total enthalpy of lipoprotein denaturation is lower for HDL_{2a} than HDL_3.

The compositional data of Anderson et al. (TABLE 2) suggest that HDL_{2a} might be produced from HDL_3 as a result of insertion of phospholipid and apoA-I into the surface of HDL_3. To investigate the changes that occur in HDL_3 following uptake of phospholipid, HDL_3 or whole plasma were incubated with unilamellar egg lecithin vesicles and then the HDL density range was analyzed by density gradient ultracentrifugation (FIGURE 9). The phospholipid-enriched HDL_3 was reisolated as a homogeneous peak of similar density to HDL_{2a} ($d \sim 1.110$) (FIGURE 9). DSC of the phospholipid-enriched HDL_3

TABLE 2

MOLECULES PER PARTICLE *

	Pro †	FC	TG	CE	PL
HDL_3 (1.125–1.200)	4	14	4	49	53
HDL_{2a} (1.100–1.125)	5	20	7	47	124
HDL_{2b} (1.063–1.100)	6	74	9	92	212

* Derived from the data of Anderson et al.[28]
† Units of 25,000.

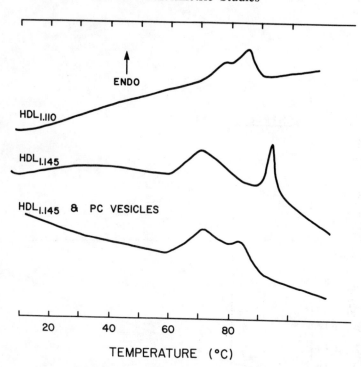

FIGURE 8. Differential scanning calorimetry heating curves of human HDL fractions obtained by NaBr density gradient ultracentrifugation. The subscripts show the density of the fractions. In the bottom curve the major fraction of HDL_3 was incubated with egg lecithin vesicles prior to examination by DSC.

showed a marked decrease in temperature of the second component of the denaturation endotherm (FIGURE 8). The total enthalpy of lipoprotein denaturation is also decreased with phospholipid enrichment. Thus, the denaturation endotherm of the phospholipid-enriched HDL_3 is altered to a pattern that resembles HDL_{2a}.

The above results raise the possibility that HDL_{2a} may be produced from HDL_3 by addition of phospholipid and apoA-I. A variety of metabolic studies are now available to show that phospholipid and apoA-I are transferred into the HDL fraction during lipolysis of chylomicrons. It is conceivable that during physiological lipolysis the surface components of the chylomicron may combine with the HDL_3 to produce a subfraction of HDL_2 of $d \sim 1.110$. This subfraction of HDL_2 may subsequently be converted into larger cholesterol ester-rich particles secondary to the acquisition of unesterified cholesterol and the action of lecithin:cholesterol acyltransferase, or by some other mechanisms such as lipoprotein fusion.

Incubation of egg lecithin vesicles with whole plasma and then re-isolation on density gradients shows that most of the phosphatidylcholine dissolving capacity of plasma depends on the uptake of phosphatidylcholine by HDL_3 with conversion to a HDL_{2a}-like particle. In these experiments the phospholipid

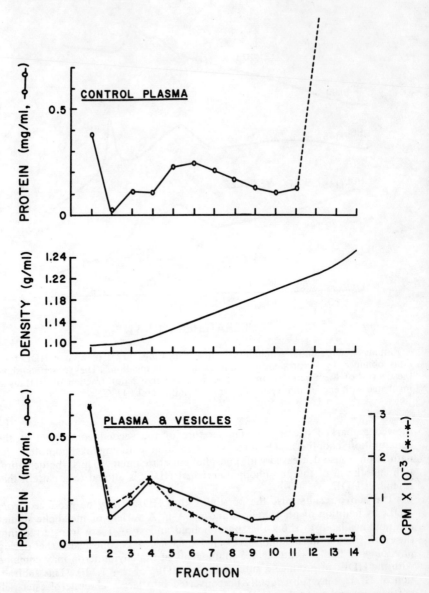

FIGURE 9. Density gradient ultracentrifugation of human plasma (0.33 ml) and of human plasma (0.33 ml) previously incubated for 4 hours at 37° C with 1.0 mg of unilamellar egg lecithin vesicles. In the middle panel the shape of the density gradient, determined by refractometry, is shown. The distribution of protein is shown with open circles and the distribution of lecithin radioactivity with crosses.

uptake capacity of HDL was found to be reduced in proportion to the period of ultracentrifugation used in preparation of the HDL, presumably due to ultracentrifugal loss of apoA-I from HDL. The amount of lecithin that could be dissolved by whole plasma was about 1 mg/ml plasma, or about 2.5 to 3.0 g/total plasma volume for humans. Assuming that 70% to 80% of chylomicron phospholipid is transferred into HDL,[16, 26] and that about 4–5 g of phospholipid are secreted on chylomicrons following ingestion of 100 g of fat,[30] about 3 to 5 g of phospholipid are probably transferred from chylomicrons into HDL following a fatty meal. Thus, the phosphatidylcholine uptake capacity of

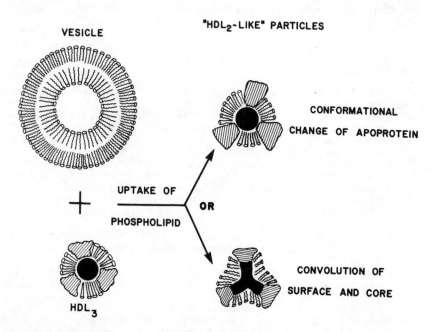

FIGURE 10. Schematic representation of potential mechanisms of incorporation of phospholipid into human HDL₃. Phospholipid molecules might be incorporated into the surface of HDL₃ as a result of a change of apoA-I from an extended conformation to a less tightly bound conformation and/or as a result of convolution in the surface and core in the HDL₃ particle. The phospholipid-enriched HDL would have a density similar to HDL₂ₐ. Alternatively, phospholipids may be taken up as a result of protein–phospholipid substitution (not shown).

plasma is concordant with the load of phospholipid transferred into HDL following a fatty meal.

How is the uptake of phospholipid by HDL₃ achieved on a molecular level? The above results suggests that under physiological circumstances, lecithin is inserted indirectly into HDL₃ and that the number of lecithin molecules can be increased from about 55 per HDL particle to about 150 per particle. Given a diameter of 90 Å of HDL₃ and a spherical shape of HDL, the total surface area of the particle is about 25,446 Å². Assume that each phospholipid molecule occupies 74 Å² at the surface of the particle. This would mean that phospholipid enrichment would produce an increase in surface area occupied by lecithin molecules from about 4,070 Å² to about 11,470 Å². How can there be such a large increase in surface area occupied by lecithin molecules? Two potential ways are illustrated in FIGURE 10. The amount of surface area occupied by protein may be reduced, as a result of a conformational change from an extended to a less tightly bound conformation. Alternately, there may be an increase in the total surface area of the particle as a result of convolution of the whole particle surface, without a major conformational change of the apoprotein (FIGURE 10). Finally, the uptake of phospholipids may occur secondary to the displacement of protein from the surface of HDL, i.e., protein–phospholipid substitution.

REFERENCES

1. FORTE, T. & A. V. NICHOLS. 1972. Plasma lipoprotein structure. Adv. Lipid Res. **10**:1–38.
2. SHIPLEY, G. G., D. ATKINSON & A. M. SCANU. 1972. Small-angle x-ray scattering of human serum high-density lipoproteins. J. Supramol. Struct. **1**:98–103.
3. ATKINSON, D., M. A. F. DAVIS & R. B. LESLIE. 1974. Proc. R. Soc. London Ser. B **186**:165–180.
4. SMALL, D. M. 1970. The physical state of lipids of biological importance: cholesteryl esters, cholesterol, triglyceride. *In* Surface Chemistry of Biological Systems. M. Blank, Ed. pp. 55–83. Publishing Corp., New York, N.Y.
5. DECKELBAUM, R. J., G. G. SHIPLEY, D. M. SMALL, R. S. LEES & P. K. GEORGE. 1975. Thermal transition in human plasma low density lipoproteins. Science **190**:392.
6. DECKELBAUM, R. J., G. G. SHIPLEY & D. M. SMALL. 1977. Structure and interactions of lipids in human plasma low density lipoproteins. J. Biol. Chem. **252**:744–754.
7. DECKELBAUM, R. J., G. G. SHIPLEY, A. R. TALL & D. M. SMALL. 1978. Lipid distribution and interaction in human plasma low density and very low density lipoproteins. Lipid core fluidity and surface properties. Protides of the Biological Fluids. Proc. 25th Colloquium. 91–98.
8. ATKINSON, D., R. J. DECKELBAUM, D. M. SMALL & G. G. SHIPLEY. 1977. Structure of human plasma low-density lipoproteins: molecular organization of the central core. Proc. Natl. Acad. Sci. USA **74**:1043–1046.
9. TALL, A. R., R. J. DECKELBAUM, D. M. SMALL & G. G. SHIPLEY. 1977. Thermal behavior of human plasma high density lipoprotein. Biochim. Biophys. Acta **487**:145–153.
10. TALL, A. R., G. G. SHIPLEY & D. M. SMALL. 1976. Conformational and thermodynamic properties of apoA-I of human plasma high density lipoproteins. J. Biol. Chem. **251**:3749–3755.
11. TALL, A. R., D. M. SMALL, G. G. SHIPLEY & R. S. LEES. 1975. Apoprotein stability and lipid–protein interactions in human plasma high density lipoproteins. Proc. Natl. Acad. Sci. USA **72**:4940–4942.
12. TALL, A. R., D. M. SMALL, R. J. DECKELBAUM & G. G. SHIPLEY. 1977. Structure and thermodynamic properties of high density lipoprotein recombinants. J. Biol. Chem. **252**:4701–4711.
13. TALL, A. R. & D. M. SMALL. 1977. Solubilisation of phospholipid membranes by human plasma high density lipoproteins. Nature **264**:163–164.
14. TALL, A. R., V. HOGAN, L. ASKINAZI & D. M. SMALL. 1978. Interaction of plasma high density lipoproteins with dimyristoyllecithin multilamellar liposomes. Biochemistry **17**:322–326.

15. TALL, A. R. 1980. Studies on the transfer of phosphatidylcholine from vesicles into plasma high density lipoproteins in the rat. J. Lipid Res. **21:**354–363.
16. TALL, A. R., P. H. R. GREEN, R. M. GLICKMAN & J. W. RILEY. 1979. Metabolic fate of chylomicron phospholipids and apoproteins in the rat. J. Clin. Invest. **64:**977–989.
17. TALL, A. R., D. ATKINSON, D. M. SMALL & R. W. MAHLEY. 1977. Characterization of the lipoproteins of atherosclerotic swine. J. Biol. Chem **252:**7288–7293.
18. TALL, A. R., D. M. SMALL, D. ATKINSON & L. RUDEL. 1978. Studies on the structure of low density lipoproteins isolated from *Macaca Fascicularis* fed an atherogenic diet. J. Clin. Invest. **62:**1354–1363.
19. DECKELBAUM, R. J., A. R. TALL & D. M. SMALL. 1977. Interaction of cholesterol ester and triglyceride in human plasma very low density lipoprotein. J. Lipid Res. **18:**164–168.
20. ATKINSON, D., A. R. TALL, D. M. SMALL & R. W. MAHLEY. 1978. The structural organization of the lipoprotein HDL$_c$ from atherosclerotic swine. Structural features relating the particle surface and core. Biochemistry **17:**3930–3933.
21. PUPPIONE, D. L., T. M. FORTE, A. V. NICHOLS & E. H. STRISOWER. 1970. Biochim. Biophys. Acta **202:**392.
22. TALL, A. R., D. L. PUPPIONE & D. M. SMALL. Submitted for publication.
23. NICHOLS, A. V., E. L. GONG, T. M. FORTE & P. J. BLANCHE. 1978. Interaction of plasma high density lipoproteins HDL$_{2b}$ (d1.063–1.100 g/ml) with single-bilayer liposomes of dimyristoylphosphatidylcholine lipids. **13:**943–950.
24. CHOBANIAN, J. V., A. R. TALL & P. I. BRECHER. 1979. Interaction between unilamellar egg yolk lecithin vesicles and human high density lipoprotein. Biochemistry **18:**180–187.
25. TALL, A. R. & D. M. SMALL. 1978. Plasma high density lipoproteins. N. Engl. J. Med. **299:**1232–1236.
26. HAVEL, R. J. 1957. Early effects of fat ingestion on lipids and lipoproteins of serum in man. J. Clin. Invest. **36:**848–854.
27. MJØS, O. D., O. FAERGEMAN, R. L. HAMILTON & R. J. HAVEL. 1975. Characterization of remnants produced during the metabolism of triglyceride-rich lipoproteins of blood plasma and intestinal lymph in the rat. J. Clin. Invest. **56:**603–615.
28. ANDERSON, D. W., A. V. NICHOLS, T. M. FORTE & F. T. LINDGREN. 1977. Particle distribution of human serum high density lipoproteins. Biochim. Biophys. Acta **493:**56–68.
29. ANDERSON, D. W., A. V. NICHOLS, S. S. PAN & F. T. LINDGREN. 1978. High density lipoprotein distribution resolution and determination of three major components in a normal population sample. Atherosclerosis **29:**161–179.
30. GREEN, P. H. R., R. M. GLICKMAN, C. SAUDEK, C. BLUM & A. R. TALL. 1979. Human intestinal lipoproteins. Studies in chyluric subjects. J. Clin. Invest. **64:**233–242.

DISCUSSION OF THE PAPER

DR. J. C. OSBORNE: Dr. Tall, that was a fine talk. I just have one comment. On your last slide you compared spectroscopic data with your calorimetric studies and I wonder if that is valid in view of the differences in concentration of plasma lipoproteins that you have to use in those two studies.

DR. A. R. TALL: The concentration is very high, as you of course know, and it is of the order of 100 mg/ml. These are intact lipoproteins of course and not apoproteins. Intact lipoproteins circulate in a concentration that is considerably higher than the concentrations at which apoproteins self-associate.

I do not believe that there is any evidence, and I would be delighted to hear a comment on it, that lipoproteins self-associate as a function of concentration. It may well happen, but I believe that the honest proof is missing. It could be that I have not seen the change in the first part of the denaturation curve because of some sort of concentration dependency. I think the clarification of that must wait for better calorimetric technology.

DR. S. EISENBERG: Dr. Tall, those are extremely important and elegant studies. As you know, when we did the change from HDL_3 to HDL_2 particles we observed about doubling the phospholipid content of the HDL_3. Interestingly enough, this was not included in our preliminary report. It is impossible to raise the amount of phospholipids in the HDL_3 above double the amount. If we change the ratio of VLDL to HDL in the lipolytic system, we generate much more phospholipids than are taken up by the system. Actually, we do find them in the bottom fraction. I was very much bothered with this doubling of phospholipids and I remember discussing this with Dr. Scanu some time ago. It is interesting that you find the same thing in your *in vitro* system.

I have two short questions: First, the table that you have shown on the HDL subfractions, is it based on David Anderson's data?

DR. TALL: It is based entirely on his data. I should say that my compositional data resembles his although I have not determined molecular weights.

In my attempts to isolate HDL_{2a} and HDL_{2b} I should say that I found there is a lot of variability, and what seems to be the most important variable is the shape of the density gradient. One needs a very shallow density gradient in the critical region to separate them. But even if you do not see them as separate peaks, if you analyze across the gradient you get the same sort of compositional information as David Anderson reported.

DR. EISENBERG: I simply might have missed it in his paper, but does the HDL_{2a} really have about double or maybe more than double the number of phospholipids per molecule without much changing the other constituents? This is something which has been isolated from plasma.

DR. TALL: That is right.

DR. EISENBERG: The second thing is, in your talk you just mentioned in one or two sentences that if you follow HDL_3 you get to a position where you cannot transform it into HDL_2 further, or did I misunderstand you?

DR. TALL: What I was talking about was the way that experiment was done. I was looking at HDL subfractions that were isolated in the regular way and then I put them on a density gradient for 2 or three days of spinning, based on what my experience had been from previous studies. In previous studies, I think we had established that most of PC residues in the d 1.25 top is in HDL. So, I isolated the 1.25 top as a function of different times up to 5 days. I then constructed a graph of PC incorporated into HDL from vesicle as a fraction of spinning time. I found a straight line that extrapolated back to zero time. From that I concluded there is a change in the HDL as a function of spinning, with a great decrease in its ability to incorporate phospholipid. The gels of those HDLs all show a loss of apoA-I.

DR. EISENBERG: I really do not want to push it further, but I think it is very important that you elaborate on this question because there are rumors of very different results obtained in different laboratories examining some of the reactions. This might also occur in the same laboratory using different conditions.

DR. R. J. HAVEL: Did you observe any change in protein?   That was not quite clear.

DR. TALL: I did not go into that. The experiments done with the large chylomicrons essentially confirmed what you showed before, namely, that apoA-I is fairly quantitatively transferred from the chylomicrons into the HDL fraction and this appears to happen during lipolysis.

DR. HAVEL: In our case, we did not observe any vesicles at all. We only observed an increase in diameter of the preexisting HDL, and there was both a protein and a lipid transfer.

DR. TALL: How did you look for vesicles?

DR. HAVEL: We looked in the microscope primarily and we did this after both gel filtration and ultracentrifugation.

DR. TALL: The vesicular particles that we observed were not numerous, I must say, but they were reproducible and we saw them as collapsed particles. To try to do that in a relatively reproducible way I added cellobiose to the sample just prior to negative staining since cellobiose is osmotically active. It causes collapse of the particles and one can see them as double bilayer-thick particles.

DR. A. M. SCANU: What is not clear to me is how far have you characterized the HDL particles upon enrichment with phospholipids. Which physicochemical techniques did you use to assess the structural features of these particles?

DR. TALL: The last slide, depicting a model of the phospholipid-enriched HDL, was shown more to suggest new ideas than actual hard facts. What I have done to date is to reisolate those particles by density gradient ultracentrifugation or by column chromatography. By electron microscopy the phospholipid-enriched HDL_3 particles appear homogeneous. Most studies I have done to date have been calorimetric. I am undertaking some spectroscopic studies which should prove useful. I think that one would expect big changes in the frictional ratio of such particles, and studies in this direction are worth undertaking.

FREEZE-ETCHING ELECTRON MICROSCOPY OF SERUM LIPOPROTEINS *

Lawrence P. Aggerbeck,† Martine Yates,‡ and
Tadeusz Gulik-Krzywicki

Centre de Génétique Moléculaire
Centre National de la Recherche Scientifique (CNRS)
91190—Gif Sur Yvette, France

INTRODUCTION

Knowledge of lipoprotein structures and understanding of the underlying organizational principles are essential for an interpretation, at the molecular level, of the physiological processes involving these particles. At present, only crystallographic techniques are capable of providing structural analyses with atomic resolution. However, in the absence of crystals suitable for such a study, biochemical, immunologic, hydrodynamic, spectroscopic, electron microscopic, x-ray, and neutron scattering methods can provide useful structural information.

Electron microscopy has often been used in the past for the study of serum lipoproteins. Fixation and shadow casting, as well as embedding techniques, have not yet provided significant structural information.[1] The technique of negative staining has been used extensively for high-density lipoproteins (HDL$_2$ and HDL$_3$). Some authors have reported substructure in the particles.[1, 2] In the case of low-density lipoproteins (LDL$_2$), apart from one report of subunit structure,[3] negative staining has revealed rather uniformly sized, quasispherical, smooth particles.[1] Furthermore, LDL$_2$ and the very-low-density lipoproteins (VLDL) have been reported to be highly deformable when visualized using negative staining techniques.[1] All these techniques involve treatments which, in the case of predominantly lipid-containing systems, can be feared to alter the structure of the sample.[4] One procedure, which seems to avoid some of the pitfalls of the other techniques, is cryofixation.[4] Yet when cryofixation is used, the sample must be quenched rapidly enough to avoid crystallization of the solvent, which leads to aggregation of the solute and possibly to morphological damage. Cryoprotectants such as glycerol may also be used to minimize freezing artifacts. However, in this case, etching (shallow freeze-drying to further expose the sample architecture) is not possible. Ultrarapid cooling of very thin samples[5] and spray freezing[6, 7] are two methods that, at present, provide satisfactory rapid quenching and avoid prefixation or antifreeze treatments. Using these procedures, we have carried out a freeze-etching electron

* This work was supported in part by a grant from the Délégation Général à la Recherche Scientifique et Technique (DGRST).

† Recipient of a DGRST fellowship, a Centre National de la Recherche Scientifique-National Science Foundation Exchange of Scientists Award, and fellowships from the Philippe Foundation and the Simone and Cino Del Duca Foundation.

‡ Recipient of DGRST fellowship.

microscopic study of serum lipoproteins in solution and, in particular, of a hyperlipidemic Rhesus monkey serum LDL$_2$.[8]

Concurrently, the Rhesus LDL$_2$ was studied in our laboratory [9] by solution x-ray scattering both above and below the thermal transition associated with the cholesteryl ester organization.[10] For the low temperature form, with which we are most concerned in this work, the following conclusions were reached: the particle is fairly isometric in shape, its outer surface is deeply corrugated, its outer region is sparsely occupied by a hydrated protein condensed in a small number of globules, and the particle lacks a coarse center of symmetry. To further pursue the analysis of the structure, assumptions concerning the symmetry of the particle were made. It was argued, on the bases of formal considerations, analysis of the x-ray scattering data, and electron microscopic observations,[8] that the particle is likely to display tetrahedral symmetry (point group 23). Assuming this symmetry, a precise model was worked out, which was characterized by an almost spherical and predominantly lipid core surrounded by four protein globules located at tetrahedral positions.

In this work, we describe a freeze-etching electron microscopic study of LDL$_2$ and its correlation with the x-ray scattering study.[9] We further describe the extension of the freeze-etching technique to the study of other serum lipoproteins in solution. We have used turnip yellow mosaic virus (TYMV), whose structure is well known, to demonstrate the performance of the technique employed.

MATERIALS AND METHODS

Human serum very-low-density lipoprotein (VLDL, density <1.006 g/ml), low-density lipoprotein (LDL$_2$, density 1.030–1.040 g/ml), and high-density lipoprotein (HDL$_3$, density 1.12–1.21 g/ml) were isolated from the blood of healthy, fasting, Caucasian male donors by preparative ultracentrifugation in aqueous NaCl and NaBr of varying density.[11] The VLDL migrated as a single broad band with pre-beta mobility on agarose electrophoresis. Agarose electrophoresis was performed according to the directions of the manufacturer with an ACI Agarose Film/Cassette System (Corning, Palo Alto, Calif.). No reaction was noted upon immunoelectrophoresis [12] or double immunodiffusion [13] against antiserum to serum albumin. For LDL$_2$, only one immunoprecipitin line was noted upon immunoelectrophoresis or double immunodiffusion using antisera raised in the rabbit against LDL$_2$ or whole human serum. Further, there was no reaction of LDL$_2$, at several concentrations of antigen and antibody, against antisera to apolipoproteins A-I, A-II, C-I, C-II, or C-III, the major apoproteins of the other serum lipoprotein classes, or against antiserum to albumin, the major serum protein constituent. Upon agarose electrophoresis, the LDL$_2$ migrated as a single well-defined band. Solution x-ray scattering and analytical ultracentrifugation suggest that the particles are relatively homogeneous with respect to mean electron density and that they possess minimal size and shape heterogeneities. The HDL$_3$ gave a single band on agarose electrophoresis and did not react against antisera to LDL$_2$ or serum albumin. Diet-induced hyperlipidemic Rhesus monkey serum LDL$_2$, (density 1.020–1.050 g/ml) the characteristics of which have been described [14] was a gift of Dr. G. Fless, of the Department of Medicine of the University of Chicago, Chicago, Ill. Prior to cryofixation, the lipoproteins were dialyzed in the dark at 4° C against four, 200-fold volumes of 10 mM sodium phosphate, pH 7.6. Although similar results were obtained at all concentrations, for convenient observation and analysis, the lipoprotein concentrations were adjusted, by dilution with dialysis buffer, to approximately 10–50 μM VLDL or LDL_2 and 100–200 μM HDL_3. Following adjustment of the concentration, the samples were filtered (Millipore filter, type HA, Millipore Filter Corp., Bedford, Mass.). The determination of lipoprotein concentration was as previously described.[15] Turnip yellow mosaic virus, prepared according to Matthews,[16] was a gift of Dr. J. Witz, IBCM, Strasbourg, France.

Three techniques were used for cryofixation of the samples. In the case of conventional freezing, a drop of the sample solution ($\sim$50 μl) was placed on a gold specimen holder and quenched in liquid Freon 22 at −160° C. Ultrarapid cooling of very thin samples [5] was carried out by compressing a small drop of the sample solution ($\sim$0.1 μl) between two thin copper plates separated by a thin (20 μm) copper washer. After quenching in liquid Freon 22 at −160° C, the upper copper plate and washer were removed. Spray freezing was carried out as described by Bachmann and Schmitt-Fumian.[7] Following cryofixation, the specimen holders were placed on a specially designed table mounted on the cold stage of a Balzers 301 freeze-etching unit. Fracturing of the samples, achieved with the microtome cutting device, was followed by etching for approximately 1 minute at −105° C under a vacuum of 10^{-6} to 10^{-7} torr. Unidirectional and rotary shadowing at several angles were used for all samples. Rotary shadowing was obtained by rotation, during shadowing, of the table upon which the sample had been fixed. After cleaning, sample replicas were examined in a Phillips 301 electron microscope.

RESULTS

Turnip Yellow Mosaic Virus

Replicas of conventionally frozen TYMV solutions viewed at low magnification show large smooth domains (probably ice) separated by domains of aggregated particles (FIGURE 1 in Reference 8). In contrast, well-isolated particles are seen in replicas of solutions frozen by ultrarapid cooling or spray freezing (FIGURES 1 & 2, also FIGURES 1 & 5 in Reference 8). The "soccer-ball" appearance and the multisubunit nature of the surface of the virus is obvious in both the unidirectionally (FIGURE 1) and rotary shadowed (FIGURE 2) specimens. Unidirectionally shadowed samples display varying degrees of surface structural detail depending upon the shadowing angle (FIGURE 1, also FIGURES 1 & 5 in Reference 8). However, the replicas of the rotary shadowed samples (FIGURE 2, also FIGURES 1 & 3 in Reference 8) show most clearly the details of the surface structure. Particles possessing 2-, 3- or 5-fold symmetry are frequently apparent in rotary shadowed specimens. The maximum diameter of the subunit displaying particles is approximately 320 Å and that of the individual subunits is approximately 70 Å. It must also be noted that some of the particles lack substructure or are exceptionally large (FIGURE 1 in Reference 8). Most likely, this is the result of denaturation or deformation occurring during the biochemical preparation or the freeze-etching procedures, aggregation of small numbers of virus particles, or fracture of the particles. Replicas of the phosphate buffer solution, rapidly frozen, fractured, etched, and shadowed under the same conditions, show smooth surfaces.

Low-Density Lipoprotein

As for TYMV, conventional freezing of LDL$_2$ solutions results in aggregation of the particles (FIGURE 2 in Reference 8), while ultrarapid freezing techniques leave most of the particles isolated in the solvent (FIGURES 1 & 2, also FIGURES 2 & 5 in Reference 8). In striking contrast to the "soccer-ball" appearance of TYMV, replicas of LDL$_2$ look markedly "knobby" and appear to contain small globules (approximately 80 Å in diameter) either isolated or clustered in small bunches approximately 300 Å wide (FIGURES 1, 2 & 3, also FIGURES 2 & 5 in Reference 8). Unidirectionally-shadowed specimens (FIGURE 1) clearly show the "knobby" surface of the particles, which is further reflected in the irregular outlines of the particle shadows. Rotary shadowing (FIGURES 2 & 3, also FIGURE 2 in Reference 8) shows most clearly the details of the particle morphology, as was also the case for TYMV. Many of the particles show coarse 2- or 3-fold symmetry (FIGURE 3). A statistical analysis of 100 particles, not obviously aggregated, showed 10 particles with one subunit, 43 with two, 31 with three, 6 with four, and 10 with more than four. However, as for TYMV, the exceptionally large objects (FIGURES 1, 2 & 3, also FIGURES 2 & 5 in Reference 8) most likely correspond to small aggregates or other types of artifacts.

High-Density and Very-Low-Density Lipoproteins

As for TYMV and serum LDL$_2$, the individual particle morphologies of HDL$_3$ and VLDL may be investigated when ultrarapid freezing techniques are employed. Replicas of HDL$_3$ obtained using either unidirectional (FIGURE 1) or rotary (FIGURE 2) shadowing show particles with an indented surface but which do not display an obvious subunit structure as in the case of the "knobby" LDL$_2$ or the "soccer-ball" TYMV (compare replicas in FIGURE 1 & in FIGURE 2). The maximum size of the particles is approximately 130–140 Å.

FIGURE 1. Freeze-etching replicas of TYMV and serum lipoproteins in 10 mM sodium phosphate buffer, pH 7, etched at −105° C, 10^{-6} to 10^{-7} torr, for approximately 1 minute, unidirectionally shadowed with platinum and coated with carbon. The shadowing direction is from the bottom of the page toward the top. The bar represents 1000Å. (TYMV) Concentration 300 μg/ml, ultrarapid cooling. Note the raspberry-like surface. (LDL$_2$) Human serum LDL$_2$, concentration 50 μM, spray freezing. Note the irregular outline of the shadows, consistent with a "knobby" surface. (HDL$_3$) Human serum HDL$_3$, concentration 100 μM, spray freezing. Small, fairly smooth particles are observed. (VLDL) Human serum VLDL, concentration 30 μM, spray freezing. Some particles appear to have been fractured with removal of part of the particle (a), others appear to possess globular subunits (b).

FIGURE 2. Freeze-etching replicas of TYMV and serum lipoproteins prepared as in FIGURE 1 except rotary shadowed with platinum and coated with carbon. The bar represents 1000 Å. (TYMV) Note the "soccer-ball" appearance reflecting the spherical shape of the particles, the regular distribution of subunits over the surface, and the presence of 2-, 3-, and 5-fold symmetry. (LDL$_2$) In contrast to TYMV, the particles are more "knobby" and look like clusters of a small number of globules (see also FIGURES 3, 4 & 5). (HDL$_3$) In contrast to both TYMV and LDL$_2$, the particles appear to have indented surfaces (especially high magnification view) but do not display an obvious subunit structure.

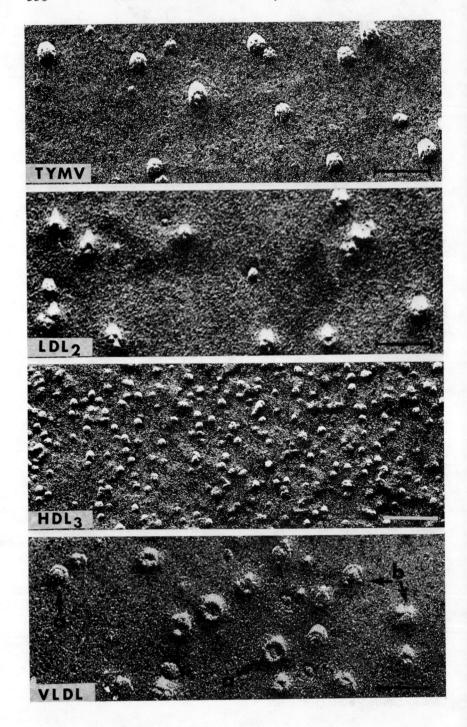

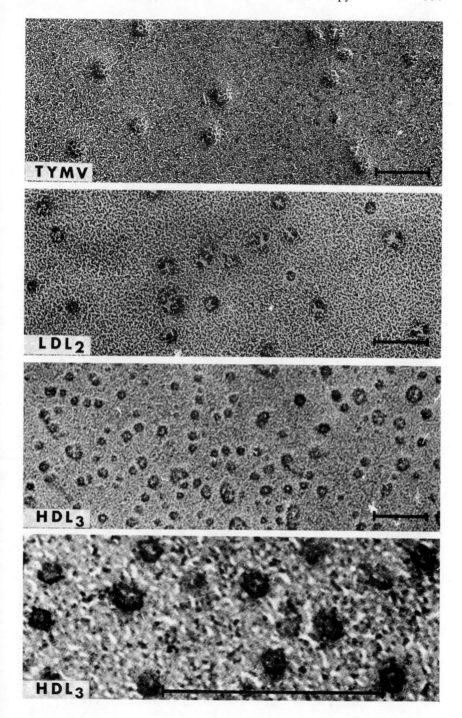

TYMV

LDL₂

HDL₃

HDL₃

Replicas of unidirectionally shadowed VLDL (FIGURE 1) show more complex images. Many particles appear roughly spherical in shape and some seem to have been fractured with removal of part of the particle (FIGURE 1, **a**). Other particles appear to possess globular subunits approximately 90 Å in diameter (FIGURE 1, **b**). The largest particles are less than 1000 Å in diameter.

DISCUSSION

Although all the micrographs reported in this paper refer to a human serum LDL_2, experiments performed with the diet-induced hyperlipidemic Rhesus monkey LDL_2 (studied by solution x-ray scattering techniques) [9] have yielded very similar results. Therefore, we feel justified in considering these particles together. It is clear that lipoproteins studied by freeze-etching electron microscopy using ultrarapid cryofixation procedures seem to have a more complex structure than when studied by other electron microscopic techniques. It must be noted that the same situation was encountered with biological membranes [4] and that, in this case, freeze-etching has supplanted the other techniques. The advantage of the cryofixation procedure is to eliminate treatments such as chemical fixation or staining which may be a source of artifacts. In addition, the freeze-etching technique offers the interesting possibilities of revealing the surface structures of unfractured particles as well as the internal structures of fractured particles.

Variations in the size and shape of the particle replicas, which reflect various aspects of the particle morphology, arise from the varying orientations with respect to shadowing and from the varying degrees of exposure of the particle above the ice background. Because the three dimensional nature of the replicated surface is retained by the replica itself,[17] stereoscopic views of the replica may give a better appreciation of the particle morphology. Furthermore, it has been suggested that three dimensional reconstruction of surface profiles may be possible from freeze-etching electron micrographs.[18]

The results obtained with TYMV demonstrate the performance of the methods employed. The 2-, 3- and 5-fold symmetry displayed by the particles and the dimensions of the particle, 320 Å, and its subunits, 70 Å, found in freeze-etching replicas correspond closely to the characteristics of the virus determined by negative staining and crystallographic techniques.[19, 20] The resolution of the freeze-etching technique, in the case of TYMV, is not worse than that of negative staining. Moreover, the freeze-etching technique reveals the morphology of only one face of the particle instead of the superposition of the two oposite faces in the case of negative staining.

The freeze-etching studies of serum LDL_2 reveal several structural features. The most striking of these is the "knobby" surface, much more deeply indented than that of TYMV indicating the presence in each particle of a small number of globules. It would be difficult to establish the number of globules per particle and their precise location on the basis of the electron microscopy alone. How-

FIGURE 3. Montage of freeze-etching replicas, such as FIGURE 2, of human serum LDL_2. The particles marked by arrows represent a few examples of the particles used in the statistical analysis (see text). Some of the particles display coarse 2- and 3-fold symmetry (arrow). The bar represents 1000 Å. (From Gulik-Krzywicki et al.[8] By permission of the *Journal of Molecular Biology*.)

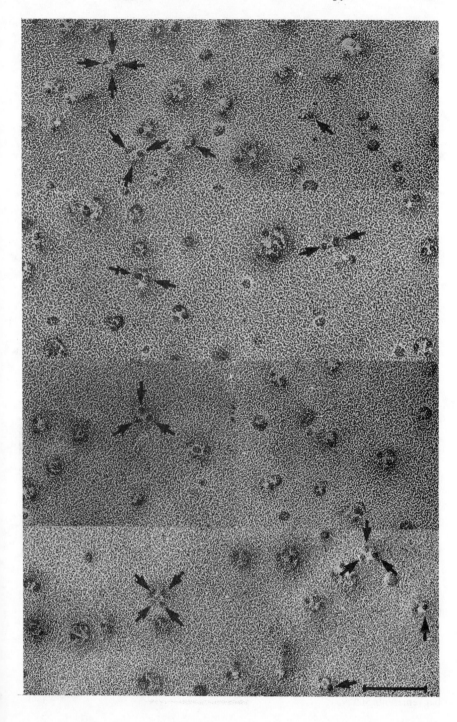

ever, the size of the globules (~80 Å), their number, the interglobular distance (~200 Å), and the overall size of the particles (~300 Å) are in remarkable agreement with the results of the solution x-ray scattering study and with the model proposed by Luzzati et al.[9] (FIGURES 4 & 5).

The chemical nature of the globular subunits can not be determined on the basis of the freeze-etching studies alone. The results of the x-ray scattering study indicate that the globules should be composed predominantly of protein. In agreement with this conclusion, preliminary freeze-etching studies of trypsin-modified LDL$_2$ have shown a reduced size of the morphological subunits.

It is worthwhile to discuss in more detail the problem of symmetry. In the case of TYMV the observation of 5-, 3- and 2-fold rotation axes in the electron microscopic pictures provides strong support for an icosahedral symmetry (point group 532).[19-21] Likewise, for LDL$_2$, the presence of 2- and 3-fold rotation axes supports tetrahedral symmetry (point group 23).[9, 21] However, in the case of TYMV, crucially important chemical information was available in support of the icosahedral symmetry; analogous chemical information is lacking in the case of LDL$_2$. This problem is discussed extensively by Luzzati et al.[9]

In the case of VLDL and HDL$_3$, the results shown here indicate that the freeze-etching technique has potential value for the study of lipoprotein classes other than LDL$_2$. We can mention, in this context, the work of Forte and Nichols[1] who have suggested the usefulness of the freeze-etching technique for studies of VLDL and chylomicrons and that of Ohtsuki et al.[2] who have investigated HDL$_3$.

We must add a few technical comments and a word of caution. We have shown that gross aggregation and/or morphological damage to the particles may be avoided if rapid cryofixation procedures are used. However, forth-

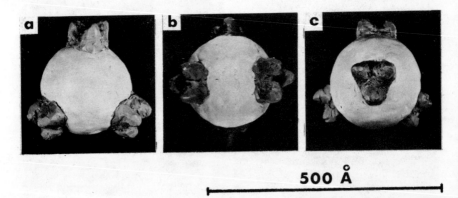

500 Å

FIGURE 4. The structure of LDL$_2$ as proposed by Luzzati et al.[9] Three photographs of a representative plasticine model. The model consists of a spherical, predominantly lipid, core (in white), diameter 205 Å, surrounded by four protein globules (in gray) at tetrahedral positions. The diameter of each protein globule is ~95 Å and the interglobular distance is ~230 Å. Note that the segregation of the protein and the lipid does not have to be complete; some of the protein may well be embedded in the lipids in the core or be located at the lipid–water interface and vice-versa. The bar represents 500 Å.

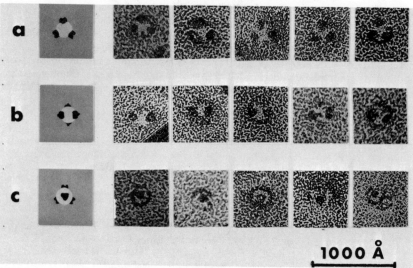

FIGURE 5. Montage of photographs of the three principal orientations of the model for LDL₂ shown in FIGURE 4 and several examples of individual LDL₂ particles taken from electron micrographs such as FIGURES 2 & 3. The bar represents 1000 Å.

coming technical improvements are expected to further diminish the danger of freezing artifacts. The fracturing process may, in some cases, result in fractures through individual particles. Although such fractures may provide insight into the internal structure, they forcibly distort the surface structure. Thus, proper interpretation will require that distinction be made among fractured and unfractured particles. The three-dimensional nature of the replica can potentially be exploited to assist in making such a distinction. Finally, with recent technical developments in the freeze-etching technique, we have been able to visualize the substructure of the TYMV morphological units. We hope that this advance will lead to additional insights into lipoprotein morphology as well.

SUMMARY

The structure of serum lipoproteins in solution has been investigated by freeze-etching electron microscopy employing rapid freezing techniques. Turnip yellow mosaic virus was used to demonstrate the performance of these techniques and their capability to provide information about the structure of particles in solution. Low-density lipoproteins appeared to deviate markedly from a smooth spherical shape. Instead, the outer layer of the particles appeared to consist of a small number of globules. The number, dimensions, and arrangements of the globules agree remarkably with the tetrahedral model proposed by Luzzati *et al.*[9] for the low temperature form of LDL₂. Further, we show that the freeze-etching electron microscopy technique may be capable of providing structural information with other lipoproteins.

ACKNOWLEDGMENTS

The authors would like to thank Dr. J. Witz for the sample of TYMV, Drs. V. Luzzati and A. Tardieu for numerous useful discussions and critical remarks, Drs. A. Scanu, R. Wissler, and G. Fless for their interest in the work and for the sample of diet induced hyperlipidemic Rhesus monkey serum LDL_2, Mr. J. C. Dedieu for excellent technical assistance, and Mrs. B. Gascard for secretarial assistance.

REFERENCES

1. FORTE, T. & A. V. NICHOLS. 1972. Adv. Lipid Res. **10**:1–41.
2. OHTSUKI, M., C. EDELSTEIN, M. SOGARD & A. M. SCANU. 1977. Proc. Natl. Acad. Sci. USA **74**:5001–5005.
3. POLLARD, H., A. M. SCANU & E. W. TAYLOR. 1969. Proc. Natl. Acad. Sci. USA **64**:304–310.
4. ZINGSHEIM, H. P. & H. PLATTNER. 1976. *In* Methods in Membrane Biology. E. D. Korn, Ed. Vol. 7: 1–146. Plenum Publishing Corp. New York, N.Y.
5. GULIK-KRZYWICKI, T. & M. J. COSTELLO. 1978. J. Microsc. **112**:103–113.
6. PLATTNER, H., W. W. SCHMITT-FUMIAN & L. BACHMANN. 1973. *In* Freeze-Etching Techniques and Applications. E. L. Benedetti & P. Favard, Eds. pp. 81–100. Société Française de Microscopie Electronique, Paris.
7. BACHMANN, L. & W. W. SCHMITT-FUMIAN. 1973. *In* Freeze-Etching Techniques and Applications. E. L. Benedetti & P. Favard, Eds. pp. 63–80. Société Française de Microscopie Electronique, Paris.
8. GULIK-KRZYWICKI, T., M. YATES & L. P. AGGERBECK. 1979. J. Mol. Biol. **131**:475–484.
9. LUZZATI, V., A. TARDIEU & L. P. AGGERBECK. 1979. J. Mol. Biol. **131**:435–473.
10. DECKELBAUM, R. J., G. G. SHIPLEY, D. M. SMALL, R. S. LEES & P. K. GEORGE. 1975. Science **190**:392–394.
11. SCANU, A. M., H. POLLARD & W. READER. 1968. J. Lipid Res. **9**:342–349.
12. NOBLE, R. P. 1968. J. Lipid Res. **9**:673–700.
13. OUCHTERLONY, O. 1949. Acta Pathol. Microbiol. Scand. **26**:507–511.
14. FLESS, G. M., R. W. WISSLER & A. M. SCANU. 1976. Biochem. **15**:5799–5805.
15. AGGERBECK, L. P., M. YATES, A. TARDIEU & V. LUZZATI. 1978. J. Appl. Cryst. **11**:466–472.
16. MATTHEWS, R. E. F. 1960. Virology **12**:521–539.
17. STEERE, R. L. 1973. *In* Freeze-Etching Techniques and Applications. E. L. Benedetti & P. Favard, Eds. pp. 223–255. Société Française de Microscopie Electronique, Paris.
18. KRBECEK, R., C. GEBHARDT, H. GRULER & E. SACKMANN. 1979. Biochim. Biophys. Acta **554**:1–22.
19. FINCH, J. T. & A. KLUG. 1966. J. Mol. Biol. **15**:344–364.
20. KLUG, A., W. LONGLEY & R. LEBERMAN. 1966. J. Mol. Biol. **15**:315–343.
21. CRICK, F. H. C. & J. D. WATSON. 1956. Nature **177**:473–475.

DISCUSSION OF THE PAPER

DR. P. LAGGNER: From what you said, I got the impression that freeze-etching alone does not allow you to deduce the model that you proposed.

On the other hand, if I read your papers in *Journal of Molecular Biology* inclusive of your recent one, on the solution of x-ray scattering study, there is a clear distinction between what is factual and what is speculative. You state that the model is supported by electron microscopy. Now, I would like to ask the question, is the model that you propose a necessary consequence of the x-ray scattering studies?

DR. L. P. AGGERBECK: I did not want to talk about small-angle x-ray scattering experiments in my presentation because of time constraints. So, I just summarized in the first five slides the solution x-ray scattering data, and those conclusions were drawn from the x-ray scattering experiments. I believe that the electron microscopic observations provide us with another set of observations, which permit conclusions by themselves. It so happens that the models constructed in each case agrees quite well with all the experimental data that we have collected.

DR. LAGGNER: That leads me to the second question. From freeze-etching electron microscopy in membranes there has been for a long time a dispute as to what one really sees. Namely, are you visualizing the surface or the inner portions? Thus, I wonder whether you can exclude the possibility that the pictures you are seeing here are a consequence of fracturing through the particle.

DR. AGGERBECK: I tried to state clearly that when we interpreted the electron microscopic images we attempted to make a distinction between fractured and nonfractured particles. About the existence of the globules I have no doubts. With the aid of the solution x-ray scattering experiments we are able to interpret the electron microscopic observations a little bit better. Also, stereoscopic views helped us in our conclusions.

DR. LAGGNER: Why do you think that these patterns do not show up in any of the other electron microscopy techniques?

DR. AGGERBECK: I think I can only speculate as to why they do not.

QUESTION: In your last summary slide you state that you will be able to visualize the internal structure of LDL or core. Do you think that any of the pictures that you showed are showing an inside structure?

DR. AGGERBECK: In the case of LDL, probably not. In the case of very-low-density lipoproteins, there are clearly particles that have been fractured. If somebody wants to see a picture of very-low-density lipoproteins I could show it to indicate that in some cases you can clearly see structures that are presumably not surface structures.

I might also mention in that respect that Forte and Nichols published in *Advances in Lipid Research* several years ago photos of chylomicrons, which I believe were prepared by the freeze-etching technique. They also suggested the utility of the freeze-etching technique to visualize chylomicrons and very-low-density lipoprotein subclasses, although they did not publish anything with respect to low-density lipoproteins.

QUESTION: The other question I have concerns the surface organization of apoB on LDL in terms of condensing it into small numbers of globules. Now, the analysis for a non-centro-symmetric component—and I do not want to discuss the x-ray scattering in too much detail—is formal and it is fine. I am perfectly happy with that. My problem with condensing the protein into such a small number of globules is this. With LDL as well as with HDL, if you do the calculations of what the surface area available in the lipoprotein is—and I have certain reservations about doing those types of calculations—you find that for both HDL and LDL the phospholipids in fact do not cover very much of the surface or are insufficient to cover the surface.

DR. AGGERBECK: That calculation necessarily depends upon the radius of the particle.

QUESTION: What about doing that for the surface of 100 Å radius, such as LDL?

DR. AGGERBECK: There is no problem. You can cover the surface with a phospholipid–cholesterol mixture quite adequately. The area in square angstroms per phospholipid or cholesterol molecule is reported in our article in the *Journal of Molecular Biology*. I think that it is 65 to 75 Å^2 per molecule.

DR. L. J. BANASZAK: I think that yours is a fairly exciting model. One question is, assuming that the surface globule represents a protein of some kind, have you calculated how far it would penetrate into the particle, assuming it is cylindrical or something like that?

DR. AGGERBECK: Naturally, we played all of those types of games. Let me summarize by saying this: On the basis of the model that I showed, there is about 70% of protein that presumably is in the form of globules on the surface and there is about 30% that is somewhere else, perhaps connecting the globules. This could be considered penetration into the particle.

DR. HUNTER: Assuming the knobs are proteins—and I am not quite sure of your conception of the fluidity of these knobs—do you actually think that these knobs are rigidly held in spheri-symmetrical position *in vivo*?

My second question would be, have you at all looked at a gluteraldehyde fixation to see if there is any association of these knobs close enough for, say, cross-linking or some sort of cross-linking study, and then looked at the freeze-etch of that?

DR. AGGERBECK: With respect to the first question, the model would indicate that the knobs would be anchored in tetrahedral position. I think there are ways we might be able to test that with cross-linking experiments as you suggested.

We have not done cross-linking experiments as yet. I think experiments of that type, not only at low temperature, which is the form that we have discussed, but also at high temperature probably would be interesting.

DR. W. A. BRADLEY: I believe that the association of the apoproteins is very possible so that the formation of globules is not beyond something that one can believe. I would like to know what that apoprotein looks like in your freeze-etched studies in VLDL. Do you see globules?

DR. AGGERBECK: We have not studied in detail the very-low-density lipoproteins. What I attempted to do was to describe a complex series of replicas. If we see replicas of these particles they appear to have a surface layer removed. We see other images and replicas of particles that appear to have a large portion of the core removed. In some cases we see particles that have globules, if you will, with a small number in the proximity to the edge of roughly spherical-appearing larger particles. These globules are about 90 Å in diameter.

I want to stress that I have absolutely no idea what the small globules are—whether they are protein or lipid, whether they are related to the VLDL structure itself or whether they represent an aggregation of protein and lipid. At the moment, all I can do is describe the images and plan further studies from there.

RATIONAL DESIGN OF SYNTHETIC MODELS FOR LIPOPROTEINS *

D. Fukushima,† E. T. Kaiser,‡ F. J. Kézdy, D. J. Kroon,
J. P. Kupferberg, and S. Yokoyama

*Departments of Chemistry and Biochemistry
University of Chicago
Chicago, Illinois 60637*

Our research on structure–function relationships in lipoproteins rests on the premise that small fragments of a protein molecule may exhibit some of the fundamental properties of the native protein itself. In enzymes, functional groups necessary for catalysis that are far apart in the linear sequence of the amino acids are brought into close proximity because of the tertiary structure. Therefore, to attempt to mimic the catalytic activity of an enzyme through the synthesis of a small portion of it around one active site residue would be naïve, in general. In contrast, structural proteins may contain smaller repeating domains on a single polypeptide chain. In the case of the principal polypeptide component of HDL, apolipoprotein A-I (apoA-I), a substantial part of the molecule has been shown by Fitch to contain a region of repeating structural units 22 amino acids in length.[1] These domains have a high helix-forming potential.[2] In the α-helical conformation, the hydrophobic and hydrophilic groups of the protein are segregated on opposite sides of the cylindrical segments. We have been engaged in testing the hypothesis that important properties of apolipoproteins such as their high collapse pressure in monolayers, their considerable tendency to aggregate, their ability to bind tightly to lipid surfaces and their activation of lecithin:cholesterol acyltransferase (LCAT) might be related to their potential for forming "amphiphilic" α-helical structures.

In our initial tests of this hypothesis, we investigated synthetic fragments of apoA-I; the sequences of the synthetic peptides corresponding to segments of apoA-I are listed in TABLE 1. The sequence of peptide I corresponds to that of residues 158–168 of apoA-I, peptide II to residues 147–168, and peptide III to residues 114–133, acetylated at the N-terminal. The numbering and amino acid composition used are those of the original sequence published by Baker *et al.*[3] Peptide I was prepared because it had been suggested by Fitch [1] that there might be 11 amino acid repeating units in apoA-I, and this fragment appeared to be a suitable prototypic peptide to test this hypothesis. Peptide II was chosen because it corresponds to the region of apoA-I with the highest helix forming potential according to Chou and Fasman analysis.[2] A terminal Pro was included because, according to Fitch's analysis,[1] Pro or Gly residues are believed to punctuate the amphiphilic helical segments of apoA-I as helix

* The studies reported in this paper were supported by U.S. Public Health Service (USPHS) Program Project HL-18577, USPHS Medical Scientist Traineeship 5TGM-07821, USPHS Cardiovascular Pathophysiology and Biochemistry Training Grant HL-7237, and USPHS Grant HL-15062 (SRC).

† Authors are listed in alphabetical order.

‡ To whom correspondence should be addressed.

breakers. Peptide III was prepared because we were not sure whether the lipid binding and surface properties of the amphiphilic helix required a straight run of helix or a sequence containing a helix breaker in the middle with helical segments on either side. Peptide IV, which has been prepared by us very recently, is a 44 amino acid segment corresponding to residues 124–167 of apoA-I, using the Baker *et al.* numbering system,[3] but with an amino acid sequence based on the revised sequence published by Brewer *et al.*[4] This peptide fragment contained two helical regions, according to Chou and Fasman analysis,[2] which are amphiphilic in this conformation.

The peptides were synthesized by the Merrifield solid phase method.[5] Typical examples of purification procedures employed for the peptides were given in a paper published from our laboratory on the syntheses of peptides I–III [6] and will not be repeated here. The criteria used to establish the purity of the

TABLE 1

SEQUENCES OF SYNTHETIC PEPTIDES

I.   158–168 (A-I)
     His-Val-Asp-Ala-Leu-Arg-Thr-His-Leu-Ala-Pro

II. 147–168 (A-I)
     Leu-Gly-Glu-Glu-Met-Arg-Asp-Arg-Ala-Arg-Ala-
     His-Val-Asp-Ala-Leu-Arg-Thr-His-Leu-Ala-Pro

III. 114–133 (A-I)
     CH₃-CO-Glu-Met-Glu-Leu-Tyr-Arg-Gln-Lys-Val-Glu-
     Pro-Leu-Arg-Ala-Glu-Leu-Gln-Glu-Gly-Ala

IV. 124–167 (A-I)
     Pro-Leu-Arg-Ala-Glu-Leu-Gln-Glu-Gly-Ala-Arg-
     Gln-Lys-Leu-His-Glu-Leu-Gln-Glu-Lys-Leu-Ser-
     Pro-Leu-Gly-Gln-Gln-Met-Arg-Asp-Arg-Ala-Arg-
     Ala-His-Val-Asp-Ala-Leu-Arg-Thr-His-Leu-Ala

V.   Synthetic Model Amphiphilic Peptide
     Pro-Lys-Leu-Glu-Glu-Leu-Lys-Glu-Lys-Leu-Lys-
     Glu-Leu-Leu-Glu-Lys-Leu-Lys-Glu-Lys-Leu-Ala

peptides included amino acid analysis, high voltage paper electrophoresis, thin layer chromatoagraphy in several solvent systems, high pressure liquid chromatography (in several instances), and automated Edman degradation. The results obtained indicated that the peptides that we used in our studies were at least 99% pure.

As can be seen from TABLE 2 which summarizes the physical properties of the peptides, the circular dichroism (CD) measurements on solutions of peptides I through IV did not indicate the presence of a great deal of α helix. There was a small progression in the amount of helix with increasing chain length, the CD spectrum of the 44 amino acid containing peptide IV showing approximately 18% helix in aqueous solution.

To examine the lipid binding ability of the peptides we employed highly purified hen egg lecithin [7] single bilayer vesicles as our model system. We used

TABLE 2

HELICITY IN SOLUTION AND VESICLE BINDING PROPERTIES OF PEPTIDES

Peptide	% α helix	$K_d \times 10^6$ for binding to PC single bilayer vesicle* (M)	$K_d \times 10^6$ for binding to mixed PC cholesterol single bilayer vesicles* (M)	N (amino acid residues bound per PC molecule)	
				PC vesicles	Mixed vesicles
I	~8[†]	>3000	—	—	—
II	15[†]	6.9	47.9	0.24	0.37
III	13[†]	~20	—	0.24	—
IV	18	3.9	8.1	0.20	0.40
V	50[‡]	1.9	2.8	0.33	0.60
apoA-I	61	0.94	0.30	0.28[‡][§]	0.60[§]

* K_d value is that measured at optimum pH.

[†] KROON, D. J., J. P. KUPFERBERG, E. T. KAISER & F. J. KÉZDY, 1978. J. Am. Chem. Soc. **100:**5975–5977.

[‡] FUKUSHIMA, D., J. P. KUPFERBERG, S. YOKOYAMA, D. J. KROON, E. T. KAISER & F. J. KÉZDY, 1979. J. Am. Chem. Soc. **101:**3703–3705.

[§] Assuming that only 2⁄3 of the apoA-I residues participate in binding.

these vesicles because of their excellent stability [8] and because of their similarity to lipoproteins with respect to the size and composition of the aliphatic chains of their lipids. Peptide binding to the vesicles was assessed by measurement of free and bound peptide, separated either by chromatography on Sepharose 6B or Cl–4B or by ultrafiltration through a 100-Å pore Amicon membrane.

The results of the binding studies are summarized in TABLE 2. Peptide I, containing 11 amino acids, bound very poorly to the vesicles. On the other hand, peptide II, which had the highest amphiphilic α-helical potential [2] of any 22 amino acid segment of apoA-I, bound to the vesicles reasonably well in acidic solution, but poorly at higher pH. The dissociation constants of the peptide II–vesicle complex as a function of pH are shown in FIGURE 1. The pH dependency observed suggested the simple equilibrium illustrated in Scheme 1, in which a single ionization governs the ability of the peptide to bind to the vesicle. In other words, only the peptide species containing the protonated form of a critical residue (PH) is able to bind to the binding site on the vesicle (B), and once the peptide is bound (BPH), the critical residue must remain protonated.

$$PH + B \overset{K_d}{=\!=\!=\!=} BPH$$

$$K_a \Big\Updownarrow$$

$$P + H^+$$

SCHEME 1

Although for the sake of simplicity we derived the binding equilibrium equation using the Langmuir isotherm, which implies the existence of discrete binding sites at the surface, it is clear that in all probability the adsorbed peptide forms a saturable mixed monolayer with the phospholipid and that mathematically the two models are equivalent. For the equilibria in Scheme 1, a simple expression describes the relationship between peptide binding and pH (Equation 1), where $K_{d(app)}$ is the apparent dissociation constant at a given pH, B_0 is the total number of binding sites on the vesicle surface (0.011 mole peptide per mole of phosphatidyl choline), P_0 is the total peptide concentration, BPH is the concentration of bound peptide, K_d is the dissociation constant when the critical residue(s) of the peptide are fully protonated, K_a is the ionization constant of the critical residue(s), and H^+ is the hydrogen ion concentration. In conformity with Equation 1, a plot of $K_{d(app)}$ versus $1/H^+$ gives a straight line (inset, FIGURE 1) with an intercept, $K_d = (6.4 \pm 2.0) \times 10^{-6}$ M and a slope $K_d K_a = (3.92 \pm 0.09) \times 10^{-12}$ M². The pK_a calculated from the slope and intercept is 6.21 (range 6.04 to 6.34). The observed pK_a value suggests that the ionization involved is that of the imidazole of histidine. The theoretical curve in FIGURE 1 was generated using Equation 1 and the above parameters.

$$K_{d(app)} = \frac{(B_0\text{-BPH})(P_0\text{-BPH})}{(\text{BPH})} = K_d + K_d K_a \frac{1}{H^+}. \tag{1}$$

A possible explanation of the observation that only the protonated peptide binds to the phospholipid vesicles is that the bound peptide is in the helical

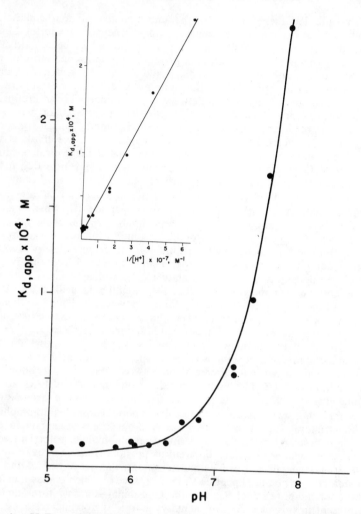

FIGURE 1. pH Dependency of the dissociation constant of the egg lecithin single bilayer vesicle–peptide complex. The theoretical curve was generated from Equation 1 using $K_d = 6.4 \times 10^{-6}$ M and $K_a = 6.17 \times 10^{-7}$ M. The binding of the peptide was measured at 25° by rapid ultrafiltration and fluorimetry. Inset: Reciprocal plot of the binding data according to Equation 1.

form and that this form is stabilized in its protonated state by the environment at the vesicle surface. In aqueous solutions the pH dependency of the molar ellipticities shows the "random-coil" to be the predominant form at all pH values, and thus the protonation of the peptide does not appreciably influence the helix-coil equilibrium. If we assume that only the protonated helix binds to the vesicle surface, this implies that K_d is actually the product of the intrinsic dissociation constant for the protonated helix–vesicle complex and the coil-to-helix ratio of the protonated peptide in solution.

The question then arises why the unprotonated random coil has a low affinity for the surface of the vesicle. A possible answer lies in the high interfacial pressure of the phospholipid vesicle, estimated to be around 30 dyn/cm.[9, 10] With such a high interfacial pressure, unfolding one mole of peptide, entailing an increase of 260 Å²/mole would require 10 kcal/mole work done against the surface pressure. Thus, the more compact helical structure is strongly favored during insertion between the phospholipid head groups. While the pH dependency of the binding of peptide II can be accounted for in terms of the favorable interaction of its protonated amphiphilic helical form with the phospholipid vesicles, an alternative explanation, which we think is unlikely but which cannot be ruled out, is that protonation of the critical residue(s) in the peptide favors formation of the complex with the vesicle due to dipole–dipole interactions of the residue(s) with the polar groups, for instance.

Studies on the lipid binding ability of peptides III and IV are much less complete than those with II. In the case of peptide III, which has its Pro residue toward the middle of the segment, binding to the phosphatidylcholine vesicles was very poor in neutral or basic solution but became appreciable in acidic solution. Finally, among the peptides we have synthesized with sequences corresponding to fragments of apoA-I, peptide IV, which contains two amphiphilic helical regions binds most tightly to the vesicles. These data and the trends observed support the idea that the amphiphilic helix is the structural feature of apoA-I involved in lipid binding. However, although we believe that the peptides are in a helical form when bound to the vesicles, we have no direct proof for this hypothesis from any studies done on the natural fragments. Furthermore, at this point we cannot dismiss the possibility that the observations made are related in some way to the specific amino acid sequences of the fragments and to particular interactions between amino acid residues and the phospholipid vesicles. The latter ambiguity is one that is hard to escape as long as modeling studies are made in which the natural sequence is employed.

A far better way, therefore, to test the hypothesis that the amphiphilic helix is the structural feature of apoA-I required for lipid binding is to design a peptide with a high potential for forming an amphiphilic helix and consisting of an amino acid sequence as different as possible from any region present in apoA-I and then to proceed with determining the properties of the peptide. Accordingly, we prepared peptide V, the sequence of which is shown in TABLE 1. Except for the N-terminal Pro and the C-terminal Ala only three amino acids are present in this peptide, Glu and Lys as the hydrophilic residues and Leu as the lipophilic residue. The C-terminal Ala is present principally because we have had extensive experience with the solid-phase synthesis of C-terminal Ala-containing peptides, and the N-terminal Pro is present because we wanted to put a helix breaker at this point, although the presence of this residue at the N-terminal is undoubtedly not crucial. The amino acid sequence was chosen to give a nearly equal distribution of acidic and basic residues on the hydrophilic side and segregation of the hydrophobic and hydrophilic residues corresponding reasonably closely with that seen in Fitch's analysis of the apoA-I sequence.[1] Estimation of the helical content of peptide V by circular dichroism showed a marked dependence of the molar ellipticity on the peptide concentration. The concentration dependency of the molar ellipticity was consistent with cooperative tetramerization of the peptide with $K_{dissoc} = 9.7 \times 10^{-16}$ M³ at pH 7.0. Gel permeation chromatography on Sephadex G-50 also demonstrated the formation of tetramers of peptide V. In 0.1 M phosphate buffer at pH 7.0, the helicity calculated for the peptide at a concentration of 1.7×10^{-4} M was 50%.

Measurements of the binding of peptide V to the egg lecithin single bilayer vesicles by rapid ultrafiltration and fluorimetric peptide assay yielded a K_d value of 1.9×10^{-6} M for the complex. Fifteen peptide molecules were bound per thousand phospholipid molecules. For comparison, measurements of apoA-I binding to the single bilayer vesicles by gel permeation chromatography and fluorimetric peptide assay yielded a K_d value of 9.4×10^{-7} M with an apoA-I to phospholipid ratio of 1.8 per 1,000 molecules. Since apoA-I is believed to have approximately six amphiphilic α-helical segments, this means that on the basis of the number of helixes present the amphiphilic peptide V binds more tightly to the phospholipid vesicles that does apoA-I. Also, the number of amphiphilic helical peptides bound is in reasonable correspondence with the number of amphiphilic helixes bound in the case of apoA-I.

Analysis of the force–area curve of insoluble monolayers of peptide V using the equation [11]

$$\pi[A\text{-}A_{00}(1 - \kappa\pi)] = C,$$

showed that the surface behavior of the monolayers corresponded closely with that of apoHDL [12] and apoA-I monolayers. [13] The compressibility measured for peptide V was $\kappa = 2.1 \times 10^2$ cm/dyne, nearly identical to that found for apoHDL, $\kappa = 1.8 \times 10^{-2}$ cm/dyne. The collapse pressures ($\pi = 22$ dynes/cm) of the peptide and protein monolayers were the same. Furthermore, the limiting area, A_{00}, of the peptide extrapolated to zero surface pressure is 23 Å² per amino acid residue, whereas it is 16.3 Å² per amino acid for apoHDL and 22 Å² for apoA-I. These results are consistent with the hypothesis that the stable form of peptide V at the air–water interface has a compact structure, presumably an amphiphilic helix. From estimates obtained from surface filling calculations, it appears reasonable to propose that the peptide molecules bind to the vesicles in the area between the lecithin head groups with the lipophilic side chains of the peptide apposed to the lipophilic free surface of the vesicle. This proposal leads to the expectation that lecithin:cholesterol single bilayer vesicles should bind more peptide than pure lecithin vesicles.

In the binding of the amphiphilic peptide V to mixed phosphatidylcholine: cholesterol (4:1) vesicles, the K_d value for peptide V (2.8×10^{-6} M) was larger than the K_d for its binding to the pure phosphatidylcholine vesicles. The converse was true for apoA-I where K_d decreased to 3×10^{-7} M for its binding to the mixed vesicles. The B_0 value for binding to the mixed vesicles was increased by 1.98×10^{-3} moles of apoA-I per mole of lecithin and by 1.21×10^{-2} moles of the peptide per mole of lecithin, respectively, as compared to the egg lecithin vesicles. The increased capacity of the mixed vesicles for the binding of apoA-I and of peptide V corresponds to 1.83 amino acid residues per cholesterol molecule in the case of apoA-I and 1.54 amino acid residues per cholesterol molecule in the case of peptide V, assuming that 70% of the phospholipid molecules are distributed in the outer layer of the vesicles and that the increased numbers of the peptide or protein molecules bound are associated with the cholesterol present. Based on the surface area occupied by the cholesterol molecule (39.1 Å²), [14] the area per amino acid for apoA-I on the mixed vesicle surface is calculated to be 21.6 Å², in good agreement with the area per amino acid of the protein in the HDL$_3$ particle. [14] (These numbers are based on the assumption that only ⅔ of the amino acid residues in apoA-I, corresponding to the helical regions,[13] are involved in lipid binding.) Consequently, most of the cholesterol molecules in the outer surface of the mixed vesicles are likely to be covered by the amino acid residues of any bound apoA-I or peptide V. Repulsion between the hydrophobic domain of peptide V and the hydroxyl group of cholesterol may account for the decrease in the affinity for the binding of peptide V to the mixed vesicles as compared to the pure egg lecithin vesicles and the increase observed in the case of apoA-I. In contrast, it may be that for a yet unexplained reason the amphiphilic helical region of apoA-I has increased affinity toward the hydroxyl of the cholesterol molecule. This aspect of the binding of amphiphilic helixes to mixed vesicles is currently under further investigation in our laboratory.

In recent experiments peptide V has been found to activate the enzyme LCAT. While a complete treatment of these findings is beyond the scope of the present article, it should be mentioned that analysis of the activation process suggests that it can be explained by a mechanism in which the binding of the peptide to mixed phosphatidylcholine:cholesterol vesicles makes the substrates available to the enzyme for reaction.

In conclusion, our experiments on the interactions of synthetic peptide fragments of apoA-I with pure egg lecithin vesicles as well as with mixed vesicles are consistent with the proposal that the amphiphilic helical regions of this protein are responsible for binding to lipid surfaces. The strongest evidence for this hypothesis comes from our experiments with peptide V, which was rationally designed to have a high degree of amphiphilic α-helical character and proved to behave very similarly to apoA-I in its surface properties at the air–water interface and binding to phosphatidylcholine vesicles. Our observation that peptide V activates LCAT is important because it demonstrates that the activation process does not require the specific amino acid sequence of apoA-I. Experiments to elucidate the mechanism of the activation process are under way.

REFERENCES

1. FITCH, W. M. 1977. Genetics **86**:623–644.
2. CHOU, P. Y. & G. D. FASMAN. 1974. Biochemistry **13**:211–222.
3. BAKER, H. N., A. M. GOTTO, JR. & R. L. JACKSON. 1975. J. Biol. Chem. **250**: 2725–2738.
4. BREWER, H. B., JR., T. FAIRWELL, A. LaRUE, R. RONAN, A. HOUSER & T. J. BRONZERT. 1978. Biochem. Biophys. Res. Commun. **80**:623–630.
5. ERICKSON, B. W. & R. B. MERRIFIELD. 1976. *In* The Proteins, H. Neurath, R. Hill & C. L. Boeder, Eds. 3rd edit. Vol. 2: 255–527. Academic Press, New York, N.Y.
6. KROON, D. J. & E. T. KAISER. 1978. J. Org. Chem. **43**:2107–2113.
7. WELLS, M. A. & D. J. HANAHAN. 1969. Methods Enzymol. **14**:178–184.
8. AUNE, K. C., K. G. GALLAGHER, A. M. GOTTO, JR. & J. D. MORRISETT. 1977. Biochemistry **16**:2151–2156.
9. DEMEL, R. A., W. S. M. GEURTS VAN KESSEL, R. F. A. ZWAAL, B. ROELOFSEN & L. L. M. VAN DEENEN. 1975. Biochim. Biophys. Acta **406**:97–107.
10. PHILLIPS, M. C. & D. CHAPMAN. 1968. Biochim. Biophys. Acta **163**:301–313.
11. FUKUSHIMA, D., J. P. KUPFERBERG, S. YOKOYAMA, D. J. KROON, E. T. KAISER & F. J. KÉZDY 1979. J. Am. Chem. Soc. **101**:3703–3704.
12. CAMEJO, G. 1969. Biochim. Biophys. Acta **175**:290–300.

13. EDELSTEIN, C., F. J. KÉZDY, A. M. SCANU & B. W. SHEN. 1979. J. Lipid Res. **20:**143–153.
14. SHEN, B. W., A. M. SCANU & F. J. KÉZDY. 1977. Proc. Natl. Acad. Sci. USA **74:**837–841.

DISCUSSION OF THE PAPER

DR. J. C. OSBORNE: One comment and then two questions. I believe that this is the first time that the molecular properties in aqueous solutions of either a synthetic peptide or a fragment of amphiphilic proteins have been addressed quantitatively. That is a step in the right direction.

First, have you found any electrostatic contribution to the interaction of these fragments with your lipid vesicles? And second, have you looked at the rates of dissociation of your fragments from vesicles?

DR. E. T. KAISER: Because of the time limitations, I could not talk about the natural sequence 22-amino-acid peptide, but let me mention something now. We have a strong pH dependency of the binding to the vesicles; you probably will not remember that there are two histidine residues that come in the wrong region of the natural sequence if you fold it up on the helical wheel. The ionization behavior of the binding is quite simple. We have done a titration of the peptide, a careful titration and the binding does not follow the titration curve. What it rather follows is apparently the ionization of essentially one functional group, which we have not established but which we think is histidine because the pK is close to 7.

Now, I hesitate a little bit to interpret that further. It is clear then that it is not a simple electrostatic interaction. I would like to think that what is happening is somehow the ionization of the histidine controls coil to helix formation associated with the binding to the vesicle. But, we cannot absolutely rule out that there may be some dipole interaction or something like that occurring which affects the binding.

So, the upshot of it is that we think that the electrostatic contribution is probably not too important, but we do not have a clear assessment in a quantitative way.

Now, as to the rate of dissociation, we have tried hard but we have not been successful in getting good measurements. We have now some radioactively labeled peptides and we will try again, but we do not have numbers at this time.

DR. D. M. SMALL: You mean it is so fast you cannot measure it.

DR. KAISER: Yes. We have not been able to get any number on it. We have run into many technical problems with it.

COMMENT: If you look at the sequence that you had on the board, as well as that of apoA-I, I would like to suggest that perhaps what one is looking at here is not an amphipathic helix, but perhaps some sort of β structure where you have alternating side chains pointing in the same direction.

DR. KAISER: Do you mean on the vesicle or in solution?

COMMENT: The structure of the peptide itself.

DR. KAISER: The solution spectrum, to the extent that one believes the circular dichroism data, makes it look as though the structure is probably α helical.

COMMENT: Is it not true that circular dichroism would also be affected by the β structure?

DR. KAISER: Yes. I think that with peptides it may be a little risky to overinterpret the circular dichroism results. But I cannot really comment about the peptide structure more than to show that the CD spectrum resembles in many ways that of apoA-I. I guess that the point that I would have to make is that we have designed the peptide with the idea that it would be an amphiphilic helix.

DR. J. A. HUNTER: You mentioned many similarities between super helix and apoA-I, and I was wondering if you looked at the increase in helicity of the super helix peptide using CD when it was bound with phospholipids.

DR. KAISER: We have now done that. The problem I think is the quantitative interpretation of what a CD spectrum looks when a peptide binds to a vesicle.

The other point is that we are already starting off with a situation where we have a considerable amount of helix. By CD measurements alone I think there is little chance for detecting small differences between peptides with and without lipids.

DR. HUNTER: Did you suspect that some discoidal complex formation might have been generated.

DR. KAISER: We do not have any evidence for that. The behavior, for example, on the gel filtration columns and the elution of the vesicles is essentially the same before and after.

DR. HUNTER: Do you think that it may be just due to concentration?

DR. KAISER: We are working with PC vesicles which we think are quite stable for these purposes. I believe that they should permit the quantitative measurement of the dissociation constants.

DR. J. T. SPARROW: It is a nice piece of work, Dr. Kaiser, but I still am worried about the lack of CD changes in the presence of lipid. We have all seen these with serum proteins, and they are particularly dramatic with apoA-III and apoC-I; apoA-I is 85% helical in the presence of lipid. So, I think it is incumbent upon you to show that this peptide, like the one we have been working with, does increase its helicity in the presence of phospholipids. My peptide is about 25% helical in the absence of lipid. In the presence of lipid, it becomes 90% in a reproducible way.

DR. KAISER: I might comment on that. First of all, I think, as everybody knows, when you bind something to a vesicle and you measure the CD, you have some light scattering problems, which one has to take into account.

DR. SPARROW: I disagree with that. If you are getting true binding, you get clarification of the lipid and your problems with recording the CD spectrum are clearly not as great as if you have unbound peptide mixed with lipid.

DR. KAISER: But, you remember that we have the intact vesicles when we have the peptide bound, and under those conditions one does have light scattering problems. We can take care of them in a sense, but in a qualitative way.

I would hesitate to place a quantitative interpretation on the CD spectra of a peptide bound to a phospholipid. But, I am not a CD expert although I must say that I have my doubts.

DR. SPARROW: I have another question or two about the LCAT activation. I would like to know how you conduct your assay with the apoA-I synthetic fragments.

DR. KAISER: The reason why I did not present the LCAT results in detail is that we are still in the middle of this work and that one has, as you know, the possibility to have a phospholipase activity in addition to the LCAT activity.

I would not like to be held to this completely now because I think we have to look at it further; but in terms of what the peptide does, the 10% activation that I referred to was measured in terms of cholesteryl ester formation. On the other hand, if one looks at the loss of the acyl group from position 2 of the phosphatidylcholine, it is quite clear that in that respect the peptide behaves somewhat better and is closer actually to the behavior of apoA-I, and we have not sorted that out. I am not sure what that means.

DR. SPARROW: Are you using an isolated peptide-cholesterol-PC complex in your LCAT assay or is this a bulk assay?

DR. KAISER: We are using phosphatylcholine:cholesterol (4:1, molar ratio) mixed vesicles—essentially the same sort of system as Dr. Scanu has recently described.

DR. SPARROW: But have you separated the unbound peptide from the bound peptide?

DR. KAISER: We have not. We have essentially used the vesicle system mixed with the peptide. Although what I am saying cannot be considered as Gospel, we think that there is a reasonable correspondence between the dissociation constant of the peptide bound to the mixed vesicles and its activation of LCAT.

DR. SMALL: I think the two of you are working on such closely related areas that you might sit down during the intermission and continue on with this.

DR. SPARROW: I just felt that the activation of LCAT by your peptide is quite interesting since we have essentially used a completely different model peptide—the peptide 4 that I showed yesterday—and with that we find 65% of the activation compared to apoA-I. We have our own ideas about how our peptide is activating LCAT, and I was wondering how his data are interpreted.

DR. KAISER: I think basically what we felt from our own results was that the amphiphilic helix *per se* is not the full answer in terms of LCAT activation and that there are other factors that come in. As I indicated, the binding to the mixed vesicles to what we call the super helix is not as good as it is to the pure vesicle, and this is in contrast to apoA-I. If one makes a structural analysis of apoA-I, one finds arginines occurring at the wrong place; in other words, in hydrophobic regions. We think that by having a more hydrophilic residue in a hydrophobic environment LCAT activation is favored.

So, one of the things that we are trying to do is to make a nonperfect amphiphilic helix by inserting an arginine residue. Actually, we have other hypotheses that are equally probable, but maybe we should discuss this in a separate context.

DR. SPARROW: I was quite interested in the apoA-I data that you presented in regard to the activation of LCAT. We have a series of peptides from apoA-I that bind lipid but do not activate LCAT. We have another series of peptides that are very similar to the ones that you have made, although longer. We find that when we get into the area between 145 and 185 we observe LCAT activation.

I would like to know in your longer fragment, which I believe was 127 through 167, what percent of the activations did you get?

DR. KAISER: It looks relatively comparable to the so-called super helix.

DR. SPARROW: We find that our 145–185 peptide has about 20% to 25% of the activity as exhibited by apoA-I, and I believe that you are probably correct when you say that the hydrophobic region with the arginine residue is responsible, because the way we identified this region of apoA-I was to compare its helix probability with apoC-I. If you do that, you see in both cases a high conservation of sequence.

DR. V. LUZZATI: As you pointed out, we all feel painfully the lack of physical information on the structure of apolipoproteins, and I was wondering whether it would not be interesting to test those ideas on systems which are far better known. I am thinking of gramicidin A, for example.

DR. KAISER: One of the questions that has come up is, if amphiphilic or amphipathic α helices occur in a variety of proteins, why doesn't every one behave the same?

I think one point one has to remember is that there may be a different balance in charge. There may be different distributions of residues, a different proportion of the balance between hydrophobic and hydrophilic residues. We have been looking, for example, at some toxins where we are quite convinced that the amphiphilic helix plays a role in their function. We think that we understand the distribution between hydrophobic and hydrophilic residues and we are testing our hypothesis by using a similar approach to what we have followed for apoA-I—take a peptide with minimum homology and build that and see what will happen.

If you follow the natural sequence synthesis approach, which is certainly very useful, you run into the ambiguity of whether or not you have something which is very sequence dependent. You can, of course, go stepwise and replace individual amino acids, but you do not always obtain a clear-cut answer. I think that is one of the problems, for instance, in a lot of the work on hormone analogs where one goes and makes a single replacement but really does not have a strong feeling of the structural aspects. In many cases, clearly biological activity is sequence dependent, and then you are going to strike out with an approach like this. Thus, it is important to use some judgment as to whether or not the secondary structure is a controlling factor in function.

DR. JACKSON: One of the things that is very important in terms of these peptides is the hydrophobic index. As we tried to point out on several occasions, apoA-I has very little hydrophobic index in each one of its helical segments, whereas in apoC-I and C-2 and C-3 the hydrophobic index is much greater. Have you made other peptides with a higher hydrophobic index?

DR. KAISER: No. We have made some related peptides, but not really appreciatively higher.

DR. JACKSON: This one is about 800 or 900 daltons?

DR. KAISER: Something like that. In regard to some of the results that Dr. Sparrow presented yesterday, although they show some interesting possibilities with the hydrophobic index, I am not convinced that they demonstrate that this index is a controlling factor.

PLASMA RETINOL-BINDING PROTEIN *

DeWitt S. Goodman

Division of Metabolism and Nutrition
Department of Medicine
Columbia University College of Physicians & Surgeons
New York, New York 10032

INTRODUCTION

Vitamin A is transported in plasma as the lipid alcohol retinol, bound to a specific transport protein, plasma retinol-binding protein (RBP).[1] This protein has been studied extensively during the past decade, and considerable information is now available about its structure, metabolism, and biological roles.

In addition to its well documented role in vision,[2] vitamin A is essential for growth, reproduction, the maintenance of differentiated epithelia, and mucus secretion in higher animals. The exact nature of the role of vitamin A in these functions has not been defined at the molecular level, except for its role in vision.

The major natural sources of vitamin A in the diet are certain plant carotenoid pigments, such as β-carotene, and the long chain retinyl esters that are found in animal tissues. In either case, retinyl esters are formed in the intestine, and are transported into the body mainly in association with lymph chylomicrons. The chylomicron remnants, containing the newly-absorbed retinyl esters, are cleared by the liver, where vitamin A is normally stored for later use.

Vitamin A is mobilized from the liver as retinol bound to RBP. This is the form in which vitamin A is transported from the liver to its peripheral sites of action. Vitamin A mobilization from the liver, and its delivery to peripheral tissues, are highly regulated processes that are particularly controlled by processes that regulate the rates of the production and secretion of RBP by the liver.

Human RBP has a molecular weight of approximately 21,000, α_1-mobility on electrophoresis, and a single binding site for one molecule of retinol. RBP interacts strongly with another protein, plasma prealbumin, and normally circulates as a 1:1 molar RBP–prealbumin complex.[1, 3, 4] The usual level of RBP in plasma is about 40–50 μg/ml and that of prealbumin is about 200–300 μg/ml.[5]

The vitamin A transport system provides an interesting model for the study of protein–protein and protein–ligand interactions, and of the characteristics of a specific lipid binding and transport system. The aim of this review will be to summarize the information currently available about this transport system, with particular emphasis upon our knowledge of the structure and chemistry of RBP and prealbumin. More extensive discussions of the biological and metabolic aspects of the plasma vitamin A transport system can be found in other reviews of this subject.[6-9]

* The studies from the author's laboratory reported and commented upon here were supported by Grants HL 21006 and AM 05968 from the National Institutes of Health.

378

PREALBUMIN STRUCTURE

A great deal of detailed information is now available about the structure of prealbumin. In addition to its role in vitamin A transport, prealbumin plays a role in the binding and plasma transport of thyroid hormones.

The prealbumin molecule is a stable and symmetrical tetramer, composed of four identical subunits, with a molecular weight of 54,980.[10] The complete amino acid sequence of human prealbumin has been reported from our laboratory.[10] Crystalline prealbumin has been studied at 6-Å,[11] at 2.5-Å,[12] and at 1.8-Å[13] resolution. These studies have shown that the subunits have extensive β-sheet structure and are linked into stable dimers, each comprising two of the four subunits. A channel runs through the center of the prealbumin molecule, in which are located two symmetry-related binding sites for iodothyronine molecules. Only one molecule of thyroxine binds to prealbumin with high affinity, however, because of negative cooperativity.[12, 14]

Recent high-resolution x-ray crystallographic studies have shown that the prealbumin molecule contains two surface sites with structural complementarity to double-helical DNA.[15] Although the binding of prealbumin to DNA has not been reported, it has been suggested that the prealbumin molecule may serve as a model for the kind of structure that may be involved in hormone receptors with nuclear effects on DNA transcription.[15]

RBP STRUCTURE

Less detailed structural information is available about RBP. RBP has been crystallized,[16] although the crystals produced were not suitable for detailed x-ray study. Studies employing circular dichroism and optical rotary dispersion have shown that RBP appears to have a relatively high content of unordered conformation, a significant but small complement of β conformation, and little or no α helix.[17, 18] The RBP molecule is a single polypeptide chain of about 185 amino acid residues and contains no bound lipid (other than retinol) and no carbohydrate.

The primary structure of human RBP has been reported very recently.[19] RBP is cleaved by cyanogen bromide into five fragments; of these, the carboxy-terminal fragment represents slightly more than half the molecule. In one recent study,[20] the five cyanogen bromide fragments were isolated and aligned, the amino acid sequences of four of the fragments were determined, and the sequence of almost two-thirds (the amino-terminal portion) of the RBP molecule was reported. Information was sought concerning the possible existence of sequence homologies between the RBP partial sequence and the amino acid sequences of other proteins whose primary structures are known. A computer search with appropriate programs failed to reveal homologies in sequence between RBP and any other known sequenced protein.[20] In another recent study, the complete primary structure of RBP was reported.[19] Slight discrepancies exist between the recent partial[20] and complete[19] sequence proposals, although in general the agreement between them is quite good. The reported complete sequence[19] consists of 182 amino acids, with the carboxy-terminal sequence: -Gly-Arg-Ser-Glu-Arg-Asn-Leu-COOH. This proposed carboxy-terminal sequence differs from those previously reported from the same[21] and other[22, 23] laboratories.

RBP–PREALBUMIN INTERACTION

The interaction of RBP with prealbumin is very sensitive to ionic strength, with dissociation of the protein–protein complex occurring at low ionic strength.[24, 25] The interaction of RBP with prealbumin is also strongly pH dependent. The maximum binding occurs near physiological pH and falls gradually at lower and higher pH values.[25]

Studies employing polarization of fluorescence [25] and equilibrium dialysis [26] have shown that there is no interdependence of the binding of thyroxine and of RBP to prealbumin. In contrast, the interaction of retinol with RBP appears to be stabilized by the formation of the RBP–prealbumin complex.[24, 27,28]

Circular dichroic spectral studies have been conducted to examine the effects of the RBP–prealbumin interaction on the secondary structures of the two proteins. In two studies,[17, 18] the results suggested that formation of the protein–protein complex results in very little if any alteration in the secondary structure of the two proteins. A third study suggested, however, that some conformational changes in one or both proteins may occur on formation of the RBP–prealbumin complex.[29] Further work is needed to fully resolve this question.

Although RBP normally circulates in plasma as a 1:1 molar complex with prealbumin, studies employing polarization of retinol fluorescence and velocity ultracentrifugation suggested that prealbumin may contain four binding sites for RBP, each with an apparent association constant of about 1.2×10^6 M^{-1}.[25] A report that the isolated prealbumin subunit showed some affinity for RBP is consistent with this conclusion.[30] In contrast, other studies employing several techniques appeared to show that one prealbumin molecule can bind only 1 to 1.35 molecules of RBP.[31]

This apparent discrepancy may have been largely resolved by fluorescence polarization studies of the interaction between RBPs and prealbumins of human and chicken.[32] The binding affinity between chicken plasma RBP and chicken prealbumin was essentially the same as between the respective human proteins. RBPs and prealbumins of human and chicken were found to cross-interact, displaying an affinity similar to that displayed by the proteins of the same species. Data analysis suggested that human prealbumin displayed approximately two binding sites for RBP, and chicken prealbumin approximately four such sites. It was suggested that prealbumin possesses four identical binding sites for RBP, but that the binding is of a negative cooperative nature, largely resulting from steric hindrance by already bound RBP molecules.

Taken together, these various studies strongly suggest that prealbumin contains four binding sites for human RBP. It seems reasonable to assume that each prealbumin subunit might contain one binding site for RBP, although additional direct evidence is needed to support this conclusion.

RBP–RETINOL INTERACTION

The structural features required for the binding of all-*trans* retinol to RBP appear to be fairly, but far from absolutely, specific. A large number of studies have explored the binding of a variety of retinoids and related compounds to apoRBP.[27, 29, 33-37] A number of isomers of retinol and of retinaldehyde, as well as retinoic acid and retinyl acetate, can bind to apoRBP with varying degrees of effectiveness. The affinity of RBP for retinoic acid is similar to its affinity for retinol.[36] A number of other retinyl derivatives and related compounds, such as some Schiff base retinylideneamines,[34] and related compounds such as a β-ionone and β-ionylideneacetic acid [37] can also bind to apoRBP. Compounds unrelated to vitamin A in structure (e.g., cholesterol, phytol) bind minimally to RBP or not at all.

Comparative Biology

During the past decade, RBP has been isolated from serum of many species other than man, including the rat, monkey, pig, dog, rabbit, cattle, and chicken (References 7–9 for earlier reviews and for references). In all of these species, RBP has been found to be a small protein of approximately 20,000 daltons, which binds one molecule of retinol per molecule of RBP. In spite of occasional reports to the contrary, the RBP of all of these species appears to circulate in plasma as a protein–protein complex together with a larger protein. In the cases where the larger protein has been isolated, it has been found to have a tetrameric structure and to generally resemble human prealbumin.

On the other hand, RBP isolated from fish (yellowtails) was somewhat smaller (16,000 daltons) and lacked binding affinity for prealbumin. The vitamin A transport system of the tadpole resembled that found in fish, but interestingly, the adult frog was found to transport vitamin A as the RBP–prealbumin complex.[38]

The comparative immunology of RBP from various species was studied using radioimmunoassays specifically developed for human and for rat RBP.[39] There was a high degree of immunological specificity within a given mammalian order. Sera from other primates cross-reacted with antiserum to human RBP, but not with antiserum to rat RBP, while sera from 4 of 5 rodents tested reacted with the antiserum to rat RBP, but not the antiserum to human RBP. Sera from other species failed to react in either assay, with the exception of a slight reactivity of canine serum in the human RBP immunoassay.

Despite these strong antigenic differences between RBPs from different mammalian orders and vertebrate classes, the structures that characterize the binding sites on RBP and prealbumin appear to be very similar across a range of species. As discussed above, RBPs and prealbumins of human and chicken cross-interact, and show interspecies affinities similar to those displayed by the proteins of the same species.[32] In addition, the affinities of human and of chicken RBP were found to be similar for both retinol and retinoic acid.[36] Rat RBP has been isolated by affinity chromatography on human prealbumin coupled to agarose,[40] and conversely rat prealbumin has been isolated by affinity chromatography on human RBP coupled to agarose.[41] These studies indicate that the binding sites on prealbumin for RBP, and on RBP for prealbumin, are structurally similar in the human, rat, and chicken proteins. Thus, it appears that the structural features that are essential for the biological roles of RBP and prealbumin were maintained during much of vertebrate evolution.

Clinical Studies: Roles of the Liver and Kidney

Many clinical studies have examined the effects of a variety of diseases on the plasma levels of RBP and prealbumin in humans. This topic is discussed in more detail in other reviews.[6-9] No disease has yet been found where RBP was totally absent or had abnormal immunological properties.

In patients with diseases of the liver, the plasma levels of vitamin A, RBP, and prealbumin have all been found to be markedly decreased.[5, 42, 43] The low levels of RBP and prealbumin reflect the facts that these proteins are both produced in the liver, and that there is presumably a reduced rate of synthesis of the proteins by the diseased liver. In patients with chronic renal disease, the level of RBP is highly elevated, while that of prealbumin remains normal.[5] The elevated levels of RBP reflect the fact that the kidney is normally the main catabolic site for RBP, so that RBP catabolism is impaired in chronic renal disease. RBP itself is small enough to be filtered by the renal glomeruli, whereas prealbumin and the RBP-prealbumin complex are not. Although very little RBP is normally present in the free state, its glomerular filtration and renal metabolism are sufficiently large to constitute the major catabolic route for RBP. Normally, very little RBP appears in the urine, as nearly all of the filtered RBP is resorbed and degraded by the renal tubules. In contrast, patients with tubular proteinuria clear RBP from plasma at a normal rate, but excrete large amounts of RBP in the urine (References 7 & 8 for reviews).

Several studies have examined the retinol transport system in patients with protein-calorie malnutrition.[44-47] Such patients have decreased concentrations of plasma RBP, prealbumin, and vitamin A. Low intake of dietary protein and calories is frequently accompanied by an inadequate intake of vitamin A. However, even in cases where there is adequate vitamin A intake, the plasma RBP and vitamin A levels are low, reflecting a functional impairment in the hepatic release of vitamin A because of defective production of RBP.

RETINOL DELIVERY: RBP RECEPTORS

RBP is responsible for the delivery of retinol from the liver to the extrahepatic sites of action of the vitamin. Information currently available suggests that the delivery process involves cell surface receptors for RBP. Thus, evidence has been reported suggesting that there are specific cell surface receptors for RBP on monkey small intestine mucosal cells[48] and on bovine pigment epithelial cells.[49, 50] With both kinds of cells, retinol was taken up (from holoRBP) by the cells without a concomitant uptake of RBP. Retinol was not taken up by the pigment epithelial cells when it was presented nonspecifically bound to bovine serum albumin.[50] Thus, RBP appears to deliver retinol to specific cell surface sites that "recognize" RBP, and to release retinol at these locations. The retinol then enters the cell for subsequent metabolism and action.

The apoRBP that results after delivery of retinol apparently has a reduced affinity for prealbumin. The fact that apoRBP definitely has affinity for prealbumin was shown by studies with serum from vitamin A-deficient rats; on gel filtration most of the apoRBP in such serum is found as the RBP-prealbumin complex.[51] Affinity chromatography studies in our laboratory, with prealbumin coupled to agarose, have shown, however, that the affinity of apoRBP for prealbumin is distinctly less than that of holoRBP. The reduced affinity of apoRBP for prealbumin results in its selective enrichment in the free RBP fraction, and its selective filtration by the renal glomeruli.

REGULATION OF RBP PRODUCTION AND SECRETION BY THE LIVER

Vitamin A mobilization from the liver, and its delivery to peripheral tissues, is highly regulated by factors that control the rates of RBP production and secretion by the liver. A major goal of our laboratory has been to try to elucidate the cellular and molecular mechanisms involved in the regulation of RBP production and secretion. These studies have employed the rat as an animal model, and a sensitive and specific radioimmunoassay for rat RBP.[51]

One factor which specifically regulates RBP secretion from the liver is the nutritional vitamin A status of the animal.[51-53] Thus, retinol deficiency specifically blocks the secretion of RBP from the liver, so that plasma RBP levels fall and liver RBP levels rise. Conversely, repletion of vitamin A-deficient rats intravenously with retinol stimulates the rapid secretion of RBP from the expanded liver pool (in the deficient rat) into the plasma. This release of RBP is not blocked by inhibitors of protein synthesis, indicating that it comes from the expanded liver pool of RBP, rather than from de novo protein synthesis.[52]

The block in RBP secretion seen after vitamin A depletion is highly specific for RBP. Thus, neither vitamin A depletion and deficiency, not retinol repletion of deficient rats, significantly altered plasma levels of prealbumin.[54] The secretion of RBP and prealbumin appear to be independently regulated processes, with formation of the RBP–prealbumin complex occurring in plasma, after secretion of the two proteins from the liver cell.

Studies are in progress in our laboratory to explore the roles of various subcellular organelles and structures in the secretion of RBP. RBP in the liver is mainly found associated with the liver microsomes,[55] and is particularly enriched in the rough microsomal fraction. The Golgi apparatus was found to contain a maximum of 22% of RBP in the liver in normal rats, and a maximum of only 9% of the expanded pool of liver RBP in vitamin A-deficient rats. Thus, the Golgi is not a major subcellular locus for RBP in either normal or deficient rats. Presumptive evidence that the microtubules are involved in the secretion of RBP has been obtained in studies with the drug colchicine. These studies, on the subcellular organelles and pathways involved in RBP secretion, are continuing with the goal of identifying and characterizing the rate-limiting steps in this overall process.

Recently, we have found two lines of differentiated rat hepatoma cells that synthesize RBP during culture in vitro.[56] When the cells were incubated in a vitamin A-free serumless medium, a relatively large proportion of the RBP synthesized was retained within the cells. Addition of retinol to the medium (at levels of 0.1 or 1 μg/ml) stimulated the release of RBP from the cells into the medium and also increased the net synthesis of RBP. In contrast, retinol had no effect on either the synthesis or secretion of rat serum albumin by these cells. Thus, these cell lines appear to respond to vitamin A depletion and repletion in a similar manner as does the intact rat liver cell in vivo. Accordingly, they should provide a good model to study the factors involved in the regulation of RBP synthesis and secretion.

Information is needed about a number of key questions relating to RBP secretion. For example, we do not know the subcellular locus where retinol normally interacts and forms a complex with RBP in the liver cell. Since RBP secretion is specifically blocked in the absence of retinol, the possibility exists that one or more of the events involved in making retinol available to RBP for complex formation may play a key role in the regulation of RBP secretion.

Nothing is known about the manner in which retinol is transported within the cell from the site(s) of retinyl ester hydrolysis [57] to a molecule of apoRBP. The intracellular cytosol binding protein for retinol (CRBP) [58] may play a role in this process. An important general question which we eventually hope to address is: What are the molecular signals from peripheral tissues that normally stimulate or depress the synthesis and secretion of RBP?

PHYSIOLOGICAL ROLES OF RBP

RBP plays a number of important physiological roles. First of all, RBP serves to solubilize the water-insoluble retinol molecule, and to provide a vehicle to transport retinol from the liver to peripheral tissues. Second, RBP also serves to protect the reactive retinol molecule from oxidative damage while it is transported in plasma.[7, 59] Third, as discussed above, RBP plays an important role in the regulation of the mobilization of vitamin A from the liver stores, and hence of its delivery to peripheral tissues. Finally, RBP also appears to direct the delivery of retinol to specific sites at the surface of cells requiring vitamin A. This directed delivery may be necessary for the proper utilization of retinol within the cell, and also may serve to prevent the toxic effects that can occur from the unregulated delivery of retinol to biological membranes.[60, 61]

SUMMARY

Vitamin A is mobilized from liver stores and transported in plasma in the form of the lipid alcohol retinol, bound to a specific transport protein, retinol-binding protein (RBP). A great deal is known about the chemical structure, metabolism, and biological roles of RBP. RBP is a single polypeptide chain with molecular weight close to 20,000. RBP interacts strongly with plasma prealbumin, and normally circulates in plasma as a 1:1 molar RBP–prealbumin complex. Both the primary and the tertiary structure of prealbumin are known, and the primary structure of RBP has recently been reported. Much information is available about the protein–protein and protein–ligand interactions that are involved in this transport system. Many clinical studies have examined the effects of a variety of diseases on the plasma levels of RBP and prealbumin in humans. Plasma RBP levels are low in patients with liver disease and are high in patients with chronic renal disease. These findings reflect the facts that RBP is produced in the liver and mainly catabolized in the kidneys. Delivery of retinol to extra-hepatic tissues appears to involve specific cell surface receptors for RBP. Vitamin A mobilization from the liver, and delivery to peripheral tissues, is highly regulated by factors that control the rates of RBP production and secretion. Retinol deficiency specifically blocks the secretion of RBP, so that plasma RBP levels fall and liver RBP levels rise. Injection of retinol into vitamin A-deficient rats stimulates the rapid secretion of RBP from the liver into the plasma. The cellular and molecular mechanisms that mediate these phenomena are under investigation. Elucidation of these mechanisms should help define the basic mechanisms that control the mobilization, transport, and delivery of vitamin A.

REFERENCES

1. KANAI, M., A. RAZ & DEW. S. GOODMAN. 1968. Retinol-binding protein: The transport protein for vitamin A in human plasma. J. Clin. Invest. **47:**2025–2044.
2. WALD, G. 1968. Molecular basis of visual excitation. Science **162:**230–239.
3. PETERSON, P. A. 1971. Characteristics of a vitamin A-transporting protein complex occurring in human serum. J. Biol. Chem. **246:**34–43.
4. RAZ, A., T. SHIRATORI & DEW. S. GOODMAN. 1970. Studies on the protein–protein and protein–ligand interactions involved in retinol transport in plasma. J. Biol. Chem. **245:**1903–1912.
5. SMITH, F. R. & DEW. S. GOODMAN. 1971. The effects of diseases of the liver, thyroid, and kidneys on the transport of vitamin A in human plasma. J. Clin. Invest. **50:**2426–2436.
6. SMITH, J. E. & DEW. S. GOODMAN. 1979. Retinol-binding protein and the regulation of vitamin A transport. Fed. Proc. **38:**2504–2509.
7. GOODMAN, DEW. S. 1976. Retinol-binding protein, prealbumin, and vitamin A transport. *In* Trace Components of Plasma: Isolation and Clinical Significance. G. A. Jamieson & T. J. Greenwalt, Eds. pp. 313–330. Alan R. Liss, New York, N.Y.
8. GOODMAN, DEW. S. 1974. Vitamin A transport and retinol-binding protein metabolism. Vitam. Horm. (N.Y.) **32:**167–180.
9. GLOVER, J. 1973. Retinol-binding proteins. Vitam. Horm. (N.Y.) **31:**1–42.
10. KANDA, Y., DEW. S. GOODMAN, R. E. CANFIELD & F. J. MORGAN. 1974. The amino acid sequence of human plasma prealbumin. J. Biol. Chem. **249:**6796–6805.
11. BLAKE, C. C. F., I. D. A. SWAN, C. RERAT, J. BERTHOU, A. LAURENT & B. RERAT. 1971. An X-ray study of the subunit structure of prealbumin. J. Mol. Biol. **61:**217–224.
12. BLAKE, C. C. F., M. J. GEISOW, I. D. A. SWAN, C. RERAT & B. RERAT. 1974. Structure of human plasma prealbumin at 2.5 Å resolution. A preliminary report on the polypeptide chain conformation, quaternary structure and thyroxine binding. J. Mol. Biol. **88:**1–12.
13. BLAKE, C. C. F., M. J. GEISOW, S. J. OATLEY, B. RÉRAT & C. RÉRAT. 1978. Structure of prealbumin: Secondary, tertiary, and quaternary interactions determined by Fourier refinement at 1.8 Å. J. Mol. Biol. **121:**339–356.
14. FERGUSON, R. N., H. EDELHOCH, H. A. SAROFF & J. ROBBINS. 1975. Negative cooperativity in the binding of thyroxine to human serum prealbumin. Biochemistry **14:**282–289.
15. BLAKE, C. C. F. & S. J. OATLEY. 1977. Protein-DNA and protein-hormone interactions in prealbumin: A model of the thyroid hormone nuclear receptor? Nature **268:**115–120.
16. HAUPT, H. & K. HEIDE. 1972. Isolierung und Kristallisation des Retinolbindenden Proteins aus Humanserum. Blut **24:**94–101.
17. RASK, L., P. A. PETERSON & I. BJÖRK. 1972. Conformational studies of the human vitamin A-transporting protein complex. Biochemistry **11:**264–268.
18. GOTTO, A. M., S. E. LUX & DEW. S. GOODMAN. 1972. Circular dichroic studies of human plasma retinol-binding protein and prealbumin. Biochim. Biophys. Acta **271:**429–435.
19. RASK, L., H. ANUNDI & P. A. PETERSON. 1979. The primary structure of the human retinol-binding protein. FEBS Lett. **104:**55–58.
20. KANDA, Y. & DEW. S. GOODMAN. 1979. Partial amino acid sequence of human retinol-binding protein. Isolation and alignment of the five cyanogen bromide fragments and the amino acid sequences of four of the fragments. J. Lipid Res. **20:**865–878.
21. RASK, L., A. VAHLQUIST & P. A. PETERSON. 1971. Studies on two physiological

forms of the human retinol-binding protein differing in vitamin A and arginine content. J. Biol. Chem. **246**:6638–6646.

22. WHITE, G. H., S. M. WESTON & J. GLOVER. 1972. Carboxy-terminal sequence of retinol-binding protein from human plasma. FEBS Lett. **27**:107–110.

23. FEX, G. & B. HANSSON. 1979. Retinol-binding protein from human urine and its interaction with retinol and prealbumin. Eur. J. Biochem. **94**:307–313.

24. PETERSON, P. A. 1971. Studies on the interaction between prealbumin, retinol-binding protein, and vitamin A. J. Biol. Chem. **246**:44–49.

25. VAN JAARSVELD, P. P., H. EDELHOCH, DEW. S. GOODMAN & J. ROBBINS. 1973. The interaction of human plasma retinol-binding protein with prealbumin. J. Biol. Chem. **248**:4698–4705.

26. RAZ, A. & DEW. S. GOODMAN. 1969. The interaction of thyroxine with human plasma prealbumin and with the prealbumin-retinol-binding protein complex. J. Biol. Chem. **244**:3230–3237.

27. GOODMAN, DEW. S. & A. RAZ. 1972. Extraction and recombination studies of the interaction of retinol with human plasma retinol-binding protein. J. Lipid Res. **13**:338–347.

28. GOODMAN, DEW. S. & R. B. LESLIE. 1972. Fluorescence studies of human plasma retinol-binding protein and of the retinol-binding protein-prealbumin complex. Biochim. Biophys. Acta **260**:670–678.

29. HELLER, J. & J. HORWITZ. 1973. Conformational changes following interaction between retinol isomers and human retinol-binding protein and between the retinol-binding protein and prealbumin. J. Biol. Chem. **248**:6308–6316.

30. NILSSON, S., L. RASK & P. A. PETERSON. 1975. Studies on thyroid hormone binding proteins II. Binding of thyroid hormones, retinol-binding protein, and fluorescent probes to prealbumin and effects of thyroxine on prealbumin subunit self-association. J. Biol. Chem. **250**:8554–8563.

31. HELLER, J. & J. HOROWITZ. 1974. The binding stoichiometry of human retinol-binding protein to prealbumin. J. Biol. Chem. **249**:5933–5938.

32. KOPELMAN, M., U. COGAN, S. MOKADY & M. SHINITZKY. 1976. The interaction between retinol-binding proteins and prealbumins studied by fluorescence polarization. Biochim. Biophys. Acta **439**:449–460.

33. HORWITZ, J. & J. HELLER. 1973. Interactions of all-*trans*-, 9-,11-, and 13-*cis*-retinal, all-*trans*-retinyl acetate, and retinoic acid with human retinol-binding protein and prealbumin. J. Biol. Chem. **248**:6317–6324.

34. HORWITZ, J. & J. HELLER. 1974. Properties of the chromophore binding site of retinol-binding protein from human plasma. J. Biol. Chem. **249**:4712–4719.

35. HELLER, J. & J. HORWITZ. 1974. Interactions of retinol-binding protein with various chromophores and with thyroxine-binding protein. A model for visual pigments. Exp. Eye Res. **18**:41–49.

36. COGAN, U., M. KOPELMAN, S. MOKADY & M. SHINITZKY. 1976. Binding affinities of retinol and related compounds to retinol binding proteins. Eur. J. Biochem. **65**:71–78.

37. HASE, J., K. KOBASHI, N. NAKAI & S. ONOSAKA. 1976. Binding of retinol-binding protein obtained from human urine with vitamin A derivatives and terpenoids. J. Biochem. (Japan) **79**:373–380.

38. SHIDOJI, Y. & Y. MUTO. 1977. Vitamin A transport in plasma of the non-mammalian vertebrates: Isolation and partial characterization of piscine retinol-binding protein. J. Lipid Res. **18**:679–691.

39. MUTO, Y., F. R. SMITH & DEW. S. GOODMAN. 1973. Comparative studies of retinol transport in plasma. J. Lipid. Res. **14**:525–532.

40. POOLE, A. R., J. T. DINGLE, A. K. MALLIA & DEW. S. GOODMAN. 1975. The localization of retinol-binding protein in rat liver by immunofluorescence microscopy. J. Cell Sci. **19**:379–394.

41. NAVAB, M., A. K. MALLIA, Y. KANDA & DEW. S. GOODMAN. 1977. Rat plasma prealbumin. Isolation and partial characterization. J. Biol. Chem. **252**:5100–5106.

42. KINDLER, U. 1972. Zur diagnostischen wertigkeit des retinolbindenden proteins (RBP) im serum bei lebererkrankungen. Dtsch. Med. Wochenschr. 97:1821–1823.

43. VAHLQUIST, A., K. SJÖLUND, Å. NORDEN, P. A. PETERSON, G. STIGMAR & B. JOHANSSON. 1978. Plasma vitamin A transport and visual dark adaptation in diseases of the intestine and liver. Scand. J. Clin. Lab. Invest. 38:301–308.

44. SMITH, F. R., DEW. S. GOODMAN, M. S. ZAKLAMA, M. K. GABR, S. EL MARAGHY & V. N. PATWARDHAN. 1973. Serum vitamin A, retinol-binding protein, and prealbumin concentrations in protein-calorie malnutrition. I. A functional defect in hepatic retinol release. Am. J. Clin. Nutr. 26:973–981.

45. SMITH, F. R., DEW. S. GOODMAN, G. ARROYAVE & F. VITERI. 1973. Serum vitamin A, retinol-binding protein, and prealbumin concentrations in protein-calorie malnutrition. II. Treatment including supplemental vitamin A. Amer. J. Clin. Nutr. 26:982–987.

46. SMITH, F. R., R. SUSKIND, O. THANANGKUL, C. LEITZMANN, DEW. S. GOODMAN & R. E. OLSON. 1975. Plasma vitamin A, retinol-binding protein and prealbumin concentrations in protein-calorie malnutrition. III. Response to varying dietary treatments. Amer. J. Clin. Nutr. 28:732–738.

47. VENKATASWAMY, G., J. GLOVER, M. COBBY & A. PIRIE. 1977. Retinol-binding protein in serum of xerophthalmic, malnourished children before and after treatment at a nutrition center. Am. J. Clin. Nutr. 30:1968–1973.

48. RASK, L. & P. A. PETERSON. 1976. In vitro uptake of vitamin A from the retinol-binding plasma protein to mucosal epithelial cells from the monkey's small intestine. J. Biol. Chem. 251:6360–6366.

49. HELLER, J. 1975. Interactions of plasma retinol-binding protein with its receptor. Specific binding of bovine and human retinol-binding protein to pigment epithelium cells from bovine eyes. J. Biol. Chem. 250:3613–3619.

50. CHEN, C.-C. & J. HELLER. 1977. Uptake of retinol and retinoic acid from serum retinol-binding protein by retinal pigment epithelial cells. J. Biol. Chem. 252:5216–5221.

51. MUTO, Y., J. E. SMITH, P. O. MILCH & DEW. S. GOODMAN. 1972. Regulation of retinol-binding protein metabolism by vitamin A status in the rat. J. Biol. Chem. 247:2542–2550.

52. SMITH, J. E., Y. MUTO, P. O. MILCH & DEW. S. GOODMAN. 1973. The effects of chylomicron vitamin A on the metabolism of retinol-binding protein in the rat. J. Biol. Chem. 248:1544–1549.

53. PETERSON, P. A., L. RASK, L. ÖSTBERG, L. ANDERSSON, F. KAMWENDO & H. PERTOFT. 1973. Studies on the transport and cellular distribution of vitamin A in normal and vitamin A-deficient rats with special reference to the vitamin A-binding plasma protein. J. Biol. Chem. 248:4009–4022.

54. NAVAB, M., J. E. SMITH & DEW. S. GOODMAN. 1977. Rat plasma prealbumin. Metabolic studies on effects of vitamin A status and on tissue distribution. J. Biol. Chem. 252:5107–5114.

55. SMITH, J. E., Y. MUTO & DEW. S. GOODMAN. 1975. Tissue distribution and subcellular localization of retinol-binding protein in normal and vitamin A-deficient rats. J. Lipid Res. 16:318–323.

56. SMITH, J. E., C. BOREK & DEW. S. GOODMAN. 1978. Regulation of retinol-binding protein metabolism in cultured rat liver cell lines. Cell 15:865–873.

57. HARRISON, E. H., J. E. SMITH & DEW. S. GOODMAN. 1979. Unusual properties of retinyl palmitate hydrolase activity in rat liver. J. Lipid Res. 20:760–771.

58. ONG, D. E. & F. CHYTIL. 1978. Cellular retinol-binding protein from rat liver. Purification and characterization. J. Biol. Chem. 253:828–832.

59. FUTTERMAN, S. & J. HELLER. 1972. The enhancement of fluorescence and the decreased susceptibility to enzymatic oxidation of retinol complexed with bovine serum albumin, β-lactoglobulin, and the retinol-binding protein of human plasma. J. Biol. Chem. 247:5168–5172.

60. DINGLE, J. T., H. B. FELL & DEW. S. GOODMAN. 1972. The effect of retinol and of retinol-binding protein on embryonic skeletal tissue in organ culture. J. Cell Sci. **11:**393–402.
61. MALLIA, A. K., J. E. SMITH & DEW. S. GOODMAN. 1975. Metabolism of retinol-binding protein and vitamin A during hypervitaminosis A in the rat. J. Lipid Res. **16:**180–188.

DISCUSSION OF THE PAPER

DR. A. JONAS: Maybe you will have to speculate on this one. You have these lipophilic substances—in this case retinol—that are transported in plasma. Do you believe, in order to be taken up by the cell membrane there has to be an internal protein?

DR. D. S. GOODMAN: Yes. In the case of retinol it is our current concept that retinol is delivered to the cell membrane by serum RBP, and then taken into the cell by the CRBP, which is a different protein.

While we do not know whether this is universal for all lipid substances, I would think that it is a very reasonable hypothesis. There is growing evidence that no water-insoluble substance is present by itself inside the cell. Virtually for every instance that has been looked at, there are specific proteins that bind these lipid substances. Our concept of the cytosolic retinol-binding protein is that it represents an intracellular transport protein, rather than from the cell membrane to some other specific site where the retinol acts. The nature of that action on a biochemical level is not really known.

DR. A. M. SCANU: You mentioned the problem of hypervitaminosis. What happens when an excess of vitamin A enters the cell? Does this excess stimulate the production of the retinol-binding protein within the cell?

DR. GOODMAN: Most of our information comes from the work done several years ago by Dr. Krishna Mallia, who is here in the audience. He and Dr. John Smith carried out extensive studies in the rat which showed that in hypervitaminosis the plasma levels of vitamin A became very high, but at the same time the RBP levels actually declined. Most of the excess circulating vitamin A turned out to be present as esterified retinol mainly associated with conventional plasma lipoproteins of density less than 1.21. We did not pursue this problem further than that, and it was our hypothesis that when that occurs, vitamin A can get delivered nonspecifically to cells all over the body and can produce damaging effects on membranes. As far as what happens inside the cell, there are no data under these circumstances.

COMMENT: You mentioned that the kidney is a principal catabolic organ for RBP and you also showed data to suggest that the plasma levels of RBP are very high in chronic renal failure. I was wondering what the levels are in the nephrotic syndrome without chronic renal failure, that is, in severe proteinuric states where the levels might be expected to be low. I also would be interested to know whether you think that this might have any effect on the synthetic rate of RBP in the liver.

DR. GOODMAN: There are data showing that in the nephrotic states indeed RBP levels are low, and the reason can be attributed to a failure in glomerular filtration. As long as glomerular filtration is normal, RBP catabolism will proceed normally.

QUESTION: Do you think that this increased catabolic pathway in nephrotic syndrome would have any effect on the synthetic rate of the liver?

DR. GOODMAN: I have no data on this although I would expect it to be the case since the synthetic rate of serum albumin and other plasma proteins is elevated.

QUESTION: Have you looked for receptor-mediated internalization of the RBP?

DR. GOODMAN: The good data that are available and that have been published come from work in Uppsala using monkey small intestinal mucosal cells and work in California on bovine pigment epithelial cells. This work has provided evidence for surface receptors for RBP which are involved in delivering retinol to the cell; however, the RBP does not enter the cell.

DR. SMALL: What happens to the protein?

DR. GOODMAN: The protein presumably delivers the retinol to the cell and then returns to the circulation. As I indicated in an earlier scheme apoRBP has a lesser affinity for prealbumin than the holo-protein so it is selectively enriched in the small fraction of free (uncomplexed) RBP. Since this is not complexed with prealbumin, it would be selectively filtered by the glomerulus and selectively catabolized.

DR. SMALL: In toxicity you said that RBP appears on lipoproteins as retinyl ester. You do not really know where that is?

DR. GOODMAN: We have not pursued that further and no one else has to my knowledge.

DR. SMALL: Do you know if the retinyl ester in the chylomicrons is transferred to other lipoproteins by the cholesterol ester transfer protein?

DR. GOODMAN: We have no information on this question. Retinyl ester goes to the liver almost quantitatively when chylomicrons are injected intravenously into rats.

DR. SMALL: Did you feel that in toxicity the retinyl ester is resecreted as an ester in VLDL coming from the liver?

DR. GOODMAN: I do not have a clear picture of what happens except the observation that it is found in the circulation. Whether it goes to the liver and is then resecreted is not clear. In vitamin A toxicity there is damage to the liver and most other organs.

DR. F. R. LANDSBERGER: The question I would like to ask really is a question of analogy—whether or not the retinol-binding protein could act as a shuttle such as the phospholipid-exchange protein does.

DR. GOODMAN: The data seem fairly clear that it does not; it is a one-way secretion of the whole of protein and peripheral catabolism.

DR. LANDSBERGER: I understand that it is not a physiologically occurring system, but more of an intellectual construction. If you had a membrane that had a large amount of retinol in it so that the likelihood is that it could pick up retinol again, would it then provide a shuttle?

DR. GOODMAN: It certainly could pick up more retinol. ApoRBP can again become holo-RBP, and there are several techniques that have been developed in the test tube for converting holo- to apoprotein without damaging the retinol binding site, and for then reconverting it to the holo-protein and regaining the original properties.

DR. LANDSBERGER: Will the apoRBP take the retinol alcohol out of the bilayered membrane system?

DR. GOODMAN: That is an interesting question and I do not think anyone has looked at that.

THE LIPID–PROTEIN INTERFACE IN BIOLOGICAL MEMBRANES *

Patricia C. Jost and O. Hayes Griffith

Institute of Molecular Biology and Department of Chemistry
University of Oregon
Eugene, Oregon 97403

INTRODUCTION

Lipid–protein associations occur in membranes as well as in serum lipo-proteins and other nonmembrane systems. At the molecular level there must be common unifying principles governing the hydrophobic, ionic, and steric interactions in all of these systems. Knowledge gained in one system about these interactions contributes to the general understanding of lipid–protein associations, just as knowledge of how lipids self-associate in aqueous solution has provided insight into the organization of lipids in both membranes and serum lipoproteins. In this paper we focus on lipid–protein associations in biological membranes, both native and reconstituted.

Over the past decade it has become generally recognized that most membranes contain fluid phospholipid bilayers, with integral membrane proteins penetrating into or through the lipids. What has not generally been emphasized is the fraction of the lipid involved at the lipid–protein interface. Most biological membranes contain a high density of integral membrane proteins, and the molecular picture more nearly resembles a crowded swimming pool than the analogy of an occasional iceberg in a sea of lipid. For example, in the rod outer segment disk membrane where 85%–90% of the protein is rhodopsin, the lipid-to-protein weight ratio is 1.35, corresponding to only about 65–75 molecules of lipid per molecule of rhodopsin. The number of lipid molecules in instantaneous contact with a rhodopsin monomer has been calculated to be 24–28 depending on the assumed geometry of the protein.[1] Therefore, 30%–45% of the lipid in this membrane may be involved at lipid–protein interfaces. In the sarcoplasmic reticulum, where the predominant protein is the calcium-dependent ATPase, the lipid-to-protein weight ratio is 0.55, corresponding to ∼100–110 molecules of lipid for each ATPase monomer.[2] Rough calculations allowing for protrusion of the headpiece, suggest that 25–30 molecules of lipid interact directly with the protein; that is, a quarter of the lipid would be involved at the interface. At the upper limit, the purple membrane of *Halobacteria halobium* has ∼10 moles lipid for each mole bacteriorhodopsin or 30 moles for each trimer, where 25–28 molecules (83%–93%) are in contact with the trimeric protein.[3] Because of the diversity of the proteins in most other intact membranes, an estimate of the molar ratio of integral membrane protein to lipids is difficult to make. However, in many functional membranes it is clear that a significant fraction of the lipid is in contact with the protein.

The lipid in contact with the hydrophobic surface of one integral membrane protein, cytochrome oxidase, was detected some years ago by spin labeling.[4]

* This work was supported by the National Institutes of Health Grant GM 25698.

Recently, a number of new experiments have been carried out by several laboratories using electron spin resonance (ESR), nuclear magnetic resonance (NMR), differential scanning calorimetry (DSC), and other techniques in an effort to characterize the lipid composition and properties at the lipid–protein interface. There is general agreement on some aspects, and controversy regarding others. There can be no controversy, however, about the existence of hydrophobic protein–lipid contacts forming an interface. We review here the present status of this field, including experimental estimates of the amount of interfacial lipid, any lipid disorganization at the protein surface, exchange between boundary and bilayer lipids, protein perturbation of the bilayer lipids, and charge selectivity by the protein.

DETECTION OF LIPID AT THE PROTEIN BOUNDARY

The principal method used for detecting lipid at the protein boundary has been electron spin resonance (ESR). Spectra of lipid spin labels serving as dilute reporter groups in membranes can be analyzed to show the presence of two components. One spectral component is characteristic of lipid bilayers, and is seen both in lipid model systems and in membranes. The other component is seen only when protein is present, is proportional to the amount of protein, and is characteristic of more restricted motion on the time scale of this technique. An example is shown in FIGURE 1, where a phospholipid spin label is present at low concentrations in bilayers containing the transmembranous protein (Na^+, K^+) ATPase. This experimental spectrum (FIGURE 1a) resembles the spectrum of the liposomes of pure lipid (FIGURE 1b) except for the broad peaks in the wings. By appropriate spectral integrations and subtractions it has been demonstrated that the membrane spectra of this type are essentially a sum of the two single components,[4, 5] fluid membrane bilayer (FIGURE 1c), and a more motionally restricted protein-associated lipid (FIGURE 1d). The membrane fluid bilayer spectrum (FIGURE 1c) resembles the bilayer of liposomes (FIGURE 1b), except that it is slightly broadened by the presence of the protein. Composite spectra have been seen in many systems in many laboratories, but the amount in each environment has been quantitated in only a few cases. In intact membranes, typical percentages of the fatty acid spin label bound at room temperature are 30%–40% in mitochondria (Jost & Griffith, unpublished data), 50%–70% in photosynthetic bacterial chromatophores,[6] 33%–41% in bovine rod outer segment membranes,[1] and 25%–30% in rabbit muscle sarcoplasmic reticulum.[2]

In order to relate the amount bound to the geometry and molecular weight of the protein, it is necessary to purify a single membrane protein and reconstitute it into lipid bilayers. For beef heart cytochrome oxidase in its naturally occurring mitochondrial lipids, 40–50 molecules of lipid are in contact with the protein.[4] A similar study of yeast cytochrome oxidase reconstituted in dimyristoyl phosphatidylcholine concludes that 50–60 molecules interact with the protein.[7] It is estimated that 60–70 molecules of lipid interact directly with the (Na^+, K^+) ATPase dimer from the electric eel.[8] The corresponding number for the calcium dependent ATPase from rabbit skeletal muscle is ~ 25[2] or ~ 30.[9] In membranes that consist primarily of one protein, an estimate can be made without further protein isolation. For example, in retinal rod outer segment membranes, rhodopsin accounts for almost all of the integral membrane present, and the estimate is that 20–30 lipids interact with each rhodopsin molecule.[1] All of these numbers correspond roughly to a layer of lipid surrounding the protein. One version of this model is sketched in FIG-URE 2. These numbers, of course, are only approximate, and may not correspond exactly to one continuous lipid layer, and there has been no direct determination of the actual geometrical relationships. Protein–protein contacts, irregular protein geometry and size of the hydrophobic region can change the calculated perimeter of the hydrophobic surfaces.

ESR spectral analyses arriving at these fractions of lipid in contact with the protein require careful quantitation. Estimates without appropriate quantitation

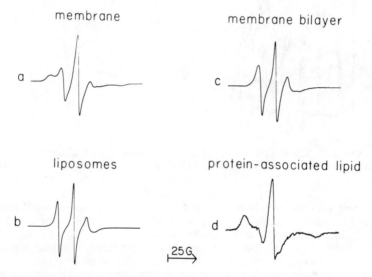

FIGURE 1. Representative ESR spectrum of a spin labeled membrane (a) and its analysis into two components (c, d). One component (c) resembles the spectrum of the liposomes (b). The samples are (a) dogfish shark rectal gland (Na^+, K^+)ATPase in α-palmitoyl-β-oleoyl-α-L-phosphatidylcholine (POPC) bilayers (0.31 mg phospholipid/mg protein), containing less than 1 mole% 14-proxylstearoylphosphate; both spectra were recorded at 25° C. The fluid bilayer component (c) and the motionally-restricted protein associated component (d) of the membrane spectrum (a) were obtained by a pairwise subtraction technique,[8] using a companion spectrum not shown.

have led to errors in interpretation. The origin of many of these difficulties is illustrated in FIGURE 3. The protein-associated component of the experimental spectrum is often largely or completely obscured by the sharper three-line bilayer component. In this example, the experimental spectrum resembles that of the bilayer (FIGURE 3c), but as shown by the integrated absorption, it actually contains more of the bound component (58%) than it does bilayer.[10] In some studies, particularly at higher temperatures or higher lipid content, the protein-associated component has not been recognized as being a significant fraction of the total lipid present. No estimate of the amount of lipid at the interface has been provided by ^{2}H-NMR, because the line shape from the lipid

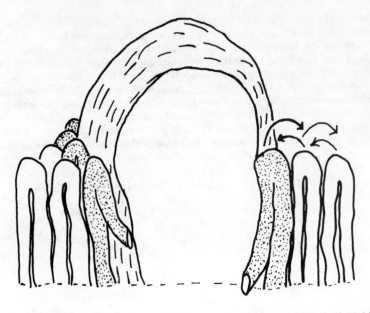

FIGURE 2. Diagrammatic sketch of a protein penetrating a phospholipid bilayer. Lipids in the boundary region (shaded) exchange with the adjacent fluid bilayer.

in contact with the protein is unknown and because exchange complicates the spectral interpretation. Proton NMR data on lipid–protein systems have proven to be rather difficult to analyze. Phosphorous NMR, although beyond the scope of this present review, shows promise for the study of phospholipid head group interactions with proteins.

It has been reported that lipid at the lipid–protein interface can be detected using differential scanning calorimetry (DSC). In this technique the excess specific heat is plotted versus increasing temperature. Peaks mark the positions of endothermic phase transitions, e.g., the gel-to-liquid crystal transition of lipids. Integration of the area under the peak and normalization to the amount of lipid in the sample gives ΔH_{cal}, the calorimetrically determined enthalpy for the transition. When membrane protein is present, the position of the peak (T_m) is essentially unchanged and the width is broadened, but the main effect is a reduction in ΔH_{cal}. This reduction in enthalpy is interpreted as due to some fraction of the lipids no longer participating in the gel-to-liquid crystal phase transition. In lipid samples containing a hydrophobic protein from human myelin, a plot of the enthalpy versus protein content gives the number of lipids removed from the phase transition as 15 per protein[11] or, more recently, 21–25[12] per protein. This is consistent with a layer of lipid in contact with a protein trimer. Several phosphatidylcholines with C–14 to C–18 chain lengths gave essentially the same result.[12] Other researchers[13, 14] have attributed this kind of extrapolated value to a constant amount of lipid trapped between proteins at the T_m. A model of patches of lipid and protein that always have the same lipid to protein ratio, i.e., eutectic patches independent of the total amount of bilayer present, is formally a two-domain model and by DSC alone is indistinguishable from the boundary bilayer equilibrium model. The distinction would lie in whether or not the protein-associated domain persists above the T_m where the proteins are randomly distributed in the plane of the bilayer (see also the discussion of effects of temperature and protein concentration).

In contrast, a similar DSC study using a hydrophobic protein fraction from beef brain myelin reports that the presence of the protein in DMPC caused a new transition about 2° C higher than that of the pure lipid. On the basis of these results, it was then suggested that the lipid at the protein boundary undergoes a phase transition and involves ~140 molecules of lipid per protein.[15] This suggests that several layers of lipid surrounding the protein were melting at the higher temperature. The lack of agreement with an earlier study in which this higher melting component was not seen [11] was attributed to differences in scan rates. Recently, however, this problem has been carefully reinvestigated and the only time a higher melting component was observed was when a small fraction of lipid decomposition products (lysoDMPC and myristic acid) were present.[16] If the presence of small amounts of lipid decomposition products provides an explanation for the conflicting results, then the DSC data in the literature indicates that a fraction of the lipid, which is constant with

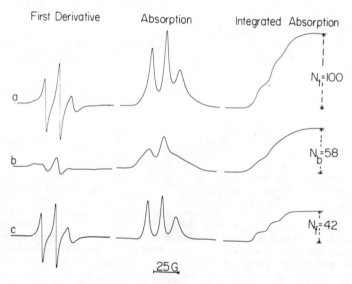

FIGURE 3. Typical ESR spectral analysis of 16-doxylphosphatidylcholine spin label in cytochrome oxidase membranes. (a) Experimental spectrum: cytochrome oxidase vesicles containing 0.32 mg of phospholipid/mg of protein. (b) Bound line shape: lipid-poor cytochrome oxidase containing 0.11 mg of phospholipid/mg of protein. (c) Difference spectrum: experimental minus bound component. Integration of the experimental first derivative spectrum (first column) yields the absorption spectrum (second column). A second integration (third column) gives the relative absorption of each first derivative spectrum and is proportional to the amount of spin label present. All spectra in each column are normalized to the relative absorption, but between columns scaling down by a constant is necessary for plotting: N_t, N_b, and N_f are the relative numbers in arbitrary units of the total, bound, and fluid spin labels, respectively. (From Jost et al.[10] By permission of Biochemistry.)

respect to the amount of protein present, does not undergo melting at the transition of the bilayer lipid, and that the T_m of the remaining lipid is similar to that of pure liposomes.

EXCHANGE OF LIPID BETWEEN BOUNDARY AND BILAYER

Information regarding the exchange of lipid between sites is derived from ESR and NMR experiments. Transfer or diffusion of lipid between different sites can have profoundly different effects on the magnetic resonance spectra

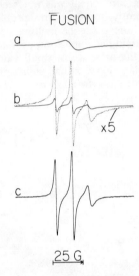

FIGURE 4. An experiment involving fusion of vesicles of a phospholipid spin label with unlabeled membranous cytochrome oxidase of high lipid content (0.50 phospholipid/mg protein). The ESR spectra (a) vesicles of 16-doxylphosphatidylcholine in buffer; (b) 2.5 hr after addition of sample a to unlabeled cytochrome oxidase vesicles and incubation at 37° C; (c) sample (b) after further incubation and discontinuous sucrose gradient centrifugation. All spectra were recorded at 24° C, and are scaled to reflect the same intergrated absorption. Spectrum (b) is also shown amplified 5 times (dotted lines) to make the line shape easier to see. (After Jost *et al.*[10].)

depending on the frequency of the process, number of sites involved and the differences in environments. One effect present in ESR, but not NMR, is electron spin exchange. Coulomb interactions between unpaired electrons are manifested as an effective weak interaction of the form $J\,\mathbf{S}_1 \cdot \mathbf{S}_2$ between two spin labels, where J is the exchange integral and $\mathbf{S}_1$ and $\mathbf{S}_2$ are the electron spin operators. In dilute solutions the spin labels exhibit the familiar three-line ESR spectrum. As the concentration of spin labels is increased, radical-radical collisions occur more frequently, the three lines broaden and then coalesce into one progressively sharper line. FIGURE 4 shows a simple application of this principle. FIGURE 4a is the exchange-narrowed spectrum of vesicles of pure phospholipid spin labels. FIGURE 4b is the spectrum obtained 2.5 hrs after incubation of unlabeled cytochrome oxidase vesicles with spin label vesicles. The appearance of the three–line spectrum indicates that a fraction of the spin label vesicles has fused with unlabeled cytochrome oxidase vesicles. Furthermore, after fusion, the patches of spin labels have diffused throughout the cytochrome oxidase preparation. The bottom spectrum (FIGURE 4c) is the cytochrome oxidase sample after removal of any remaining unincorporated phospholipid spin label vesicles. The bound component is not obvious in either b or c because of the high lipid content, but it is there. Computer analysis shows that 32% of the label is in association with the protein, corresponding to 40–50 moles of phospholipid per mole of protein, consistent with the values obtained by other methods of introducing lipid spin labels. The diffusion of the phospholipid spin label and the resulting equilibrium between boundary and bilayer are clear evidence of exchange between these two domains. This sets a lower limit on the exchange rate of 1 hr^{-1}, i.e., the first time the incubation mixture was sampled.[10] The exchange rate is undoubtedly very much faster than this.

Another approach, applicable in both ESR and NMR, is to consider the effect of lipids randomly hopping back and forth between the boundary layer and the adjacent bilayer at equilibrium. This is an example of the classical two-site chemical exchange model that was treated some years ago by solving modified Bloch equations.[17] To apply this method, some knowledge is needed of the line positions of each site in the absence of exchange. With slow exchange, the lines associated with each site broaden and in the fast exchange limit only a single line spectrum is observed. The criterion for two spectra to be resolved is that the residence time in each site must be much greater than $1/(2\pi\delta\nu)$ where $\delta\nu$ is the difference in corresponding line positions in frequency units.

In ESR, two spectral components are clearly resolved, so by definition the exchange process is slow in the ESR time scale. However, the ESR time scale itself is very short so that the exchange could be quite rapid and still be consistent with the two component ESR spectra. The differences in corresponding line positions are typically 2–10 G (5.6–28 MHz) so the upper limit of the exchange frequency is 10^7–10^8 sec^{-1}. For comparison, the lateral diffusion constant of bilayer lipid is typically 10^{-8} cm^2/sec corresponding to a hopping frequency in the range of 10^7 sec^{-1}.[18, 19] Thus, exchange rates approaching that of pure lipid would still be slow by this criterion. The upper limit of the exchange rate is evidently lower, however, since exchange effects are not evident on the individual line shapes in the two component spectra (the bilayer component is somewhat broader when protein is present but the dominant effect is almost certainly reduction in segmental motion of the lipid chains when protein is present). Different lipids can have different exchange rates, providing that the fastest rate does not exceed this upper limit.

The time scale of NMR is much longer than ESR, offering the potential of providing new information about exchange rates. Recently, specifically deuterated phosphatidylcholines have been studied by ^{2}H-NMR, with many studies using the quadrupolar echo technique.[20] This is a relatively new development and the conclusions are somewhat tentative. The general observation is that only one component is seen when the lipid is above the T_m, even when a substantial amount of protein is present. This result has been reproduced in several laboratories with the deuterium label at different positions along the lipid chain.

Samples containing protein exhibit a small decrease in the quadrupole splitting and usually an increase in the apparent line width.[21-25]

An example is shown in FIGURE 5 where the phospholipid is labeled at the C–6 position of one acyl chain. All spectra are above the lipid transition temperature of −5° C. The three spectra at the top are from lipid vesicles, and the corresponding three spectra at the bottom show the effect of 67 wt% cyto-

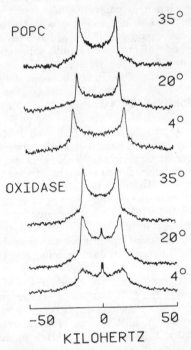

FIGURE 5. ^{2}H-NMR spectra of phospholipid vesicles deuterated at the C_6 position on one acyl side chain, with and without cytochrome oxidase (67 wt%), POPC, 1-palmitoyl-2-oleyl-sn-glycero-3-phosphatidylcholine, prepared from 6,6-d_2 palmitic acid. For best fits, the spectral simulation parameters for the quadrupole splitting ($\Delta\nu_Q$) and line widths (δ) of the pure lipids are: $\Delta\nu_Q$ of 26, 29, and 36 kHz; and δ of 300, 300, and 360 Hz for 35°, 20°, and 4° C, respectively. Comparable parameters for the protein-containing sample are: $\Delta\nu_Q$ of 24, 27, and 30 kHz; and δ of 600, 1,000, and 3,000 Hz at 35°, 20°, and 4° C, respectively. The samples above the lipid transition temperature ($T_m = -5$° C). (From Rice et al.[26] By permission of Biochemistry)

chrome oxidase (~125 molecules of lipid for each protein). By spectral simulation the quadrupole splittings have been shown to decrease slightly and the apparent line widths increase appreciably in the presence of protein.[26] The observation of a single component is evidence for exchange between boundary and bilayer that is rapid on the ^{2}H-NMR time scale. Similar results have been obtained when the deuterium label is on the terminal methyl group, using either cytochrome oxidase or (Ca^{2+})ATPase.[26, 27]

CONFORMATION AND MOTION OF LIPID AT THE PROTEIN INTERFACE

Information concerning molecular motion and configuration of lipids in the boundary layer is available, in principle, from both ESR and NMR. With ESR, changes in the environment of the unpaired electron associated with the N-O group are being detected. The magnetic interaction between the unpaired electron and ^{14}N nucleus ($I = 1$) of the nitroxide moiety gives rise to $2I + 1 = 3$ lines of equal intensity, with the distance between two adjacent lines being the coupling constant or splitting A (or T). Since there is a moderately large dipolar contribution, the magnitude of the splitting varies with the orientation of the N-O group in the magnetic field. The largest splitting A_{zz} occurs when the magnetic field is parallel to the $2pz$ orbital associated with the unpaired electron. In an all *trans* configuration of the lipid spin labels, this corresponds to a direction parallel to the long molecular axis. The use of oriented samples provides the most direct way to assess the influence of protein on spatial order. The spectra of oriented lipid bilayers have been analyzed using a Gaussian distribution of orientations, and there is substantial spatial alignment of the lipid chains.[28] Introduction of cytochrome oxidase largely preserves the spatial order of the bilayer regions, although the distribution of orientations is somewhat broader. In contrast, little or no orientation is seen for the lipids in contact with the protein.[29] Similar experiments with the specialized purple membrane patches of *Halobacterium halobium* also suggest a much lower spatial order on the surface of the protein.[3] This is the main evidence that the lipid chains undergo many *gauche-trans* isomerizations in conforming to the highly irregular protein surface. This is also the most physically plausible picture of spatial arrangements at the lipid–protein interface.

The ESR line shape of the protein-associated lipid has many of the features of a powder pattern. Therefore, ESR spectroscopists refer to it as immobilized. This has turned out to be an unfortunate choice of terms, since some workers outside the ESR field have interpreted this technical description as indicating a rigid long-lived specialized class of lipids at the protein boundary. Actually, some motion is present in the protein-associated lipid, even on the ESR time scale, although this motion is highly restricted relative to the bilayer motion. The motion of lipids has been evaluated in terms of a rapid random walk about a molecular axis, with the amplitude related to the motion.[30] Typically, the overall splitting of the protein-associated component is reduced by 5–10 G from the powder pattern (no motion) limit, over the temperature range of 5°–35° C.[8] This corresponds to motion of the reporter group within a cone of half-angle γ ranging from ~25° to ~36°. The values of γ for the bilayer are much larger, e.g., 60°–75° (and for isotropic motion $\gamma = 90°$). However, this model is less appropriate for characterizing the very high amplitude of motion near the center of the bilayer because of the role that frequency, as well as amplitude, plays.

A common term used to describe ESR and NMR data is the order parameter. In the current magnetic resonance literature, the term order parameter refers to amplitude of molecular motion within a given frequency or time domain. The most common form of the order parameter $S = 1/2(3 < \cos^2 \theta > -1)$, where the brackets indicate an average over a range of angles that the director axis can sample during a given time interval. The limits are $S = 1$ for no motion and $S = 0$ for complete averaging. The order parameter as it is often used does not imply spatial order in the crystallographic sense. For example, molecules in a perfect single crystal or a random powder both can correspond to an order parameter of $S = 1$ if no motion is present. This has led to some confusion in the literature. For example, the ESR results on protein-associated lipid are sometimes quoted as indicating that lipid in the boundary layer is "highly ordered" (because of the reduced motion), whereas, in fact, the ESR experiments show just the opposite, with both restricted motion and spatial disordering present.

In the ²H-NMR experiment, the dominant field gradient occurs along the C–D bond and the order parameter (S_{CD}) time-averages the angular excursions of the C–D bond about the director axis. For a randomly oriented sample, S_{CD} is calculated from the residual quadrupole splitting $\Delta\nu = 3/4(e^2qQ/h)S_{CD}$, where the deuteron quadrupole splitting constant (e^2qQ/h) has been determined in paraffin hydrocarbons to be ~170 kHz.[31] Thus, if no motion is present, the observed quadrupole splitting would be ~127 kHz. The parameter S_{CD} is often converted into a molecular order parameter S_{mol} in order to relate the order parameter to the motion about the long chain molecular axis. There are several possible cases depending on assumptions about the anisotropy of the motion, so that values of S_{mol} are model dependent.[27, 31] Frequently only the S_{CD} values are reported and these can include the time averages over chain isomerization (i.e., trans-gauche), chain reorientation including changes in tilt and rotation, diffusion, and, if protein is present, exchange between the boundary and the bilayer regions (also contributions from protein rotation, if any). It will understandably take time to sort out all these contributions. As seen in the last section, the main observation by ²H-NMR is that above the T_m of the lipids, the quadrupole splitting is slightly decreased in the presence of protein, accompanied by line broadening. Only a single-component spectrum is seen. These observations are consistent with rapid exchange of the lipid (phosphatidylcholine) between magnetically non-equivalent sites. Several different models fit these data, all assuming exchange between the protein surface and the bilayer that is rapid on the NMR time scale. In one model, the lipid in contact with the protein executes larger amplitude motion (motional disorder) than lipid in the bulk bilayer phase. In another model, the lipid in contact with the protein is forced to conform to the irregular protein surface and therefore undergoes many gauche-trans isomerizations (spatial disorder). The exchange, therefore, involves two states of the lipid differing greatly in conformation. In this model the motion of the lipid could be substantially reduced in the boundary layer, and this would be entirely consistent with the ESR data. A third model, not plausible but formally acceptable, is that the lipids in contact with the protein are spatially highly ordered (e.g., all trans configuration) but have various angles of tilt with respect to the bilayer plane and undergo rapid exchange with the bilayer lipids. Further line shape analyses and relaxation data should help to sort out the various models. For phosphatidylcholine and the proteins examined thus far, the exchange rate is $>10^4$ sec^{-1} above T_m. However, the NMR line shape characteristic of the protein-associated lipid has not yet been characterized, and until this is done, the exchange rate cannot be quantitated. The advantage of the NMR technique is that the probes are non-perturbing. The disadvantages are the reduced sensitivity (some high binding sites may be difficult to observe), and the multiple contributions to the line shape that are encountered in the longer time frame of the experiment. The advantages of spin labeling are the shorter time frame and relative ease of spectral interpretation and high sensitivity. The disadvantage is in evaluating the perturbation that is introduced by the reporter group. Because of the com-

bination of advantages and limitations, information from both magnetic resonance techniques are needed to characterize the lipid at the protein interface
and to determine the relative binding affinities of different classes of lipids.

There have been relatively few quantitative studies of the amount of lipid
that is protein-associated as a function of temperature. Two recent spin labeling
studies of rhodopsin reach very different conclusions. One study involves
rhodopsin covalently labeled and reconstituted in vesicles of egg yolk phosphatidylcholine at several protein concentrations. The conclusion reached was
that the broad spectral component vanishes at temperatures and lipid-to-protein
ratios of physiological relevance.[32] This is formally equivalent to a melting of
the boundary layer, or exchange of the labeled hydrocarbon segment with a
rate that is rapid on the ESR time scale. In contrast, the other study is of
spin labeled rod outer segment membranes, where rhodopsin represents the
major membrane protein. The conclusions reached in this case are that, in the
native membrane, there is little or no temperature dependence of the amount
of bound component over the range of 3° to 37° C.[1] In a third study, membranous (Na^+,K^+)ATPase in a native lipid background was examined over the
temperature range of 5° to 35° C. The amount of bound component reported
by negatively and positively charged lipid spin labels was very nearly constant,
although different for the two labels (charge selectivity) as shown in FIGURE 6.
There is a small systematic trend with the negatively charged lipid, but this
change is within the experimental error.[8] In the upper right hand corner are
the same data, analyzed using the assumption of a temperature-independent
broad line shape, i.e., invariant $2A_{max}$, which is an assumption made in the
data analysis of the covalently-labeled rhodopsin study.[32] This assumption,
which has been shown to be invalid for the (Na^+,K^+)ATPase,[8] produces an
artificial appearance of a melting away of the bound component (inset, FIG-
URE 6). This type of artifact could account for the differences between the
two rhodopsin studies, but the experimental designs and samples are somewhat
different and this artifact may not account for all the differences observed.

Considerable confusion in the literature has been generated by qualitative
interpretations of ESR data as a function of temperature or extent of the bilayer.
With the reporter group near the center of the bilayer, the line width differences
between the broad protein-associated line shape and the narrow bilayer line
shape are marked. The prominence of the narrow lines can give a visual impression that the bound component is disappearing as the bilayer line narrows,
either with temperature or with increases in the extent of the bilayer. Careful
analysis of the digitized data, however, shows that this visual effect is not due
to any significant decrease in the protein-associated component in the cytochrome oxidase and (Na^+,K^+)ATPase studies. Equilibrium constants for specific
lipids could, of course, be temperature dependent.

EQUILIBRIUM BINDING CONSTANTS AND CHARGE PREFERENCE

One of the interesting questions is whether the membrane protein influences
the composition of its nearest-neighbor lipids rather than accepting a solvation

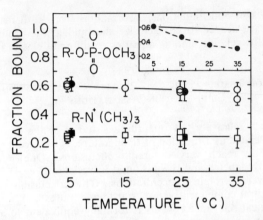

FIGURE 6. Fractions of negatively and positively charged lipid spin labels bound to (Na$^+$,K$^+$)ATPase as a function of temperature. R is an 18-carbon chain with the proxyl group at the C-14 position near the hydrocarbon terminus. Open and closed symbols indicate two different methods of analysis.[8] *Inset:* The circles and dashed line show the artifactual decrease in the bound fraction of the methylphosphate label with increased temperature, caused by using a single low temperature (5° C) spectrum for all subtractions. The error introduced by neglecting the changes in 2A$_{max}$ of the bound spectrum as a function of temperature can be seen by comparing the results to the appropriate spectral subtractions indicated by the solid line. (From Brotherus *et al.*[8] By permission of the *Proceedings of the National Academy of Sciences.*)

layer that reflects the bulk lipid composition. To estimate the equilibrium binding constants, it is convenient to treat lipid–protein association as an exchange reaction. For one binding site the reaction is

$$L^* + LP \rightleftharpoons L + L^*P,$$

where L* and L are the labeled and unlabeled lipids occupying a hydrophobic binding site on the membrane protein, P. A useful approximate solution for n equivalent accessible binding sites is [33]

$$y = x/nK - 1/K.$$

Thus, a plot of the lipid/protein ratio, x, versus the ratio of bilayer/bound label, y, should yield a straight line with a y-intercept of $-1/K$, an x-intercept of n binding sites, and a slope of $1/nK$. An application of this approach is shown in FIGURE 7. In this case, a labeled stearic acid was diffused into cytochrome oxidase containing a mixture of native lipids. The value of $n \simeq 48$ and K is near unity, indicating that the lipid spin label mimics the behavior of the natural unlabeled lipids. It also indicates that there is apparently no strong interaction between the nitroxide moiety and the protein surface, i.e., any hydrogen bonding does not have a measurable effect on the equilibrium constant. It is probable that there are high affinity lipid binding sites for which this label does not compete. This can be tested by using labeled phospholipids (e.g., diphosphatidylglycerol). For some proteins, there is biochemical evidence for a specific lipid requirement, which may mean that some of these lipids have a higher binding affinity.

Recently, a definite charge selectivity has been demonstrated for the transmembranous (Na^+,K^+)ATPase (electric eel) in vesicles of the native lipids. This enzyme exhibits a relative binding affinity for a negatively charged label that is four-fold higher than that for an analogous positively charged label and two and a half-fold higher than for no charge on the head group.[8] This charge selectivity can be reversibly abolished by high salt concentrations, confirming that the effect is due to electrostatic interactions between the polar head group and the protein. The number of sites involved in this charge selectivity has not yet been determined. These experiments used a series of labeled lipids, where the chain length and label position were held constant and the polar head group varied. Thus, any influence of the label on the relative binding constants is largely factored out. In contrast, retinal rod outer segment membrane protein, predominantly rhodopsin, was not observed to preferentially bind more negatively charged phospholipid spin label than neutral analogs, although the data suggest the possibility of a small preferential binding of phosphatidylserine.[1]

There is also DSC evidence that the myelin proteolipid, lipophilin, interacts preferentially with acidic lipids in a binary mixture of neutral and acidic lipids, removing more of the acidic lipids from the lipid undergoing melting, as judged by DSC.[34]

SUMMARY

A significant fraction of the lipid in many biological membranes is at the lipid–protein interface. The ESR and NMR data are in basic agreement that

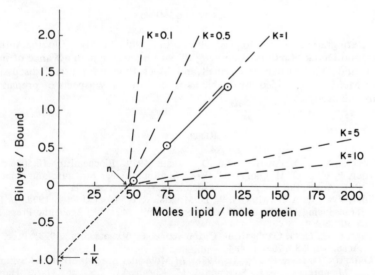

FIGURE 7. A plot of the equilibrium binding equations for n equivalent sites with relative equilibrium constant K. The three circles are experimental values of the ratio of bilayer/bound spectral components from cytochrome oxidase vesicles as a function of lipid content. Calculated slopes are shown for $n=48$, and relative equilibrium binding constants ranging from 0.1 to 10. (From Griffith & Jost.[33] By permission of Elsevier/North Holland Biomedical Press.)

there is a dynamic equilibrium between lipid at the interface and the bulk bilayer. The lipid in contact with the hydrophobic surfaces of the protein is spatially disordered compared to the bilayer lipids. The spatial disordering on the protein surface leads to the prediction that cooperative chain melting would not occur between lipid tails directly contacting the protein. This is in agreement with most, but not all of the DSC data. While there are some disagreements in the ESR studies, most of the quantitative data support the conclusion that the protein-associated lipid is motionally restricted under physiologically relevant conditions. In general, the NMR data are in agreement that exchange between boundary and bilayer regions is rapid on the NMR time scale at physiological temperatures, although there are some differences in interpretation of the lipid dynamics. From the available data, several kinds of lipid binding sites may be involved. Most of these sites are probably nonspecific, but with some additional sites exhibiting specificity for the chemical properties of the polar head group. The relative binding constants can vary within the boundary layer with several exchange rates applying. Although most of the exchange rates are rapid, perhaps more rapid than specific mechanistic steps in the enzyme reaction, there is a characterizable set of thermodynamic parameters for the boundary and bilayer equilibrium. Although many of the lipid binding sites may have very low relative binding constants, they must be higher than the binding constants for nonspecific protein–protein contacts. One probable function of the boundary is to act as a molecular spacer, preventing indiscriminate protein–protein aggregation in the two-dimensional lipid solvent. Other roles are suggested by the higher relative binding constants of some specific lipids.

ACKNOWLEDGMENTS

We are grateful to Drs. Joan M. Boggs, Eric Oldfield, Myer Bloom, Anthony Watts, and Derek Marsh for supplying us with manuscripts in advance of publication, and Drs. Harden McConnell and Myer Bloom for useful discussions. Debra McMillen provided invaluable assistance in many aspects of preparation of this manuscript.

REFERENCES

1. WATTS, A., I. D. VOLOTOVSKI & D. MARSH. 1979. Biochemistry **18:**5006–5013.
2. JOST, P. C. & O. H. GRIFFITH. 1978. *In* Biomolecular Structure and Function, P. F. AGRIS, Ed., pp. 25–56. Academic Press, New York, NY.
3. JOST, P. C., D. A. MCMILLEN, W. D. MORGAN & W. STOECKENIUS. 1978. *In* Light Transducing Membranes, D. Deamer, Ed., pp. 141–155. Academic Press, New York, N.Y.
4. JOST, P. C., O. H. GRIFFITH, R. C. CAPALDI & G. VANDERKOOI. 1973. Proc. Nat. Acad. Sci. USA **70:**480–484.
5. GRIFFITH, O. H. & P. C. JOST. 1978. *In* Molecular Specialization and Symmetry in Membranes. A. K. Solomon & M. Karnovsky, Eds., pp. 31–60, Harvard University Press, Cambridge, Mass.
6. BIRRELL, G. B., W. R. SISTROM & O. H. GRIFFITH. 1978. Biochemistry **17:**3768–3773.
7. KNOWLES, P. F., A. WATTS & D. MARSH. 1979. Biochemistry **18:**4480–4487.
8. BROTHERUS, J. R., P. C. JOST, O. H. GRIFFITH, J. F. W. KEANA & L. E. HOKIN. 1979. Proc. Natl. Acad. Sci. USA **77:**272–276.

9. HESKETH, T. R., G. A. SMITH, M. D. HOUSLAY, K. A. McGILL, N. J. M. BIRDSALL,
    J. C. METCALFE & G. WARREN. 1976. Biochemistry 15:4145–4151.
10. JOST, P. C., K. K. NADAKAVUKAREN & O. H. GRIFFITH. 1977. Biochemistry 16:
    3110–3114.
11. PAPAHADJOPOULOS, D., W. J. VAIL & M. A. MOSCARELLO. 1975. J. Membr. Biol.
    22:143–164.
12. BOGGS, J. M. & M. A. MOSCARELLO. 1978. Biochemistry 17:5734–5739.
13. CHAPMAN, D., B. A. CORNELL, A. W. ELIASZ & A. PERRY. 1977. J. Mol. Biol.
    113:517–538.
14. CORNELL, B. A., M. M. SACRÉ, W. E. PEEL & D. CHAPMAN. 1978. FEBS Lett.
    90:29–35.
15. CURATOLO, W., J. D. SAKURA, D. M. SMALL & G. G. SHIPLEY. 1977. Biochemistry
    16:2313–2319.
16. BOGGS, J. M. & M. A. MOSCARELLO. 1980. Biochim. Biophys. Acta. In press.
17. POPLE, J. A., G. W. SCHNEIDER & H. J. BERNSTEIN. 1959. High-Resolution
    Nuclear Magnetic Resonance. McGraw-Hill, New York, N.Y.
18. DEVAUX, P. & H. M. McCONNELL. 1972. J. Am. Chem. Soc. 94:4475–4481.
19. SACKMANN, E. & H. TRAUBLE. 1972. J. Am. Chem. Soc. 94:4492–4498.
20. DAVIS, J. H., K. R. JEFFREY, M. BLOOM, M. I. VALIC & T. P. HIGGS. 1976. Chem.
    Phys. Lett. 42:390–394.
21. SEELIG, A. & J. SEELIG. 1978. Hoppe-Seyler's Z. Physiol. Chem. 359(S):1747–
    1756.
22. OLDFIELD, E., R. GILMORE, M. GLASER, H. G. GUTOWSKY, J. C. HSUNG, S. Y.
    KANG, T. E. KING, M. MEADOWS & D. RICE. 1978. Proc. Natl. Acad. Sci.
    USA 75:4657.
23. KANG, S. Y., H. S. GUTOWSKY, J. C. HSUNG, R. JACOBS, T. E. KING, D. RICE &
    E. OLDFIELD. 1979. Biochemistry 15:3257–3267.
24. SMITH, I. C. P., K. W. BUTLER, A. P. TULLOCH, J. H. DAVIS & M. BLOOM. 1979.
    FEBS Lett. 100:57–61.
25. DAHLQUIST, F. W. & M. BLOOM. 1979. Personal communication.
26. RICE, D., J. C. HSUNG, T. E. KING & E. OLDFIELD. 1979. Biochemistry 18:
    5585–5891.
27. RICE, D. M., M. D. MEADOWS, A. O. SHEINMAN, F. M. GOÑI, J. C. GOMÉZ,
    M. A. MOSCARELLO, D. CHAPMAN & E. OLDFIELD. 1979. Biochemistry 18:
    5893–5903.
28. LIBERTINI, L. J., C. A. BURKE, P. C. JOST & O. H. GRIFFITH. 1974. J. Mag. Res.
    15:460–474.
29. JOST, P. C., O. H. GRIFFITH, R. A. CAPALDI & G. VANDERKOOI. 1973. Biochim.
    Biophys. Acta 311:141–152.
30. GRIFFITH, O. H. & P. C. JOST. 1976. In Spin Labeling: Theory and Applica-
    tions. L. Berliner, Ed. Vol. 1:454–523. Academic Press, New York, N.Y.
31. SEELIG, J. 1977. Quart. Rev. Biophys. 10:353–418.
32. DAVOUST, J., B. M. SCHOOT & P. F. DEVAUX. 1979. Proc. Natl. Acad. Sci. USA
    76:2755–2759.
33. GRIFFITH, O. H. & P. C. JOST. 1979. In Cytochrome Oxidase. T. E. KING,
    B. Chance, K. Okunuki & Y. Orii, Eds. pp. 207–218. Elsevier/North-Holland
    Biomedical Press, The Netherlands.
34. BOGGS, J. M., D. D. WOOD, M. A. MOSCARELLO & D. PAPAHADJOPOULOS. 1977.
    Biochemistry 16:2325–2329.

DISCUSSION OF THE PAPER

DR. G. G. SHIPLEY (*Boston University, Boston, Mass.*): Is there a boundary gradient of lipid?

DR. JOST: You are talking about a second tail or second shell effect. We have some recent evidence from a photolabeling experiment, where we have tied the lipid to the protein, suggesting that the gradient is relatively small. That is, by the second tail or shell you have relatively little perturbation. There is a slightly broader bilayer line width in this second shell lipid and this is in agreement with unpublished data of Knowles, Watts, and Marsh † where they have used difference spectra to demonstrate this point.

DR. SHIPLEY: These data would suggest that the adjacent lipids are modified.

DR. P. C. JOST: Yes, although we think that this effect is actually less than it is usually thought to be, and it is dependent upon the lipid content. Chapman has been making a point that the line shapes in ESR are dependent on the content of the lipid and it is a very good point; we believe this effect is not due to the lipid directly associated with the protein, but to the lipids in the second shell and beyond.

DR. LUZZATI: I remember discussing this point of the interaction of lipids and proteins in membranes with Richard Henderson. He pointed out to me that in his diffraction diagrams there was a concentration of intensity located in the 4.5 reciprocal Å region, meaning that the hydrocarbon chains are of the liquid kind, but that they were localized in spots. In other words, he meant that you had a glass structure, in other words, a frozen liquid.

DR. JOST: Yes. We had occasion to look at that in collaboration with Walter Stoeckenius and, in fact, there is a small pool of hindered bilayer, which is consistent with the compositional data and with Henderson's data.

DR. TALL: I seem to recall seeing some data that indicated that there was a decrease in quadrupole splitting as a function of the lipid:protein ratio, which would indicate a positive evidence for increased disordering, the more protein there was. I am not sure that you really addressed that. I believe that you said that they could not see the boundary lipid, but that evidence would seem to support a disordering effect.

DR. JOST: There are some technicalities involved here. I think you are referring to Dr. Seelig's paper in which he got a pronounced decrease in the coupling constant, and there is some suggestion from some unpublished data ‡ that I received from Dr. Odfield that this may partially be due to cholate. Nevertheless, it is a consistent observation that in the presence of protein above the transition temperature of the lipid that the quadrupole splitting is decreased.

† KNOWLES, P. F., A. WATTS & D. MARSH. 1979. Lipid immobilization in dimyristoylphosphatidylcholine-substituted cytochrome oxidase. Biochemistry **18:** 4480–4487.

‡ RICE, D., J. C. HSUNG, T. E. KING & E. OLDFIELD. 1979. Biochemistry **18:** 5885–5891.

This is consistent with several models, the most plausible of which has been advanced by Seelig that the lipid in contact with the protein is forced to conform to an irregular surface.

DR. LANDSBERGER: I would just like to make a comment on magnetic resonance spectroscopy in general and deuterium NMR specifically. The line shape one gets from deuterium NMR particularly at high protein-to-lipid ratios is not evidence of a great change in what was referred to as a quadrupole coupling constant. What you see are divergences in spectra so that areas that are supposed to be very sharp become very broad, and the broadening that you observe is consistent with the model that you are seeing in many different environments, each characterized by a different coupling constant. Thus, simply analyzing data in terms of coupling constants is a bit treacherous because you happened to pick out a component that gives rise to the peak, but there are a lot of different environments contributing to the spectrum.

DR. JOST: I agree. There are several models. When you talk about the order parameter, there is a semantic issue involved. For example, if you say a lot of disorder and you are just talking about the order parameter, you mean high motion. You do not mean spacial disorder. When you are talking about a lot of order, you do not necessarily mean special order. You are talking about less motion. The ESR and NMR semantics on this are slightly different, so you get into communication problems. I think that is what happened with the NMR data versus the ESR data, and that is the reason that some people have been tempted to call what we had earlier named boundary lipid as highly ordered. That is, it shows restricted motion, but this lipid is spatially disordered. We have been able to show this effect with oriented samples, and what you see is what you would expect of lipid that is forced to conform to a protein that has an irregular surface, with hydrophobic amino acid residues projecting.

DR. SMALL: So we really have a tremendous range, from lipids that are extremely loosely associated with protein such as those discussed by Dr. Goodman and Dr. Wirtz, to lipids that are highly immobilized and specifically bound.

DR. JOST: For example, in cytochrome oxidase there have been estimated to be 45 to 55 contact sites. It looks as if at least six of these may be specific for certain phospholipids.

LIPID DOMAINS IN THE YOLK LIPOPROTEIN COMPLEX *

Joe Ross,† Richard F. Wrenn,‡ Douglas H. Ohlendorf,§ and
Leonard J. Banaszak

*Department of Biological Chemistry
Division of Biology and Biomedical Sciences
Washington University
St. Louis, Missouri 63110*

Because of the size and complexity of the serum lipoproteins, a variety of "model" lipid–protein systems have been studied with the goal of understanding their organization. One such model system is the yolk lipoprotein complex found in oocytes from oviparous animals. This yolk system in amphibian eggs is present in microcrystalline form,[1] and hence can be studied by diffraction methods. To the extent that similarities exist in the overall assembly of lipid and protein between the yolk, serum, and other soluble lipoproteins, simple ordered model systems can propide a wealth of structural data.

The yolk system from *Xenopus laevis* and other amphibia, birds, and insects contains two major components: a lipoprotein called lipovitellin and a phosphoprotein named phosvitin. This complex is derived from a precursor protein called lipovitellogenin, produced in the liver. Lipovitellogenin is transported in the serum in a form that is thought to contain two copies of a single polypeptide chain having a molecular weight in the range of 180,000–200,000.[2, 3] This single chain polypeptide precursor is believed to be cleaved during uptake by the ovaries into phosvitin and the three different polypeptïdes in lipovitellin.

Biochemical analysis of the yolk lipoprotein from *Xenopus,* combined with earlier estimates of its size, showed that it is a dimeric complex of MW 456,000.[4] Each monomeric unit contains four different polypeptide chains called LV-A (MW 105,000), LV-B (MW 35,500), and LV-C (MW 32,000).[4] Phosvitin, the other protein component, was found to have a molecular weight of 17,000.[4] The complex contains about 17% lipid, which, by further analysis, is equivalent to a stoichiometry of about 35 molecules of phospholipid and 15 molecules of neutral lipid in each subunit of lipovitellin.[4]

THE EM MODEL

Although it has not been possible to obtain large single crystals of the yolk lipoprotein complex, the use of electron microscopy and image reconstruction methods has resulted in a low resolution map of the complex as seen in nega-

* This work was supported by the National Institutes of Health Grant GM 13925 and by the National Science Foundation Grant PCM 74–03397.

† Postdoctoral fellow of the Missouri Heart Association and the National Institutes of Health.

‡ Recipient of the Biomedical Engineering Training Grant at Washington University.

§ Present address: Institute of Molecular Biology, University of Oregon, Eugene, Oregon 94703.

tively stained fragments of the microcrystals.[5] Interpretation of the map reveals a molecule with an ellipsoidal shape of dimensions about $55 \times 115 \times 250$ Å.[5]

In the crystalline form, the component subunits, each of about 228,000 daltons, appear to be related by two-fold rotational symmetry. This symmetry was used to average the two component subunits in the EM map.[5] A schematic view of the yolk complex is shown in FIGURE 1. The surface features in the EM map are sufficiently visible to permit the tentative identification of several different domains. However, it must be emphasized that the domains indicated in FIGURE 1 are based only on these low resolution surface features and that

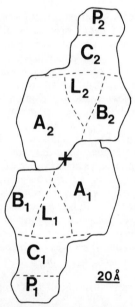

FIGURE 1. Schematic representation of the yolk lipoprotein complex. The schematic representation of the yolk lipoprotein complex is based on a map derived from electron micrographs and image reconstruction methods. Details of these results can be found in Reference 5. The cross marks the position of the local two-fold axis of the lipoprotein dimer. This symmetry dyad would be perpendicular to the plane of the drawing. The dotted lines outline crude surface domains which are marked by the letters A, B, C, D, and L. Subscripts to each lettered domain suggest how each might interact to form a subunit in the dimeric lipoprotein.

there is a need to identify these structural components by some experimental means. Though it is tempting to assign them to the known chemical components, at this point it is sufficient to conclude that the lipovitellin–phosvitin complex has a subunit structure typical of globular proteins.

Foremost in identifying the domains in the EM model is the problem of finding the location(s) of the lipid in the overall complex. It was felt that if the lipid were aggregated into two domains (one lipid domain/lipovitellin monomer), then it would probably be centrally located in each monomer. Such a location would shield the hydrocarbon chains of the lipid from the aqueous environment. One such region is visible in the EM model and is labeled L in FIGURE 1.[5] An alternative lipid site in the complex would be the central-most region of the dimer itself, near the two-fold symmetry element in FIGURE 1. However, earlier chemical studies have shown that lipovitellin will dissociate into two stable monomers at alkaline pH.[1] It is difficult to see how such a dissociation would be possible if the lipid were organized around the local two-fold axis.

THE EXPERIMENTAL LOCATION OF STRUCTURAL DOMAINS IN THE EM MODEL

One obvious method for locating structural components within a low resolution map of the complex would be to produce specific modifications of the microcrystals and then to locate the sites of such changes using crystallographic techniques. This could be done with either electron microscopy and three-dimensional image reconstruction or x-ray powder diffraction. Although EM and 3-D image reconstruction can produce an image of the modified complex, the x-ray powder technique is easier and the chances of finding suitable modifications from which data can be collected are greater, and thus this approach was taken.

Early attempts to mark the lipid domain focused on removing the lipid from the microcrystals in a manner that did not affect crystallinity.[13] To extract the lipid, lyophilized microcrystals were treated with acetone and other solvents at low temperatures. After the microcrystals were returned to temperatures above 0° C, they were washed to remove residual solvent. X-ray photographs were then obtained from tightly packed specimens of such material. These extraction studies showed that the crystalline lipoprotein would survive short exposures to organic solvents at low temperatures. However, if an exhaustive lipid extraction was carried out, there was a comcomitant loss in crystallinity as judged by the x-ray exposure needed to obtain suitable powder photographs. Because of the detrimental effect of complete lipid extraction on lipoprotein crystallinity, these studies were abandoned and another property of lipid domains was exploited.

A characteristic of most packed lipid systems which might be used as a natural marker is the relatively low electron density in the region of the hydrocarbon chains. For example, low electron density can be seen at the midpoint of one-dimensional electron density profiles from phospholipid bilayers. This is the so-called terminal methyl region or bilayer midline. Similar regions of low electron density are thought to exist in other lipid forms such as the serum lipoproteins. Data suggest that the core of these complexes is less electron dense than the surface.

CONTRAST MATCHING

If the hydrocarbon chains contained in the yolk lipoprotein are present in the form of a low electron density domain, then this fact can be used to locate their physical position in the crystalline lipoprotein lattice. To visualize how this might work, consider x-ray scattering from a multicomponent system with each component having a notable difference in electron density. The scattering is a weighted sum of contributions from each component or domain, and the weighting is proportional to the difference between its own electron density and that of the solvent. By changing the electron density of the solvent, domains of different electron density can be made to contribute more or less to the scattered radiation. This principle, often called contrast matching, has been used most elegantly to study the quaternary structure of macromolecules using neutron scattering.[7] It has also been used successfully to study the relative distribution of lipid and protein in both high and low density serum lipoproteins.[8, 9] In these lipoprotein experiments, changes in the solvent scattering density are used to enhance the contrast of the pertinent low electron density region.[8] In both the x-ray and neutron experiments, the Patterson function calculated from small angle solution scattering data was used to obtain the distance between scattering elements in spherically averaged particles.

With crystalline diffraction data, the Patterson analysis yields not only the length of the vector separating the structural elements, but the orientation of that vector. With enough additional symmetry in the crystal array, the origin of that vector can be determined and thus the coordinates of any major scattering domain in the unit cell can be found. This is ideally true if contributions from all other domains can be matched with a solvent of equal electron density. Determining the crystal coordinates of scattering components using Patterson maps is a problem frequently encountered by both protein and small molecule crystallographers. For those interested in how such methods are applied, a description can be found in most x-ray crystallography texts.

CONTRAST MATCHING OF YOLK LIPOPROTEIN CRYSTALS

Since the yolk lipoprotein crystals dissolve in the presence of high concentrations of salt, solvent electron density changes were made by the addition of glycerol. By varying the concentration of glycerol from 0% to 80% (vol/vol), the solvent electron density can be changed from 0.335 electrons/Å^3 (e/Å^3) to 0.393 e/Å^3. FIGURE 2 illustrates the changes in the electron density contrast between the solvent and three different structural components within the lipoprotein as the glycerol concentration is increased. The polar head group and hydrocarbon regions of phospholipids were assumed to have electron densities of 0.49 and 0.29 e/Å^3, respectively.[9] For the protein, a value of 0.41 e/Å^3 was used, which is equal to that described for the high electron density region of the serum lipoproteins.[9] It is also similar to the value of 0.45 e/Å^3 used for protein by other workers.[10] FIGURE 2 illustrates the two important experimental aspects of contrast matching in x-ray experiments with lipoproteins. The first requirement is that a sizeable difference in electron density must exist between the protein and the lipid. Assuming that the aforementioned electron densities taken from the literature are applicable to the yolk system, the first requirement is fulfilled. The second prerequisite is that it must be possible to nearly "match" the protein electron density with the solvent. FIGURE 2 shows that this can be done with glycerol–water solutions.

X–RAY METHODS

Since no large single crystals of the yolk lipoprotein complex had yet been obtained, it was necessary to devise a method for collecting x-ray data from

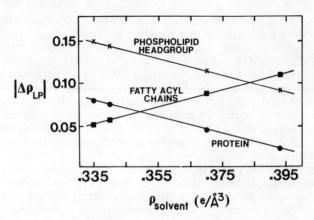

FIGURE 2. Contrast matching effects in lipoproteins. In the graph, electron density contrast is plotted versus solvent electron density beginning at the left with water. The other points are calculated for solutions containing 10, 50, and 80% (vol/vol) glycerol. The ordinate, $|\Delta\rho_{LP}|$, is the absolute value of electron density contrast estimated for structural elements within the yolk lipoprotein starting with literature values as described in the text. For example, in a solvent of pure water (0.335 e/Å³), loosely packed hydrocarbon chains have a contrast $|\Delta\rho_{LP}|$ equal to the absolute value of 0.335–0.29 e/Å³ and this is the lowest point in the left hand corner of the plot.

microcrystals. X-ray powder diffraction data for the lipoprotein crystals in each of four solvent electron densities were recorded on film with a Huxley-Brown x-ray camera.[6, 11] After densitometry of the powder photographs, the structure factors of the low angle Bragg reflections, to a resolution of about 45 Å (20 x-ray reflections), were estimated by a numerical procedure which separates overlapping reflections and utilizes the entire ring profile as recorded on the film.[11] By using the centric reflections at varying solvent electron densities, the data were scaled so that the scattering due to the molecule remained constant and the scattering due to the solvent varied linearly with solvent electron density.[11] Using such scaled estimates of the x-ray data at each solvent density, three-dimensional Patterson functions were calculated and inspected for peaks that changed most rapidly between data sets.

To analyze the Patterson maps, a careful comparison of the sections containing Harker peaks was first made. Harker peaks are the result of vectors between symmetry-related positions in the crystal unit cell and can be used directly to obtain the position of the scattering element. In Patterson maps from the yolk lipoprotein crystals, one expects peaks due to the low electron dense lipid to become more dominant as the solvent electron density approaches that of the protein. One set of mutually consistent Harker peaks was more prominent on the 80% glycerol Patterson map than on the other three maps. Specifically, one of these Harker peaks changes from 12% to 40% of the origin peak as the solvent density was increased. Several such changes were visible and, as already noted, it was possible to locate a mutually consistent set of Harker peaks on the 80% glycerol map which was not recognizable on the corresponding map obtained with water.

This initial position will hereafter be referred to as a low electron density site (LED). To some degree, the presence of a region of low electron density could be verified by using the known two-fold symmetry of the lipoprotein dimer.[5] A second LED site should exist in a position related to the first by the known dyad symmetry of the lipoprotein molecule. In fact, a set of Harker peaks was identified in the Patterson map obtained from the crystals in 80% glycerol, corresponding to this symmetry-related position.

A POSSIBLE LIPID–CONTAINING REGION—THE LED SITE

Two orthogonal views of the lipoprotein complex are shown in FIGURE 3 with the observed LED positions marked by the large crosses. Note that these

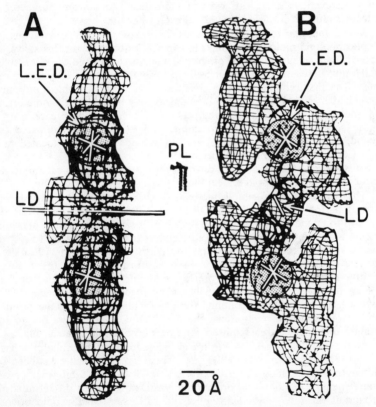

FIGURE 3. The location of the low electron density site in the yolk lipoprotein map. The contour map of the yolk lipoprotein shown here is very similar to that first described in Reference 5 and was photographed directly from a molecular graphics system called the MMS-X. Two approximately orthogonal views of the molecular envelope are shown. The map shown in FIGURE 3B is nearly oriented such that the viewer is looking down the local dyad marked by the symbol, *LD*. The low electron density regions are marked by the white crosses labeled LED. In the center of the drawing is a scaled stick model of dipalmitoyl phosphatidylcholine. It has been included outside the map so that the reader can obtain perspective of the relative sizes of lipid and lipoprotein.

positions correspond to a central location in the L regions of the EM model. The small difference in appearance between the schematic drawing given earlier in FIGURE 1 and the contour map in FIGURE 3 is partly due to the use of a higher contour level and should be ignored. As can be seen in FIGURE 3, the distance between the LED regions in the two subunits of the dimeric lipoprotein is about 60 Å. This relatively large separation can be taken as evidence for two unique non-interacting lipid domains in the lipoprotein.

Before discussing the significance of the LED site in terms of lipid packing, one factor should be emphasized. Because the resolution of the x-ray data is only 45 Å, the LED sites must be interpreted as regions. This can be explained as follows. At low resolution, a site detectable by contrast matching must either be very large or have very high contrast. Since the contrast between the lipid and the solvent is not great, we conclude that a significant number of lipid molecules must be clustered together at each LED site.

Model building techniques were used to explore possible arrangements of the phospholipid molecules within the two LED domains. In this study, knowledge of lipid arrangements in other systems was combined with the structural data found here using several criteria to limit the number of possible orientations. The first requirement was that the lipid must fit within the boundaries of the EM map. Although these boundaries may be subject to some errors, the final molecular volume of the lipoprotein model was based on careful estimates of the components and their volumes,[5] and hence is a reasonable criteria. Second, the methyl ends of the fatty acyl chains should be located near the LED site and away from the surface of the molecule that is exposed to the aqueous solvent. Third, because of the known stoichiometry, each lipid domain must contain about 50 lipid molecules.

The results of these simple modeling tests produce many possible orientations of the phospholipid in the EM map. Only a few will be described here. The two top panels, FIGURE 4A and 4B, show a single dipalmitoyl phosphatidylcholine molecule aligned with the acyl chains parallel to the narrowest dimension of the lipoprotein complex and the methyl end near the LED site. The phosphatidylcholine head group is in a conformation with the positive and negative charges of the head group approximately perpendicular to the fatty acyl chains [12] and the head group has been placed at the aqueous surface of the complex. FIGURE 4B contains the phospholipid in the same position but now viewed almost directly down the acyl chains. This allows one to roughly estimate the surface area required for one phospholipid head group.

In the bottom panels of FIGURE 4, an additional phospholipid has been added to the region near the LED site. This second molecule has been rotated relative to the one shown in FIGURE 4A and 4B to start a bilayer type of lipid arrangement. The tail-to-tail orientation was arranged with the terminal methyl carbons of the fatty acyl chains near the LED site. In the lipid orientations that are shown in FIGURE 4C and 4D, the head groups are again placed near the solvent region with the fatty acyl chains parallel to the narrowest dimension of the lipoprotein complex. As can be seen in the illustration, such a bilayer-like orientation does indeed fit into the low resolution model. However, a bilayer-like packing arrangement suggests that the primary lipid, that is, those molecules that are interacting directly with the protein, are doing so in a roughly symmetrical way. This can be described in more detail as follows. A tail-to-tail bilayer arrangement can have approximately two-fold rotational symmetry between the acyl chains. If such symmetry is then extended to primary lipid binding sites on the apoprotein, a similar symmetry in the underlying conformation of the protein is implied. Such conformational symmetry is difficult to envision because of the general asymmetrical nature of single globular proteins.

Using the same model building methods or volume calculations, it is also possible to test whether or not a micellar arrangement of lipid would satisfac-

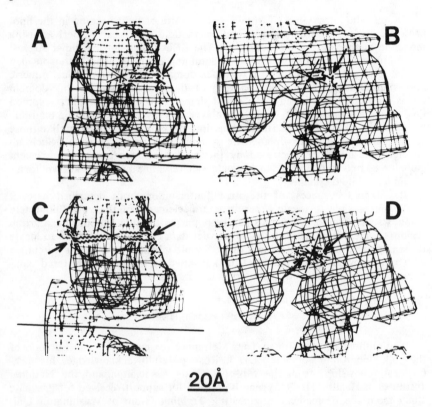

20Å

FIGURE 4. Phospholipid in the LED region. The contoured maps were prepared in the same way as FIGURE 3 and contain a scaled stick model of dipalmitoyl phosphatidylcholine within the boundaries of the yolk lipoprotein complex. Each phospholipid molecule is marked by an arrow and the positions of the LED sites are again marked by crosses. FIGURES 4A and B, and 4C and D are roughly orthogonal views. The phospholipid(s) in views 4B and D are seen down a line of sight that is almost parallel to their hydrocarbon chains. In FIGURE 4D the two head groups appear very close together but are in fact on opposite sides of the molecule.

torily fulfill the aforementioned criteria. The overall size of a micelle is limited by the packing of the hydrocarbon chains near the core. By simply requiring that the 100 fatty acyl chains be no closer than about 4.5 Å, the radius of the core must be at least 12 Å and the radius of the micelle itself must be greater than 27 Å. Such a structure would protrude beyond the boundaries of the EM model. Furthermore, in any micellar phospholipid arrangement, many of the head groups would have to be placed in an inner region of the lipoprotein complex, and because of these chemical arguments and the volume considerations, micellar domains were rejected.

Summary

Despite the importance of knowing the nature of lipid packing in the lipoprotein complex, the trial phospholipid orientations which can be derived using modeling methods are still speculative. The LED regions in the dimer suggest the approximate positions of the lipid-containing domains. The Patterson map at 80% glycerol is consistent with two such domains in the symmetrical dimeric lipoprotein molecule. Micellar packing of the phospholipid in this domain seems highly unlikely based on size and shape considerations. Other common lipid packing arrangements, either monolayer or bilayer-like, would be plausible based on the LED location. However, a lipid packing arrangement unlike those so far observed in only lipid–water systems also seems possible. Such an arrangement might be nucleated by the lipid binding sites on the adjacent globular components and as such would not resemble presently known forms of condensed lipid systems.

Based on the success of the x-ray Patterson methods described here, it should be possible to locate other structural elements of the yolk lipoprotein complex. For example, if metals can be bound to the phospholipid head group region(s), measurement of the x-ray powder data could again be used to locate those positions in the crystalline lattice. Simple labeling experiments combined with x-ray powder measurements could be used to locate any clustered component of the complex, and such work is in progress.

Acknowledgments

The authors are grateful to Tom Meininger for his help in the isolation of the yolk lipoprotein complex. Dr. J. Ross gratefully acknowledges his postdoctoral fellowships from the Missouri Heart Association and the National Institutes of Health. Dr. R. Wrenn is grateful for support received for graduate study from the Biomedical Engineering Training Grant at Washington University.

References

1. Wallace, R. A. & J. N. Dumont. 1968. The induced synthesis and transport of yolk proteins and their accumulation by the oocytes in *Xenopus laevis*. J. Cell. Physiol. **72**:73–89.
2. Bergink, E. W. & R. A. Wallace. 1974. Precursor-product relationship between amphibian lipovitellogenin and the yolk proteins, lipovitellin and phosvitin. J. Biol. Chem. **249**:2897–2903.
3. Clemens, M. J., R. Lofthouse & J. R. Tata. 1975. Sequential changes in the protein synthetic activity of male *Xenopus laevis* liver following induction of egg yolk lipoproteins by estradiol-17 β. J. Biol. Chem. **250**:2213–2218.
4. Ohlendorf, D. H., G. R. Barbarash, A. Trout, C. Kent & L. J. Banaszak. 1977. Lipid and polypeptide components of the crystalline yolk system from *Xenopus laevis*. J. Biol. Chem. **252**:7992–8001.

5. OHLENDORF, D. H., R. F. WRENN & L. J. BANASZAK. 1978. Three dimensional structure of the lipovitellin-phosvitin complex from amphibian oocytes. Nature **272**:28–32.
6. OHLENDORF, D. H., M. L. COLLINS, E. O. PURONEN, L. J. BANASZAK & S. C. HARRISON. 1975. Crystalline lipoprotein-phosphoprotein complex in oocytes from *Xenopus laevis:* Determination of lattice parameters by x-ray crystallography and electron microscopy. J. Mol. Biol. **99**:153–165.
7. ENGELMAN, D. M. & P. B. MOORE. 1975. Determination of quaternary structure by small angle neutron scattering. Ann. Rev. Biophys. Bioeng. **4**:219–241.
8. LUZZATI, V., A. TARDIEU, L. MATEU & H. B. STUHRMANN. 1976. Structure of human serum lipoproteins in solution. I. Theory and techniques of an x-ray scattering approach using solvents of variable density. J. Mol. Biol. **101**:115–127.
9. TARDIEU, A., L. MATEU, C. SARDET, B. WEISS, V. LUZZATI, L. AGGERBECK & A. M. SCANU. 1976. Structure of human serum lipoproteins in solution. II. Small angle scattering study of HDL$_3$ and LDL. J. Mol. Biol. **101**:129–153.
10. MULLER, K., P. LAGGNER, O. GLATTER & G. KOSTNER. 1978. The structure of human-plasma low-density lipoprotein B. An x-ray small angle scattering study. Eur. J. Biochem. **82**:73–90.
11. WRENN, R. 1979. Ph.D. Thesis, Washington University, St. Louis, Mo. Manuscript in preparation.
12. FRANKS, N. P. 1976. Structural analysis of hydrated egg lecithin and cholesterol bilayers. I. X-ray diffraction. J. Mol. Biol. **100**:345–358.
13. COLLINS, M. 1977. Ph.D. Thesis, Washington University, St. Louis, Mo.

DISCUSSION OF THE PAPER

DR. D. M. SMALL: I wonder whether it would be possible to remove the lipids, and then put them back and restore the structure. This could be tried with deuterated lipids, and then you might conduct the neutron scattering studies. Have you done that?

DR. L. J. BANASZAK: We have been considering the possibility that replacing the phospholipid with deuterated phospholipids, which would give an enormous contrast factor between the lipid binding region and the protein. The problem is that it may not be possible to get many crystal reflections because of the nature of our system. I think we would be limited to three or four reflections, and the neutron camera may not be able to resolve them satisfactorily.

DR. G. G. SHIPLEY: Dr. Banaszak, you are trying to pack 40 or so phospholipids per protein subunit—you also mentioned there was a neutral lipid component which I think accounts for about 15 or 20 molecules per subunit. Could you remind us what those neutral lipids are?

DR. BANASZAK: There are some triglycerides and I think we measured some cholesterol too. If you remember the slide that I presented earlier, I think that there are about 30 molecules of neutral lipid, and that is one of the reasons that lead me to believe that the whole thing must be a condensed lipid domain. I would suggest that as the structure builds up it somehow accepts neutral lipids into the central region of the lipid binding domain, but this is just pure speculation.

QUESTION: Have you ever tried to hydrolyze the phospholipids in your complex enzymatically?

DR. BANASZAK: No.

COMMENT: It may be a gentle way to remove the components from your crystal system.

DR. BANASZAK: I agree. We intend to do some more work along that line.

LIPID–PROTEIN INTERACTIONS IN ENVELOPED VIRUSES *

Frank R. Landsberger † and Larry D. Altstiel

Rockefeller University
New York, New York 10021

The influenza, parainfluenza, and rhabdoviruses are enveloped, negative-strand RNA viruses that mature by a process of budding at the host cell plasma membrane.[1-3] During virus maturation, virus proteins associate with regions of the host cell plasma membrane, and host cell proteins are excluded from areas of the plasma membrane containing virus proteins.[1-3] During virus assembly, there is continuity between the lipid bilayers of the host cell and the envelope of the maturing virus particle.[1-3] The lipid composition of the virion reflects that of the host cell plasma membrane, while the protein composition of the virus envelope is determined by the viral genome.[4-9]

The outer surface of a typical enveloped virus particle contains glycoproteins, which form spike-like projections on the virus envelope. The rhabdovirus, vesicular stomatitis virus (VSV), contains a surface glycoprotein (G-protein), which is responsible for virus binding to cell surface receptors.[10-12] Influenza virus contains two surface glycoproteins: a hemagglutinin (HA), which is responsible for virus-induced hemagglutinating of erythrocytes and virus binding to neuraminic-acid-containing receptors on the host cell surface; and a neuraminidase, which can catalyze the removal of neuraminic acid from glycoprotein virus receptors.[2] Paramyxoviruses such as Sendai virus contain a surface glycoprotein (HN), which has both hemagglutinating and neuraminidase activity and an envelope-associated glycoprotein (F), which promotes fusion of the virus envelope with the plasma membrane of the target cells.[1] Associated with the inner surface of the lipid bilayer of many enveloped viruses is the nonglycosylated matrix or membrane protein (M-protein).[1-3]

The lipids of the enveloped viruses appear to have an asymmetric distribution in the lipid bilayer.[13]

MEMBRANE STRUCTURE OF ENVELOPED VIRUSES

In our studies of the structure of enveloped viruses and their interaction with the cell surface, we have used spin label electron spin resonance (ESR) techniques. Spin labels that have proved to be useful in probing the structure of the lipid bilayer are diagramed below.

An ESR spectrum of the C_5 stearic acid spin label incorporated into the lipid bilayer of VSV is shown in FIGURE 1. The distance between the outermost peaks of the spectrum $2A'_{zz}$ is a measure of the motion of the probe. An increase in $2A'_{zz}$ indicates that the spin label is in a more rigid environment whereas a

* This work was supported by United States Public Health Service Grant AI-14040 from the National Institute of Health and National Science Foundation Grants PCM 78–09346 and PCM 79–22956.

† Andrew W. Mellon Foundation Fellow.

$$CH_3(CH_2)_{17-n}—C—(CH_2)_{n-2}COOH \qquad (C_n)$$

$$CH_3(CH_2)_{17-n}—C—(CH_2)_{n-2}—C—O—CH \qquad (PC_n)$$

decrease in $2A'_{zz}$ indicates that the spin label is in a more fluid environment.[14, 15] Because the motion of the probe is governed by the motion of the surrounding molecules, the spin label spectrum provides information about the relative fluidity or rigidity of the matrix in which the probe is located.

The lipid bilayer of all enveloped virus examined is more rigid than that of the host cell plasma membrane from which it is derived.[16] Similarly, lipid bilayers prepared from lipids extracted from virus envelopes are less rigid than the intact virion envelope.[16, 17] These results suggest that interactions between envelope-associated proteins and lipids can increase the rigidity of the lipid bilayer.

The ESR data obtained in the study of enveloped viruses indicate that changes in lipid–protein interactions can result in changes in the ESR spectrum of spin labels incorporated into the lipid bilayer.[16-19] In the case of a simple one-component lipid bilayer, a spin label such as a C_5 stearic acid probe is

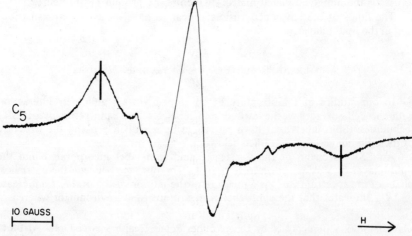

FIGURE 1. C_5 spin labeled vesicular stomatitis virus. The vertical lines are drawn through the extrema of the outermost peaks. The distance between these two lines is defined as $2A'_{zz}$.

homogeneously distributed in the plane of the bilayer. The observed ESR spectrum is thus characterized by the motional properties of the fatty acyl chains of membrane lipids. In a multicomponent lipid bilayer, such as found in enveloped viruses or in the plasma membrane of cells, it is likely that there is heterogeneity in the lateral composition of the plasma membrane in addition to the asymmetric distribution of lipids between the inner and outer monolayers of the bilayer. In this case, the spin labels are distributed among the various domains in accordance with the extent of these domains and with the relative solubility of the probe in these regions of different lipid composition. The observed ESR spectrum in a bilayer having a complex composition represents the sum of the environments probed by the spin label, weighted according to the fraction of spin labels in each domain. Thus, the measured ESR splitting $(2A'_{zz})$ represents what can be described as an effective rigidity of the lipid bilayer. Therefore, the changes that we have observed upon alterations in the lipid–protein interactions reflect changes in the effective environment observed by the spin labels.

To assess the nature of the interaction between the G-protein of VSV and the lipid bilayer, the G-protein extracted from VSV with lysolecithin, which can be quantitatively removed with bovine serum albumin, was reconstituted in liposomes composed of egg yolk lecithin. Like intact virions, the lecithin vesicles that were reconstituted with G-protein were found to agglutinate goose erythrocytes and bind to tissue culture cells. The molar ratio of G-protein to lipid in the reconstituted vesicles is similar to intact virus. Using the C_5 spin label we found that insertion of G-protein into a lipid bilayer causes a small increase in the rigidity of the lipid bilayer. Cross-linking of G-protein in the lipid bilayer was investigated by cross-linking the G-protein reconstituted in lecithin liposomes with antibody directed against G. The ESR spectra of C_5-labeled lecithin vesicles containing G-protein indicate that cross-linking of the G-protein does increase the rigidity of the lipid bilayer.

VIRUS ATTACHMENT AND PENETRATION

The initial step in a virus infection is the attachment of the virus particle to the host cell plasma membrane.[20, 21] Enveloped viruses possess a net negative surface charge as do the host cells.[22, 38] Two such negative surfaces could be expected to repel each other, thereby preventing attachment of the virus to the cell surface. The negative charges on the virus and cell surfaces are screened by positive counterions in the surrounding solution, which in turn are partially screened by their counterions. This results in an ionic double layer, one layer being the charges on the membrane surface and the other being counterions in solution near the membrane surface.[23] Spin label ESR techniques were used to investigate the properties of this ionic double layer.

A series of head-group phospholipid spin labels having a nitroxide group separated from the phosphate ester moiety by spacer groups of different lengths was used to measure properties associated with the electrical double layer. The fatty acids of the lipid spin labels intercalate into the membrane lipid bilayer and the nitroxide spin label probes regions at varying distances from the surface of the membrane. The isotropic hyperfine coupling constant of the spin label, which can be directly measured from the ESR spectrum, is proportional to the local electric field.[24-26] Therefore these labels can be used to measure the electrical field at varying distances from a membrane surface. ESR data obtained from these spin labels incorporated into lecithin vesicles containing 10% phosphatidic acid and into VSV indicate that the change in the isotropic hyperfine coupling constant with distance from the surface of these membranes has the functional form predicted by the Gouy-Chapman theory. The Gouy-Chapman theory predicts that the width of the ionic double layer at a charged surface increases as the ionic strength of the surrounding medium decreases.[23] This suggests that at low ionic strength the ability of a virus particle to bind to a cell surface will be diminished by the interaction between the extended double layers surrounding both the virus and cell membrane. It was found that the efficiency of infection of VSV decreased with decreasing ionic strength, thereby suggesting that interactions between ionic double layers on the virus and cell surfaces are involved in virus attachment.

As summarized in TABLE 1, adsorption of VSV particles to BHK cells results in an increase in the rigidity of the cell plasma membrane lipid bilayer. As was shown by Lyles and Landsberger,[27, 28] the adsorption of influenza and parainfluenza viruses to the surface of avian erythrocytes similarly results in a structural change in the plasma membrane as a result of the cross-linking of the membrane receptors.

VSV-infected cells secrete a water soluble form of the G-protein (G_s),[29-31] which appears to be monovalent. Addition of G_s to the cell surface does not cause an increase in the rigidity of the plasma membrane lipid bilayer of BHK cells. However, addition of anti-G IgG to cells pretreated with G_s results in an increase in bilayer rigidity as shown in TABLE 1. These results suggest that the cross-linking of virus receptors in the plane of the plasma membrane results

TABLE 1

THE EFFECT OF VSV ON THE FLUIDITY OF THE BHK-21 CELL PLASMA MEMBRANE LABELED WITH C_5 *

Experiment	$2A'_{zz}$ (experiment) $-2A'_{zz}$ (control) (Gauss)
BHK	0.0
BHK+VSV	1.3
BHK+G_s	0.0
BHK+G_s+IgG	1.0
BHK+colchicine	0.0
BHK+colchicine+VSV	0.3

* The order of the reagents, e.g., BHK+G_s+IgG, is the order in which they were added to the cells prior to harvesting and spin labeling. A change in $2A'_{zz}$ (experiment) $-2A'_{zz}$ (control) greater than 0.3 gauss indicates the treatment indicated in the table entry caused an increase in the rigidity of the cell plasma membrane lipid bilayer.

in a structural change in the plasma membrane. From TABLE 1, it is seen that the VSV-adsorption-induced change in lipid bilayer structure is inhibited by colchicine. Since microtubules can modulate the lateral mobility of membrane proteins, these results suggest that VSV receptors may be linked to microtubules.

Fusion of spin labeled Sendai virus with human erythrocytes has been investigated as a model for virus penetration. As fusion occurs, the viral and erythrocyte lipid bilayers mix, and the ESR spectrum changes with time from a spectrum characteristic of a spin label in a virus envelope to that of the probe in the erythrocyte membrane. The kinetics of the structural change in the the erythrocyte lipid bilayer resulting from virus-induced hemolysis has also been measured.[32] The fusion kinetics appear to be independent of virus concentration. The rates of fusion induced by early and late harvest Sendai virus, which differ only in that the early harvest virus lacks hemolytic activity, are the same, indicating that hemolytic activity is not required for virus fusion. Fusion of the viral envelope with the erythrocyte lipid bilayer occurs at a similar rate to that of membrane structural changes induced by hemolysis. These results suggest that fusion may be the rate-limiting step under conditions of active hemolysis.

MEMBRANE STRUCTURAL CHANGES DURING VIRUS MATURATION

The assembly of the enveloped viruses in the infected cell appear to share several common features. In the infected cell, the negative strand virus genome is transcribed by viral RNA polymerase into messenger RNAs coding for virus polypeptides. Envelope glycoproteins appear to be synthesized on membrane-bound ribosomes, whereas the M-proteins and proteins that form the virus nucleocapsid are translated on free ribosomes. It is likely that the glycoproteins are inserted into the plasma membrane by fusion of glycoprotein-containing vesicles, derived from cytoplasmic membranes, with the plasma membrane. M-protein preferentially associates with regions of the plasma membrane containing glycoprotein. Upon association of the M-protein with the cytoplasmic side of the plasma membrane, the nucleocapsid binds to areas of the membrane containing M-protein and glycoprotein, and the budding process is initiated.[33-37]

We have used spin label ESR techniques to measure changes in host cell plasma membrane structure during the replicative cycle of VSV. Cells infected with VSV were harvested at various times after infection, spin labeled, and examined by ESR spectroscopy. The results indicate that there is an increase in plasma membrane rigidity caused by the addition of virus and also an additional increase in membrane rigidity over control cells, which coincides with the period of maximal virus release. These results may suggest that the association of viral proteins with the host cell plasma membrane results in a local bilayer rigidity increase. It was also found that colchicine, while not inhibiting intracellular synthesis of viral polypeptides, delayed both the appearance of virus particles and membrane structural changes associated with virus assembly in the infected cell. These data suggest that microtubules may be associated with virus assembly and release.

ACKNOWLEDGMENT

Mrs. Caryn Doktor is acknowledged for her expert assistance in the preparation of the manuscript.

REFERENCES

1. CHOPPIN, P. W. & R. W. COMPANS. 1975. *In* Comprehensive Virology. H. Fraenkel-Conrat & R. R. Wagner, Eds. Vol. 4: 95. Plenum Press, New York, N.Y.
2. COMPANS, R. W. & P. W. CHOPPIN. *Ibid.* Vol. 4: 179.

3. WAGNER, R. R. *Ibid.* Vol. 4: 1.
4. KLENK, H.-D. & P. W. CHOPPIN. 1969. Virology **38**:255.
5. KLENK, H.-D. & P. W. CHOPPIN. 1970. *Ibid.* **40**:939.
6. KLENK, H.-D. & P. W. CHOPPIN. 1970. Proc. Natl. Acad. Sci. USA **66**:57.
7. CHOPPIN, P. W., H.-D. KLENK, R. W. COMPANS & L. A. CALIGUIRI. 1971. Perspect. Virol. **7**:127.
8. CHOPPIN, P. W., R. W. COMPANS, A. SCHEID, J. V. MCSHARRY & S. G. LAZAROWITZ. 1972. *In* Membrane Research. C. F. Fox, Ed. p. 163. Academic Press, New York, N.Y.
9. MCSHARRY, J. J. & R. R. WAGNER. 1971. J. Virol. **7**:59.
10. BISHOP, D. H. L., P. REPIK, J. F. OBIJESKI, N. F. MOORE & R. R. WAGNER. 1975. J. Virol. **16**:75.
11. CARTWRIGHT, B., C. J. SMALE & F. BROWN. 1969. J. Gen. Virol. **5**:1.
12. CARTWRIGHT, G., P. TALBOT & F. BROWN. 1970. J. Gen. Virol. **7**:267.
13. PATZER, E. J., R. R. WAGNER & E. J. DUBOVI. 1979. CRC Crit. Rev. Biochem. **6**:165.
14. HUBBELL, W. L. & H. M. MCCONNELL. 1971. J. Amer. Chem. Soc. **93**:314.
15. JOST, P., L. J. LIBERTINI, V. C. HEBERT & O. H. GRIFFITH. 1971. J. Mol. Biol. **59**:77.
16. LANDSBERGER, F. R., D. S. LYLES & P. W. CHOPPIN. 1978. *In* Negative Strand Viruses and the Host Cell. B. W. J. Mahy & R. D. Barry, Eds. p. 787. Academic Press, New York, N.Y.
17. SEFTON, B. M. & B. J. GAFFNEY. 1974. J. Mol. Biol. **90**:343.
18. LANDSBERGER, F. R., R. W. COMPANS, P. W. CHOPPIN & J. LENARD. 1973. Biochemistry **12**:4498.
19. LANDSBERGER, F. R. & R. W. COMPANS. 1976. Biochemistry **15**:2356.
20. DALES, S. 1973. Bact. Rev. **37**:103.
21. LONBERG-HOLM, K. & L. PHILLIPSON. 1974. Monogr. Virol. **5**.
22. SHERBERT, G. V. 1978. The Biophysical Characterization of the Cell Surface. Academic Press, New York, N.Y.
23. VERWEY, E. J. W. & J. T. G. OVERBECK. 1948. Theory of Lyophobic Colloids. Elsevier Publishing Co., Amsterdam.
24. GRIFFITH, O. H., P. J. DEHLINGER & S. P. VAN. 1974. J. Membrane Biol. **15**:159.
25. SEELIG, J., H. LIMACHER & P. BADER. 1972. J. Amer. Chem. Soc. **94**:6364.
26. GRIFFITH, O. H. & P. C. JOST. 1976. *In* Spin Labelling Theory and Applications. L. J. Berliner, Ed. p. 454. Academic Press, New York, N.Y.
27. LYLES, D. S. & F. R. LANDSBERGER. 1976. Proc. Natl. Acad. Sci. USA **73**:3497.
28. LYLES, D. S. & F. R. LANDSBERGER. 1978. Virology **88**:25.
29. KANG, C. Y. & L. PREVEC. 1971. Virology **46**:678.
30. LITTLE, S. P. & A. S. HUANG. 1977. Virology **81**:37.
31. LITTLE, S. P. & A. S. HUANG. 1978. J. Virol. **27**:330.
32. LYLES, D. S. & F. R. LANDSBERGER. 1979. Biochemistry **18**:5088.
33. ROTHMAN, J. E. & H. LODISH. 1977. Nature 269:775.
34. KATZ, F., J. E. ROTHMAN, V. R. LINGAPPA, G. BLOBEL & H. LODISH. 1977. Proc. Natl. Acad. Sci. USA **74**:3278.
35. KNIPE, D. M., H. F. LODISH & D. BALTIMORE. 1977. J. Virol. **21**:1121.
36. KNIPE, D. M., D. BALTIMORE & H. F. LODISH. 1977. J. Virol. **21**:1128.
37. KNIPE, D. M., D. BALTIMORE & H. F. LODISH. 1977. J. Virol. **21**:1149.
38. BRINTON, C. C. & M. A. LAUFFER. 1959. *In* Electrophoresis Theory, Methods, and Applications. M. Bier, Ed. Vol. 2:427. Academic Press, New York, N.Y.

◄►

DISCUSSION OF THE PAPER

DR. D. M. SMALL: Dr. Landsberger, in the ESR data that you showed, it seemed as if there were fairly small changes in the splitting. What does that correspond to in terms of a change in temperature? Several degrees?

DR. F. R. LANDSBERGER: This is an old problem. With most of the magnetic resonance techniques you report changes whether it is a coupling constant in NMR or deuterium NMR or splittings in ESR, and the question that none of us have really satisfactorily resolved is how much of a physical change would correspond to a given spectral change. We really do not have an answer to it except expressing perhaps such changes in degrees. In our case it may mean several degrees.

DR. R. BLUMENTHAL: Could you speculate about the reasons why cross linking of proteins would change bilayer fluidity and are there other systems known like capping in lymphocytes that change bilayer fluidity?

DR. LANDSBERGER: Just to speculate and that is the best that I can do, the visual model that I have in mind is basically the following: if you have a set of barges in a river floating along they will not change the current greatly, but if you now chain them all together and you have a lot of barges, you are going to change the flow of the water.

DR. P. C. JOST: Do you not think it is conceptually equally probable that if your aggregated protein is in the plane of the bilayer and there is a secondary effect on the protein in the bilayer itself, you should see an apparent increase in fluidity rather than a decrease?

DR. LANDSBERGER: From the arguments that I presented, I could not tell you the sign of the change. It could be greater fluidity or lesser fluidity. In the way we have presented spin labeling here it is used as an empirical assay. I will go one step further. I do not know how many different fluidities there are in the membrane and what kind of average we observe.

DR. JOST: Is it possible that the reporter group is sensing one more or another environment? In other words, you do not have an homogeneous distribution in the bilayer; if you get aggregation it is the equilibrium between those domains that you are sensing.

DR. LANDSBERGER: I agree. That is our mental picture of it as well.

COMMENT: In a number of systems such as herpes simplex virus there is an increased amount of saturated fatty acids as compared to the plasma membrane of the host cell. I wonder whether in your change in fluidity you are just seeing the reflection of the change in the basal chain composition.

DR. LANDSBERGER: I said that the lipid composition of the virus closely reflects that of the plasma membrane. The reason for that phrasing is that the accuracy of the comparison between the plasma membrane and the virus particle rests on the ability to obtain extremely pure plasma membrane preparations. The statement that the lipid composition closely reflects the plasma membrane also rests on the observation that the virus lipid composition follows the change predicted by a change of the host cell.

GENERAL DISCUSSION

D. M. Small, *Moderator*

Boston University
Boston, Massachusetts 02215

DR. D. M. SMALL: Historically, the interest in serum albumin has arisen because of the wide variety of ligands to which this molecule is able to bind. Many years ago, Karusch proposed that this might be explained on the basis of conformational adaptability, that is to say, that there might be conformational changes that allow albumin to bind different ligands. Instead, the studies presented by Dr. J. R. Brown show a very constrained structure for albumin, and thus the conformational flexibility would be rather small in this molecule. Moreover, the model proposed by Dr. Brown indicates that while fatty acids do not compete with the binding of bilirubin, there is some kind of interaction whereby the bilirubin binding is enhanced. This might be perhaps interpreted as conformational influence by both fatty acids upon the binding site of bilirubin.

So, my question to Dr. Brown would be, do you believe that conformational flexibility plays any part in the binding of ligands?

DR. J. R. BROWN (*University of Texas, Austin, Texas*): I think so. As I envision the subdomains, half of the domain would appear to be a rather rigid structure, but the two subdomains appear to be somewhat independent and connected by a flexible peptide. In consequence it is easy to imagine the subdomains being able to wobble a bit to one side or the other or front to back and change their shape a little bit. This may be considered adaptability.

DR. SMALL: Someone mentioned a crystalline structure of albumin being published in abstract form. I know that Craven and other people in Pittsburgh were working on this a couple of years ago, but can anyone give us any details concerning those studies?

COMMENT: I know that particular group has not solved the structure.

DR. SMALL: The microcalorimetric tracing of human serum albumin has been obtained by several people and found to be very complex. There are at least three peaks, as if there are three separate units that might be undergoing a different transition.

LIPOPROTEIN BIOSYNTHESIS: THE AVIAN MODEL *

L. Chan,† W. A. Bradley, A. Dugaiczyk, and A. R. Means

Departments of Cell Biology and Medicine
Baylor College of Medicine
Houston, Texas 77030

Over the past decade, a lot of progress has been made on the primary and secondary structure of eukaryotic apolipoproteins, and the physical chemistry of the lipid–protein interactions of these interesting molecules. However, relatively little is known of the biosynthesis of these proteins at a subcellular and molecular level. In the past five years, our laboratory has used the estrogen-treated cockerel as a model to study the biosynthesis of eukaryotic apolipo-proteins. In this animal, estrogen acutely stimulates the synthesis of the major apolipoproteins in very-low-density lipoproteins (VLDL), without significantly affecting the synthesis of two other major proteins, albumin and apolipoprotein A-I (apoA-I), the major apolipoprotein in high-density lipoproteins (HDL).[1] We have purified and characterized a major VLDL apoprotein, apoVLDL-II. This protein contains two identical polypeptide chains of 82 amino acids each, which are linked by a single disulfide bond at residue 76. The primary amino acid sequence of apoVLDL-II has been determined.[2] Estrogen was found to selectively stimulate the accumulation of the mRNA for apoVLDL-II in the cockerel liver.[1] Analysis of the *in vitro* translation product of apoVLDL-II mRNA by slab gel electrophoresis demonstrated that apoVLDL-II was initially synthesized as a larger putative precursor, pre-apoVLDL-II. Automated N-terminal sequencing of the pre-apoVLDL-II synthesized *in vitro* using various labeled amino acids revealed a 23-amino-acid residue extension consisting of the following sequence: Met-Gln-Tyr-Arg-Ala-Leu-Val-Ile-Ala-Val-Ile-Leu-Leu-Leu-Ser-Thr-Thr-Val-Pro-Glu-Val-X-Ser-Lys . . ., where Lys is the N-terminal amino acid of plasma apoVLDL-II. Hence, a major apolipoprotein in avian VLDL is synthesized initially with a highly hydrophobic signal peptide attached to its N-terminal. This signal peptide is probably cleaved off before the completion of translation. Hence, apoVLDL-II appears to be synthesized and processed by a mechanism similar to that of secretory protein biosynthesis in general.[3] Since apoA-I in the cockerel also appeared to be initially syn-thesized as a putative precursor,[1] it is likely that this biochemical pathway is common to all secreted eukaryotic apolipoproteins.

To understand the modulation of apoVLDL-II synthesis at the DNA level, we have partially purified apoVLDL-II mRNA by various biochemical tech-niques and have prepared a double-stranded (ds) cDNA to the RNA, using the enzyme reverse transcriptase. The ds-cDNA was tailed with about 14 deoxycytidine nucleotides, and was inserted into the *Pst*I site of the plasmid pBR322, which had been tailed with about 14 deoxyguanosine nucleotides. The chimeric plasmid was amplified in *E. coli* strain RRI. Clones were initially selected by hybridization *in situ* to apoVLDL-II cDNA. Confirmation that the

* This work was supported by Grant HL-16512 from the National Institutes of Health and Grant-in-Aid 78–1102 from the American Heart Association.
† Established Investigator of the American Heart Association.

correct sequence was amplified was obtained by the technique of hybrid-arrested cell-free translation.[4] One of the clones selected by these procedures (pVL10) was further analyzed by direct DNA sequencing by the technique of Maxam and Gilbert.[5] In the *Hin*fI fragment of pVL10, we detected a stretch of 42 nucleotides which were the corresponding codons for amino acids 62–75 of apoVLDL-II.[2]

We have thus successfully cloned the structural gene for a major apoprotein in avian VLDL. Using the cloned DNA as a probe, we will be able to answer a number of basic questions on the control of apolipoprotein biosynthesis at the genomic level. Studies are currently in progress to determine the structure of the natural gene for apoVLDL-II, and the regulation of the expression of this gene by various hormonal manipulations.

ACKNOWLEDGMENT

The authors would like to thank Mr. J. P. Moore for excellent technical assistance.

REFERENCES

1. CHAN, L., W. A. BRADLEY, R. L. JACKSON & A. R. MEANS. 1980. Endocrinology **106:**275–283.
2. JACKSON, R. L., H.-Y. LIN, L. CHAN & A. R. MEANS. 1977. J. Biol. Chem. **252:** 250–253.
3 . BLOBEL, G. & B. DOBBERSTEIN. 1975. J. Cell Biol. **67:**835–851.
4. PATERSON, B. M., B. E. ROBERTS & E. L. KUFF. 1977. Proc. Natl. Acad. Sci. USA **74:**4370–4374.
5. MAXAM, A. M. & W. GILBERT. 1977. Proc. Natl. Acad. Sci. USA **74:**560–563.

INTERACTION OF HDL SUBCLASSES
WITH PHOSPHOLIPID

J. A. Hunter, P. J. Blanche, T. M. Forte, and A. V. Nichols

Donner Laboratory
University of California at Berkeley
Berkeley, California 94720

Studies by Havel *et al.* (1973) on human subjects showed phospholipid increases in the HDL_2 range (1.063–1.125 g/ml) and HDL_3 range (1.125–1.200 g/ml) 3 hours following fat ingestion. These *in vivo* observations could be accounted for, singly or in combination, by phospholipid uptake by the HDL subclasses, by increases in their concentration, or by the appearance of phospholipid–apolipoprotein complexes in the HDL density range. *In vivo* studies on rats by Redgrave and Small (1979) and Tall (1979) also showed phospholipid increases in the HDL fraction during chylomicron catabolism.

As a model system for possible interaction of HDL with surface components released during catabolism of triglyceride-rich lipoproteins, we have examined phospholipid uptake by human HDL subclasses, HDL_3 (1.125–1.200 g/ml) and HDL_{2b} (1.063–1.100 g/ml), during *in vitro* incubation (37° C for 4.5 hours) with increasing amounts of sonicated dispersions of human lipoprotein phosphatidylcholine (HL-PC). We also investigated possible changes in HDL size and transfer of apolipoproteins.

Preparative density ultracentrifugation of HDL_3 incubation mixtures showed a maximal increase of 41% in HDL_3 phospholipid (HDL_3-PL) content, at an initial incubation weight ratio of 2.5/1 (HL-PC/HDL_3-PL). Equilibrium density gradient ultracentrifugation of HDL_{2b}, after incubation with HL-PC at a weight ratio of 1.6/1, showed a maximal increase of 26%. To determine whether the increases in phospholipid actually reflected uptake by the HDL subclasses, fractions were analyzed by negative stain electron microscopy and polyacrylamide gradient (4%–30%) gel electrophoresis. At maximal phospholipid uptake, electron microscopy of product HDL showed spherical particles without stacking discoidal complexes or vesicular structures. Gradient gel electrophoresis (GGE), for both HDL_3 and HDL_{2b}, indicated particle-size distributions similar to those noted by electron microscopy. The mean particle diameter obtained by GGE of HDL_3 increased from 9.2 to 9.6 nm with increasing concentrations of HL-PC. The increase in mean particle diameter for HDL_{2b} from 10.9 to 11.1 nm was not statistically significant.

In summary, the HDL subclasses, HDL_3 and HDL_{2b}, show a capacity for direct uptake of HL-PC. Using HDL compositional data of Anderson *et al.* (1977), we estimate a maximal uptake of about 32 phospholipid molecules per HDL_3 and 47 per HDL_{2b}. Under the conditions used, the size increase associated with HL-PC uptake by HDL_3 was not sufficient to shift it into the HDL_{2a} size range (9.7–10.7 nm).

During uptake of HL-PC, a redistribution of HDL apolipoprotein to lower density fractions occurred. The redistribution increased with increasing concentrations of HL-PC and reached a maximal value of about 15% for both HDL subclasses. For HDL_3, redistributed apolipoprotein appeared in discoidal and possibly vesicular form. Tetramethylurea (TMU) electrophoresis of these product complexes for HDL_3 showed apoA-I, apoA-II, and apoC. For HDL_{2b}, some apolipoprotein was associated with both the discoidal complex fractions and the HL-PC vesicle fractions. TMU electrophoresis showed transfer of apoA-I from HDL_{2b} to lower density fractions. Information on the transfer of other apolipoproteins was equivocal due to insufficient banding intensity.

We have considered two possible interaction pathways to explain the results described above. The first would involve a substitution of phospholipid for apolipoprotein transferred from the HDL surface to lower density fractions. The second would also involve HL-PC uptake by HDL but without a corresponding apolipoprotein transfer from the HDL surface. In this case, the observed redistribution of apolipoprotein would require some form of incorporation of intact HDL_3 into liposomes, giving rise to complexes containing all of the HDL_3 apolipoproteins. In view of data by Havel *et al.* (1973) on the transfer of apoprotein from HDL to triglyceride emulsions, transfer of lipid-free apoA-II from HDL_3 to HL-PC vesicles appears unlikely, and hence, we consider the results more consistent with the second rather than the first pathway. Further work is in progress on the molecular mechanisms of phospholipid uptake, and associated HDL structural and compositional changes.

REFERENCES

1. HAVEL, R. J., J. P. KANE & M. L. KASHYAP. 1973. J. Clin. Invest. **52:**32–38.
2. REDGRAVE, T. G. & D M. SMALL. 1979. J. Clin. Invest. **64:**162–171.
3. TALL, A. R., P. H. R. GREEN, R. M. GLICKMAN & J. W. RILEY. 1979. J. Clin. Invest. **64:**977–989.
4. ANDERSON, D. W., A. V. NICHOLS & T. M. FORTE. 1977. Biochim. Biophys. Acta **493:**55–68.

STRUCTURAL STUDIES ON AN INSECT
HIGH-DENSITY LIPOPROTEIN *

Eric C. Mundall, Nikhil M. Pattnaik, Bruno G. Trambusti,
George Hromnak, Ferenc J. Kézdy, and John H. Law

Department of Biochemistry
University of Chicago
Chicago, Illinois 60637

Lipoproteins isolated from pupal or adult flying insects [2, 6] are high-density particles characterized by a high content of diglycerides. Diglycerides are derived from the fat body triglycerides and released, under the influence of the adipokinetic hormone,[4] into the hemolymph where they are picked up by the HDL and transported to the flight muscle to power locomotion. Diglycerides may also be the principal form of absorbed fat in the gut.[1]

We have isolated the HDL that represents the major lipid carrier of the hemolymph of the tobacco hornworm, *Manduca sexta*. The particle, which is essentially the same in all life stages (caterpillar, pupa, and adult), has the properties shown in TABLE 1.[5]

The particle contains two apoproteins: 2.85×10^5 daltons (AL_L) and 8.1×10^4 daltons (AL_s). The amino acid composition of AL_L and AL_s are very similar. When the intact particle is digested with trypsin, AL_L is completely degraded to smaller peptides, while AL_s is completely resistant to attack.[5]

If the particle is subjected to iodination with radioactive iodide and a solid-phase oxidant,[3] the particle becomes extensively labeled. After precipitation of the labeled lipoprotein with antibodies raised to *Manduca* HDL, polyacrylamide gel electrophoresis was used to separate the apoproteins. AL_L was heavily labeled, while AL_s was labeled only to a small extent. These results illustrate that the structure of the insect HDL particle is quite different from that of mammalian lipoproteins and that one of the apoprotein chains is protected from the external environment in such a way that the basic amino acid residues and tyrosine are not accessible to enzymatic or chemical attack. Calculations based upon the size and composition of the particle suggest that the small apoprotein, AL_s may occupy the center of the particle.[5]

We have isolated the HDL from hemolymph of *M. sexta* pupae and adults, where it is present in much higher concentrations than in larval hemolymph. Semiquantitative analysis of the lipid components and apoproteins indicates that the composition is virtually identical at all life stages. Furthermore, the overall composition of the *M. sexta* lipoprotein is very similar to the HDL isolated from pupal or adult silkmoths and locusts. This indicates that diglyceride transport is universal in insects at all life stages, and the same type of particle is used for transport of diglyceride from the gut to the fat body, and from the fat body to the muscle.

* This work was supported by the National Institutes of Health Grants GM 13863 and HL 15062 and a postdoctoral fellowship AM 05350 (for E. Mundall).

431

TABLE 1

PHYSICAL PROPERTIES AND COMPOSITION OF THE HDL FROM THE LARVAL HEMOLYMPH
OF THE TOBACCO HORNWORM, *Manduca sexta*

Molecular weight (centrifugation, compositional analysis)	6×10^5
Density, g/ml	1.115
Diameter, Å (electron microscope)	122 ± 13
Stokes radius, Å (gel filtration)	63
Sedimentation coefficient, svedbergs	8.7
Composition:	
Protein, %	61
Total lipids, %	37
Phospholipids, %	14
Neutral lipids, % *	23
Carbohydrates, %	2

* More than half of the neutral lipids are diglycerides, while only 10% are triglycerides.

REFERENCES

1. CHINO, H. & R. G. H. DOWNER. 1979. The role of diacylglycerol in absorption of dietary glyceride in the American cockroach, *Periplaneta americana* L. Insect Biochem. **9**:379.
2. CHINO, H., S. MURAKAMI & K. HARASHIMA. 1969. Diglyceride-carrying lipoproteins in insect hemolymph. Isolation, purification and properties. Biochim. Biophys. Acta **176**:1.
3. FRAKER, R. J. & J. C. SPECK, JR. 1978. Protein and cell membrane iodinations with a sparingly soluble chloramide, 1,3,4,6-tetrachloro-3α,6α-diphenylglycoluril. Biochem. Biophys. Res. Commun. **80**:849.
4. MAYER, R. J. & D. J. CANDY. 1969. Control of hemolymph lipid concentration during locust flight: An adipokinetic hormone from the corpora cardiaca. J. Insect Physiol. **15**:611.
5. PATTNAIK, N. M., E. C. MUNDALL, B. G. TRAMBUSTI, J. H. LAW & F. J. KÉZDY. 1979. Isolation and characterization of a larval lipoprotein from the hemolymph of *Manduca sexta*. Comp. Biochem. Physiol. **63B**:469.
6. PELED, Y. & A. TIETZ. 1975. Isolation and properties of a lipoprotein from the hemolymph of the locust, *Locusta migratoria*. Insect Biochem. **5**:61.

HUMAN MACROPHAGES AND THEIR INTERACTIONS WITH SERUM LIPOPROTEINS: MORPHOLOGICAL AND BIOCHEMICAL CHANGES

M. G. Traber and H. J. Kayden

New York University School of Medicine
Department of Medicine
New York, New York 10016

Lipid-laden, cholesterol-rich macrophages are found in atheromatous and xanthomatous lesions. The circulating monocyte is a precursor of these macrophages. Freshly isolated blood monocytes have been shown to have a relatively low cholesterol content and to have few high affinity receptors for low-density lipoprotein (LDL). In this study we evaluated various functions of human monocytes as they are transformed into actively phagocytizing macrophages in culture.

Specifically, we determined whether: (1) the cholesterol metabolism of macrophages is similar to that of other cell types in culture, (2) the high-affinity receptor for LDL can be demonstrated, and (3) how various lipoprotein fractions affect these parameters.

Morphological observations were made by phase contrast microscopy and transmission electron microscopy. Biochemical determinations included: (1) cellular cholesterol and cholesteryl ester, (2) cholesterol biosynthesis and esterification, and (3) quantitation of the binding, internalization, and degradation of [^{125}I]LDL at 37° C.

Large numbers of human monocytes, obtained from a white cell concentrate, were cultured, and thus transformed into macrophages. The macrophages were grown in medium containing different lipoprotein fractions and were studied for up to 17 days. The lipoprotein fractions used were very low density (VLDL), low density (LDL), and high density (HDL), as well as lipoprotein-deficient serum (LPDS) and fetal calf serum (FCS).

Macrophages cultured with VLDL accumulate lipid droplets, as shown by phase and electron microscopy and Oil Red O staining.

Macrophages cultured with LDL or VLDL have a two- to threefold increase in total cholesterol content compared with those cultured with LPDS or FCS. The increase in cholesterol content is mainly as unesterified cholesterol. Cholesterol esterification, as measured by labeled oleic acid incorporation into cholesteryl oleate was not stimulated. Cholesterol biosynthesis, as measured by incorporation of labeled acetate into sterols, was inhibited in macrophages cultured with VLDL and LDL as compared to those cells cultured with LPDS.

Macrophages apparently develop high-affinity receptors for LDL, as measured by degradation of [^{125}I]LDL. These receptors increase in number in cells cultured with LPDS for 10 days. The number of the high affinity receptors is reduced in cells cultured with LDL, VLDL, or in FCS compared to cells cultured in LPDS.

Human monocyte-derived macrophages, when cultured in LPDS and then incubated with LDL, degrade LDL with high affinity kinetics. When exposed to high levels of LDL or VLDL, macrophages will accumulate 2 to 3 times as much cholesterol as they usually contain, and cells grown with VLDL will also become lipid-laden. The study of these macrophages is important in evaluating the role of scavenger cells in the degradation of lipoproteins and the evolution of atheromatous and xanthomatous lesions.

Index of Contributors

(Italicized page numbers refer to comments made in Discussions)

435